Epilepsy and the interictal state

Co-morbidities and quality of life

Epilepsy and the interictal state

Co-morbidities and quality of life

EDITED BY

Erik K. St. Louis
Department of Neurology
Mayo Clinic and Foundation
USA

David M. Ficker
University of Cincinnati Neuroscience Institute Epilepsy Center
Department of Neurology
University of Cincinnati Academic Health Center
USA

Terence J. O'Brien
Professor of Medicine
Royal Melbourne Hospital
Australia

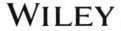

Library of Congress Cataloging-in-Publication Data

The interictal state in epilepsy : comorbidities and quality of life / [edited by] Erik K. St. Louis, David Ficker, Terence J. O'Brien.
     p. ; cm.
Includes bibliographical references and index.
ISBN 978-0-470-65623-5 (cloth)
I. St. Louis, Erik K., 1965- editor. II. Ficker, David (David M.), 1965- editor. III. O'Brien, Terence J. (Terence John), 1964- editor.
[DNLM: 1. Epilepsy–complications. 2. Epilepsy–psychology. 3. Cognition–physiology. 4. Comorbidity.
5. Quality of Life. 6. Seizures. WL 385] RC372
616.85'3–dc23

                                                                                                    2014018401

A catalogue record for this book is available from the British Library.

Wiley also publishes its books in a variety of electronic formats. Some content that appears in print may not be available in electronic books.

Typeset in 8.5/12pt MeridienLTStd by Laserwords Private Limited, Chennai, India

Printed in Singapore by C.O.S. Printers Pte Ltd

1 2015

The Editors wish to dedicate this book foremost to our families (Kerith, Aren, Kjersti, Siri, Ken and Karen St. Louis; Angela, Lauren, Anna and Kerstin Ficker; and Louise, William, Patrick, Lawrence and Alice O'Brien); to our epilepsy care mentors (Gregory D. Cascino, Frank W. Sharbrough, and Elson L. So); to all the chapter authors; and especially, to our patients.

Contents

List of contributors

Sophia J. Adams
Melbourne Neuropsychiatry Centre
University of Melbourne
and
Neuropsychiatry Unit
Royal Melbourne Hospital
Australia

Gus Baker
Walton Centre for Neurology & Neurosurgery
University of Liverpool
UK

Yvan A. Bamps
Department of Behavioral Sciences and
    Health Education
Rollins School of Public Health
Emory University
USA

Selim R. Benbadis
Department of Neurology & Neurosurgery
University of South Florida
and
Tampa General Hospital
USA

Frank M.C. Besag
South Essex Partnership University
    NHS Foundation Trust
Twinwoods Health Resource Centre
Bedford and Institute of Psychiatry
UK

Colleen K. Dilorio
Department of Behavioral Sciences and
    Health Education
Rollins School of Public Health
Emory University
USA

Joe Drazkowski
Department of Neurology
Mayo Clinic
USA

David W. Dunn
Department of Psychiatry and Neurology
Indiana University School of Medicine
USA

Jonathan C. Edwards
Department of Neurosciences
Medical University of South Carolina
USA

Dana Ekstein
Epilepsy Center
Department of Neurology
Hadassah University Medical Center
Israel

John O. Elliott
Department of Medical Education
Ohio Health Riverside Methodist Hospital
and
College of Social Work
Ohio State University
USA

Ashley M. Enke
Creighton University
USA

David M. Ficker
University of Cincinnati Neuroscience Institute
    Epilepsy Center
Department of Neurology
University of Cincinnati Academic Health Center
USA

Frank G. Gilliam
Department of Neurology, Penn State University
Hershey, USA

Keith D. Hill
School of Physiotherapy and Exercise Science
Curtin University
and
Department of Allied Health
La Trobe University
Northern Health and National Ageing
    Research Institute
Australia

R. Edward Hogan
Washington University in St. Louis
Adult Epilepsy Section, Department of Neurology
USA

Ann Jacoby
Department of Public Health and Policy
Institute of Psychology, Health and Society
University of Liverpool
UK

Robert D. Jones
Department of Neurology
University of Iowa
USA

Simon Jones
Melbourne Neuropsychiatry Centre
University of Melbourne
and
Neuropsychiatry Unit
Royal Melbourne Hospital
Australia

Irakli Kaolani
Department of Neurology
Mayo Clinic
USA

Rosemarie Kobau
Division of Population Health
Centers for Disease Control and Prevention
USA

Vladimír Komárek
Department of Pediatric Neurology
2nd Faculty of Medicine
Charles University
Motol University Hospital
Czech Republic

William G. Kronenberger
Department of Psychiatry
Indiana University School of Medicine
USA

Ekrem Kutluay
Department of Neurosciences
Medical University of South Carolina
USA

Beth A. Leeman
Department of Neurology
Emory University
USA

Esmeralda L. Park
Rush Epilepsy Center
Rush University Medical Center
USA

Luigi Maccotta
Washington University in St. Louis
Adult Epilepsy Section, Department of Neurology
USA

Bláthnaid McCoy
Division of Neurology
The Hospital for Sick Children
Canada

Kimford J. Meador
Department of Neurology
Emory University
USA

J. Layne Moore
Department of Neurology
Wright State University Boonshoft
    School of Medicine
USA

Katherine H. Noe
Department of Neurology
Mayo Clinic
USA

Terence J. O'Brien
Royal Melbourne Hospital
Australia

Alison M. Pack
Neurological Institute
Columbia University
USA

Philip N. Patsalos
Department of Clinical and Experimental Epilepsy
UCL Institute of Neurology
UK

Piero Perucca
The Montreal Neurological Institute
Canada

Sandra J. Petty
The Florey Institute of Neuroscience and Mental Health
and
Ormond College
and
Department of Medicine
Royal Melbourne Hospital
University of Melbourne
Australia

Michael Salzberg
Department of Psychiatry
St. Vincent's Hospital
University of Melbourne
Australia

Steven C. Schachter
Departments of Neurology
Beth Israel Deaconess Medical Center
Massachusetts General Hospital
and
Harvard Medical School
Consortia for Improving Medicine with Innovation and
Technology
Boston
MA

Joseph I. Sirven
Department of Neurology
Mayo Clinic
USA

Michael Smith
Rush Epilepsy Center
Rush University Medical Center
USA

Dee Snape
Department of Public Health and Policy
Institute of Psychology, Health and Society
University of Liverpool
UK

Laura S. Snavely
Department of Neurology, Penn State University
Hershey, USA

Cher Stephenson
Stephenson Counseling LLC
USA

Erik K. St. Louis
Department of Neurology
Mayo Clinic
USA

Nancy J. Thompson
Department of Behavioral Sciences and Health Education
Rollins School of Public Health
Emory University
USA

Lily H. Tran
Department of Pediatrics and Neurology
University of California at Irvine
and
Children's Hospital of Orange County
USA

Christopher Turnbull
Melbourne Neuropsychiatry Centre
University of Melbourne
and
Neuropsychiatry Unit
Royal Melbourne Hospital
Australia

Frank J.E. Vajda
Department of Medicine and Neuroscience
University of Melbourne
Royal Melbourne Hospital
Australia

Clemente Vega
Division of Epilepsy and Clinical Neurophysiology
Children's Hospital Boston and Harvard University
USA

Dennis Velakoulis
Melbourne Neuropsychiatry Centre
University of Melbourne
and
Neuropsychiatry Unit
Royal Melbourne Hospital
Australia

John D. Wark
Department of Medicine
University of Melbourne
and
Bone & Mineral Medicine
Royal Melbourne Hospital
Australia

Elizabeth Waterhouse
Department of Neurology
Virginia Commonwealth University School of Medicine
USA

Kristine Ziemba
Department of Neurology
Mayo Clinic
USA

Mary L. Zupanc
Department of Pediatrics and Neurology
University of California at Irvine
and
Children's Hospital of Orange County
USA

Foreword

According to the International League Against Epilepsy (ILAE) and the International Bureau for Epilepsy (IBE), epilepsy is a disorder of the brain characterized by an enduring predisposition to generate epileptic seizures, and by the neurobiologic, cognitive, psychological, and social consequences of this condition [1]. This conceptual definition explicitly states that there is more to epilepsy than seizures. The ILAE and IBE conclude that for some people with epilepsy, "behavioural disturbances, such as interictal and postictal cognitive problems can be part of the epileptic condition ... " and that "patients with epilepsy may suffer stigma, exclusion, restrictions, overprotection, and isolation, which also become part of the epileptic condition" [1].

Although it has long been known, increasing attention has recently been directed to the fact that comorbidities often add significantly to the burden of epilepsy, whether they are causative (e.g., cerebrovascular conditions or traumatic brain injuries causing epilepsy), resultant (caused by seizure, epilepsy, or its treatment), or related to a common cause underlying both the epilepsy and the comorbidity (e.g., learning disabilities or some psychiatric conditions). Such comorbidities not only add to the burden of epilepsy, but can also lead to poorer response to treatment with antiepileptic drugs, increased risk of adverse drug reactions, and even increased risk of death [2].

The theme of this book, "Epilepsy and The Interictal State: Co-Morbidities and Quality of Life," is therefore very timely, and it addresses some of the most urgent issues for the successful management of people with epilepsy.

This volume takes a very broad approach to the Co-Morbidity and Quality of Life theme. Some emphasis is on cognitive impairments in epilepsy, including chapters on difficulties caused by neurodevelopmental disorders and other co-morbidities, as well as on cognitive impairments caused by the treatment of epilepsy. Several chapters address other aspects of adverse effects of epilepsy therapies, ranging from idiosyncratic to dose/serum concentration-related, and even to second-generation effects on the unborn child. A particular strength of this book is that, in addition to identifying and describing these aspects of the burden of epilepsy, several chapters discuss ways to prevent, reduce, or manage adverse consequences of epilepsy and its treatment. Chapters on rehabilitation and the use of complementary medicine make this overview of possible interventions to improve everyday life for people with epilepsy most comprehensive. In conclusion, this book reminds us of the wider implications of the diagnosis of epilepsy, of the burden beyond seizures, and of our opportunities to assist in easing this burden. The editors have assembled world-renowned experts as authors to each of the 24 chapters, which contributes to making this book a most useful read for every physician involved in the management of people with epilepsy.

Torbjörn Tomson, MD, PhD
Professor in Neurology and Epileptology
Department of Clinical Neuroscience
Karolinska Institutet
Stockholm, Sweden

References

1 Fisher RS, van Emde Boas W, Blume W et al: Epileptic seizures and epilepsy: definitions proposed by the International League Against Epilepsy (ILAE) and the International Bureau for Epilepsy (IBE). *Epilepsia* 2005; **46**:470–472.
2 Moshé SL, Perucca E, Ryvlin P, Tomson T: Epilepsy: new advances. *Lancet* 2014 (Sep 23). pii: S0140-6736(14)60456-6, doi: 10.1016/S0140-6736(14)60456-6.

SECTION I
Quality of life and the interictal state in epilepsy

CHAPTER 1

Quality of life in epilepsy: the key importance of the interictal state

David M. Ficker

University of Cincinnati Neuroscience Institute Epilepsy Center, Department of Neurology, University of Cincinnati Academic Health Center, USA

Introduction

Quality of life (QOL) has become recognized as a critical concept in a wide range of disease states in medicine over the last several decades, especially in chronic medical conditions such as epilepsy. The traditional clinical measures used by clinicians in treating patients with epilepsy are seizure frequency and medication adverse effects. A patient with epilepsy is considered to be controlled when they are seizure-free and are having few or no adverse effects from their antiepileptic drugs (AEDs). Patients, however, may be more concerned about psychosocial issues such as driving, independence, and employment than about AED adverse effects or seizure unpredictability [1]. These aspects of QOL are infrequently assessed in routine clinical care. Although epilepsy is a disorder that only produces neurologic symptoms on an intermittent basis (i.e., only during the seizure), psychosocial problems, AED therapy, and side effects may be the major factors that a patient perceives as interfering with daily living. Other interictal factors have been explored as potential contributors to QOL and will be briefly reviewed here.

QOL is clearly subjective in nature and may be difficult to measure. In the simplest terms, QOL can be defined as how a patient feels and functions. There are three essential elements [2,3]: 1) physical health, 2) psychological health, and 3) social health. Physical health includes aspects such as daily function, general health, pain, endurance, and specific epilepsy-related variables such as seizure frequency, severity, and medication-related side effects. Psychological health includes aspects such as emotional well-being, psychiatric and emotional health, self-esteem, and cognition. Social health includes aspects of relationships with friends and family, occupational status, and issues pertaining to independence.

Tools for measuring QOL

Because QOL is difficult to quantify in everyday practice, research instruments have been developed with which to assess it. Measurement tools can be either generic or disease-specific.

Generic assessments such as the RAND 36-Item Health Survey [4] (also known as the SF-36) can be applied to many different patient populations and may allow for comparisons among different disease states. However, they may not measure important features in patients with epilepsy, such as fear of seizures or social embarrassment.

Epilepsy-specific measures of QOL have been developed over the past several years. The Quality of Life in Epilepsy (QOLIE) instruments were designed for use in a wide range of epilepsy patients, including those who with both benign and severe disease [3]. Three tools have been developed: QOLIE-89 [5], QOLIE-31 [6], and QOLIE-10 [7]. The QOLIE-89 contains 89 items in 17 scales, the QOLIE-31 contains 31 items in 7 scales, and the QOLIE-10 contains 10 items from the 7 QOLIE-31 scales and is intended as a screening tool. The scales represented in each survey are outlined in Table 1.1. All of the QOLIE inventories have been

Epilepsy and the Interictal State: Co-Morbidities and Quality of Life, First Edition.
Edited by Erik K. St. Louis, David M. Ficker, and Terence J. O'Brien.

Table 1.1 Comparison of epilepsy-specific quality-of-life (QOL) tools.

Scale	QOLIE-89	QOLIE-31	QOLIE-10
Health perceptions	×		
Seizure worry	×	×	×
Physical function	×		
Role limitation, physical	×		
Role limitation, emotional	×		
Pain	×		
Overall QOL	×	×	×
Emotional well-being	×	×	×
Energy/fatigue	×	×	×
Attention/concentration	×	×	×
Memory	×		
Language	×		
Medication effects	×	×	×
Social function, work, driving	×	×	×
Social support	×		
Social isolation	×		
Health discouragement	×		

validated in studies of patients with epilepsy [5–7]. The questionnaires are simple to complete and have a standardized scoring system; however, they may be challenging to use in routine clinical practice. A QOL tool for newly diagnosed epilepsy patients (NEWQOL) has also been developed [8].

These tools have been used in many epilepsy QOL studies, and several important findings that impact the clinical practice of epilepsy have been reported. In particular, it seems that *interictal* factors rather than the ictal state have the greatest impact on QOL in epilepsy patients. While these findings may impact clinical practice, unfortunately interictal factors are often not routinely assessed in the clinic setting.

Ictal factors: seizure frequency and severity

It is relatively intuitive that seizures should affect QOL; large-scale surveys suggest that they have a negative impact. Seizure frequency, seizure type, and seizure severity each have an effect. A European study of 5000 epilepsy patients showed that those who experienced at least one seizure per month had poorer QOL than those who were seizure-free in the past year [9]. Another

study suggested that patients who had a minimum of six seizures over the previous 6 months had poorer QOL than those who had fewer seizures and those who were seizure-free [10]. In addition, patients who achieved seizure freedom had QOL similar to the general population [10]. A study analyzing different degrees of seizure control showed that QOL improved only when seizure freedom was attained, while lesser degrees of seizure reduction (i.e., 75–99%, 50–74%, or 0–50%) were not associated with improvement in QOL [11]. Recent seizures also seem to have a greater impact on QOL than more remote seizures [12] and have bearing on how patients with epilepsy prioritize the perceived impact of seizure control or medication adverse effects on QOL; in particular, patients who had recent seizures tended to be more sensitive toward medication adverse effects, while patients who had more remote seizures (but who had not experienced a recent seizure) were more concerned about seizure control [13]. Longer periods of seizure freedom were associated with better QOL in a cohort of over 600 people with epilepsy [14]. Seizure severity has also been shown to impact QOL in a number of studies [15–18]. Epilepsy surgery, especially when resulting in seizure freedom, results in improved QOL [19–21].

Interictal factors

While seizures and seizure severity may negatively impact QOL, when multivariate studies are performed there are other factors that have a greater effect. In particular, mood and medication adverse effects make a significant contribution to QOL.

The presence of medication adverse effects has been shown in several studies to negatively impact QOL. These studies utilized a standardized checklist of medication adverse effects: the Adverse Events Profile (AEP) [22]. In a cohort of 200 patients with epilepsy, higher AEP scores were associated with a worse QOL [23]. Use of the AEP in a randomized controlled trial resulted in improvements in QOL scores when clinicians were presented with AEP scores, compared to standard clinical practice without AEP review [24]. In this study, seizure frequency did not correlate with QOL but the presence of higher AEP scores was associated with a poorer QOL, suggesting the importance of interictal symptoms to QOL.

Comorbid mood disorders are very common in people with epilepsy [25], with both anxiety and depression being highly prevalent. Both depression and anxiety significantly impact QOL. A study of refractory epilepsy patients shows that depression is an important contributor to QOL, yet seizure-related factors are not [26]. Other studies suggest that depression and anxiety significantly impact QOL [27–30].

Conclusion

Although it is important to assess ictal factors such as seizure frequency, severity, and recency in the clinic, interictal factors should be prioritized in order to maximize patient QOL. A conceptual model (Figure 1.1) can be used to elucidate the relationship between ictal and interictal factors in epilepsy QOL. There are many interrelated contributions; our traditional clinical assessments of seizure frequency and a cursory assessment of side effects may not be sufficient and other measures – including mood and more systematic and quantitative screening for adverse effects with validated tools such as the AEP – may be needed. In our epilepsy specialty clinics, we routinely include assessment of anxiety with the Generalized Anxiety Disorder 7-Item (GAD-7) scale [31] and of depression with the Neurological Disorders Depression Inventory for Epilepsy (NDDI-E) [32]. Use of these instruments may aid the clinician and patient in identifying otherwise subtle problems caused by mood, anxiety, or adverse

medication effects that have important bearing on QOL, leading to improved dialogue and proactive discussions that aid clinical decision-making in epilepsy care.

References

1 Gilliam F, Kuzniecky R, Faught E et al.: Patient-validated content of epilepsy-specific quality-of-life measurement. *Epilepsia* 1997; **38(2)**:233–236.

2 Dodrill CB, Batzel LW: Issues in quality of life assessment. In: Engel J Jr, Pedley TA (eds): *Epilepsy: A Comprehensive Textbook*. Lippincott-Raven: Philadelphia, PA, 1997, pp. 2227–2231.

3 Devinsky O: Quality of life with epilepsy. In: Wylie E (ed.): *The Treatment of Epilepsy: Principles and Practice*. Lippincott Williams & Wilkins: Baltimore, MD, 1996, pp. 1145–1150.

4 Hays RD, Sherbourne C, Mazel E: The RAND 36-item health survey 1.0. *Health Econ* 1993; **2**:217–227.

5 Devinsky O, Vickrey BG, Cramer J et al.: Development of the quality of life in epilepsy inventory. *Epilepsia* 1995; **36(11)**: 1089–1104.

6 Cramer JA, Perrine K, Devinsky O et al.: Development and cross-cultural translations of a 31-item quality of life in epilepsy inventory. *Epilepsia* 1998; **39(1)**:81–88.

7 Cramer JA, Perrine K, Devinsky O, Meador K: A brief questionnaire to screen for quality of life in epilepsy: the QOLIE-10. *Epilepsia* 1996; **37(6)**:577–582.

8 Abetz L, Jacoby A, Baker GA, McNulty P: Patient-based assessments of quality of life in newly diagnosed epilepsy patients: validation of the NEWQOL. *Epilepsia* 2000; **41(9)**: 1119–1128.

9 Baker GA, Jacoby A, Buck D et al.: Quality of life of people with epilepsy: a European study. *Epilepsia* 1997; **38(3)**: 353–362.

10 Leidy NK, Elixhauser A, Vickrey B et al.: Seizure frequency and the health-related quality of life of adults with epilepsy. *Neurology* 1999; **53(1)**:162.

11 Birbeck GL, Hays RD, Cui X, Vickrey BG: Seizure reduction and quality of life improvements in people with epilepsy. *Epilepsia* 2002; **43(5)**:535–538.

12 Kobau R, Zahran H, Grant D et al.: Prevalence of active epilepsy and health-related quality of life among adults with self-reported epilepsy in California: California Health Interview Survey, 2003. *Epilepsia* 2007; **48(10)**:1904–1913.

13 Cramer JA, Brandenburg NA, Xu X et al.: The impact of seizures and adverse effects on global health ratings. *Epilepsy Behav* 2007; **11(2)**:179–184.

14 Jacoby A: Epilepsy and the quality of everyday life. findings from a study of people with well-controlled epilepsy. *Soc Sci Med* 1992; **34(6)**:657–666.

15 Sancho J, Ivanez V, Molins A et al.: Changes in seizure severity and quality of life in patients with refractory partial epilepsy. *Epilepsy Behav* 2010; **19(3)**:409–413.

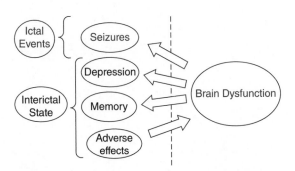

Figure 1.1 Conceptual model of quality of life (QOL) and epilepsy. It is crucial to address both ictal and interictal factors in epilepsy care; recent evidence has shown that interictal factors such as mood state, cognitive problems, and adverse medication effects have a crucial influence on epilepsy QOL.

16 Bautista RE, Glen ET: Seizure severity is associated with quality of life independent of seizure frequency. *Epilepsy Behav* 2009; **16(2)**:325–329.

17 Harden CL, Maroof DA, Nikolov B et al.: The effect of seizure severity on quality of life in epilepsy. *Epilepsy Behav* 2007; **11(2)**:208–211.

18 Vickrey BG, Berg AT, Sperling MR et al.: Relationships between seizure severity and health-related quality of life in refractory localization-related epilepsy. *Epilepsia* 2000; **41(6)**:760–764.

19 Bien CG, Schulze-Bonhage A, Soeder BM et al.: Assessment of the long-term effects of epilepsy surgery with three different reference groups. *Epilepsia* 2006; **47(11)**:1865–1869.

20 Spencer SS, Berg AT, Vickrey BG et al.: Health-related quality of life over time since resective epilepsy surgery. *Ann Neurol* 2007; **62(4)**:327–334.

21 Mikati MA, Comair YG, Rahi A: Normalization of quality of life three years after temporal lobectomy: a controlled study. *Epilepsia* 2006; **47(5)**:928–933.

22 Baker G, Middleton A, Jacoby A et al.: Initial development, reliability, and validity of a patient-based adverse event scale. *Epilepsia* 1994; **35(Suppl. 7)**:80.

23 Perucca P, Carter J, Vahle V, Gilliam FG: Adverse antiepileptic drug effects: toward a clinically and neurobiologically relevant taxonomy. *Neurology* 2009; **72(14)**:1223–1229.

24 Gilliam FG, Fessler AJ, Baker G et al.: Systematic screening allows reduction of adverse antiepileptic drug effects: a randomized trial. *Neurology* 2004; **62(1)**:23–27.

25 Tellez-Zenteno JF, Patten SB, Jette N et al. Psychiatric comorbidity in epilepsy: a population-based analysis. *Epilepsia* 2007; **48(12)**:2336–2344.

26 Boylan LS, Flint LA, Labovitz DL et al.: Depression but not seizure frequency predicts quality of life in treatment-resistant epilepsy. *Neurology* 2004; **62(2)**:258–261.

27 Johnson EK, Jones JE, Seidenberg M, Hermann BP: The relative impact of anxiety, depression, and clinical seizure features on health-related quality of life in epilepsy. *Epilepsia* 2004; **45(5)**:544–550.

28 Tracy JI, Dechant V, Sperling MR et al.: The association of mood with quality of life ratings in epilepsy. *Neurology* 2007; **68(14)**:1101–1107.

29 Loring DW, Meador KJ, Lee GP: Determinants of quality of life in epilepsy. *Epilepsy Behav* 2004; **5(6)**:976–980.

30 Zeber JE, Copeland LA, Amuan M et al.: The role of comorbid psychiatric conditions in health status in epilepsy. *Epilepsy Behav* 2007; **10(4)**:539–546.

31 Spitzer RL, Kroenke K, Williams JB, Lowe B: A brief measure for assessing generalized anxiety disorder: the GAD-7. *Arch Intern Med* 2006; **166(10)**:1092–1097.

32 Gilliam FG, Barry JJ, Hermann BP et al.: Rapid detection of major depression in epilepsy: a multicentre study. *Lancet Neurol* 2006; **5(5)**:399–405.

CHAPTER 2

Comorbidities in epilepsy: range and impact

J. Layne Moore[1] and John O. Elliott[2]

[1] *Department of Neurology, Wright State University Boonshoft School of Medicine, USA*
[2] *Department of Medical Education, Ohio Health Riverside Methodist Hospital and College of Social Work, Ohio State University, USA*

Introduction

Although rendering patients "seizure-free" is the first goal of treating persons with epilepsy, many other factors affect their quality of life (QOL), including mental health and social, vocational, and somatic health issues [1].

The US government report *Healthy People 2010* sought to increase quality and years of healthy life and to diminish health disparities [2]. Recognition of comorbid conditions in persons with epilepsy may assist in selecting treatments and in identifying future goals and objectives for improving overall QOL.

A recent seminal article examining psychiatric and somatic comorbidities reported huge disparities in disease prevalence for persons with epilepsy in the United Kingdom [3]. Since this study, smaller-scale data have been reported from the United States in the 2003 California Health Interview Survey (CHIS).

Psychosocial factors

Persons with epilepsy are at higher risk for symptoms of depression and anxiety than people suffering from many other chronic diseases [4]. Psychiatric disorders occur in persons with epilepsy almost twice as much as in the non-epilepsy population, including obsessive–compulsive disorder (OCD; rate ratio (RR) = 2.7), anxiety (RR = 2.2), depression (RR = 2.0), schizophrenia (RR = 3.8), and dementia (RR = 25.2) [3].

Persons with epilepsy and their families suffer from stigma that may impact how they are perceived and how they view themselves [5]. Stigma may be worse when the diagnosis occurs early in life [6] and may be present even in incident epilepsy, especially in those with poor health or history of depression [7].

Patients who develop healthy attitudes are active and flexible, focusing on possibilities and planning how to handle negative emotions. In contrast, a "handicapped" group is passive and resigned to epilepsy in a negative way, is fearful of being exposed, and tends to focus on obstacles and negative emotions [8]. Persons with epilepsy report higher scores on measures of learned helplessness [9,10]. Persons with uncontrolled seizures are also prone to a greater sense of external locus of control [11].

However, an improved sense of self-efficacy (beliefs in one's capabilities) to organize and execute action to produce attainments can assist persons with epilepsy in coping with their psychosocial difficulties [12]. Self-efficacy approaches may reduce disability and increase emotional well-being [13]. Such applications of neuropsychological and psychosocial interventions as treatment for epilepsy can also improve a person's QOL [14].

Poor QOL is associated with greater utilization of medical resources (number of clinic visits, ER visits, and in-patient admissions) [15]. In one study, 90% of the variance in QOL was explained by a combination of disease severity, epilepsy self-efficacy, social support, and locus of control [16].

Socially isolated people are more likely to rate their health status as poor [17]. Poor community-level social connection results in poor self-rated health status [18]. Persons with epilepsy tend to lack an adequate primary support group and have problems related to the social environment, education, occupation, housing, economic issues, and access to health care services.

Social support

Unhealthy people are less likely to establish and maintain social relationships that provide social support [19]. An extensive body of literature suggests that poor social support is a major risk factor for morbidity and mortality, with statistical effect sizes comparable to established risk factors such as smoking, hypertension, high cholesterol, obesity, and physical activity [19].

A recent meta-analysis of 148 studies examining social relationships and mortality risk found a weighted average effect size odds ratio (OR) of 1.50 (95% CI 1.42–1.59), indicating a 50% increased likelihood of survival in persons with stronger integration in social networks providing social support [20]. This effect remained consistent across age, gender, initial health status, cause of death, and follow-up period.

In a 30-year longitudinal study from Finland, childhood onset seizures were found to have a long-term adverse impact on education, employment, marriage, and having children [21]. This negative impact was still present even when persons were seizure-free without medication for many years [21,22].

Socioeconomic factors

Investigations have found that the incidence and prevalence of epilepsy in adults increases with socioeconomic deprivation [23–26]. Population studies from the United States show persons with a history of epilepsy report poorer health status, lower educational attainment, and lower household income compared to those without [27–29]. Persons with epilepsy are known to have significant difficulties in obtaining and maintaining employment [30]. These human capital factors improve health both directly and indirectly through work and economic conditions, psychosocial resources, and a healthy lifestyle [31]. For persons with epilepsy, limited education and employment impact health care access and environmental and lifestyle risk factors.

Poverty

Poverty imposes constraints on the material conditions of everyday life through limitations on the fundamentals of health: housing, good nutrition, and societal participation [32]. Material asset indicators such as home ownership are significantly associated with health outcomes after controlling for age, gender, and income [33].

People living in poverty who have difficulty paying for affordable housing and utility bills are less likely to have a usual source of care, more likely to postpone treatment, and more likely to use emergency-room services [34]. Persons with epilepsy living in poverty are half as likely to report taking medication for their seizures [35].

Income inadequacy adversely impacts the ability of persons with epilepsy to obtain not only medications but also basic resources such as food. Food insecurity is defined by the United States Department of Agriculture (USDA) as "when people do not have adequate physical, social, or economic access to sufficient, safe, and nutritious food that meets their dietary needs and food preferences for an active and healthy life" [36]. Adults in households with food insecurity are more likely to report poor or fair health status, as well as poor physical and mental health [37]. One recent Canadian study found persons with epilepsy were significantly more likely to report food insecurity [38].

Persons in poor environments experience significantly higher amounts of stress and poor mental health [39,40] and are more likely to adopt unhealthy coping behaviors such as smoking or drug and alcohol use [41].

Somatic health issues

Somatic disorders are significantly increased in persons with epilepsy, including stroke (RR = 14.2), Alzheimer's disease (RR = 39.8), Parkinson's disease (RR = 2.5), migraine (RR = 1.6), heart disease (RR = 1.6), heart failure (RR = 2.4), diabetes (RR = 1.8), asthma (RR = 1.4), emphysema (RR = 2.9), peptic ulcer (RR = 2.2), and fractures (RR = 2.2) [3].

Based on the 2003 and 2005 CHIS data, persons with epilepsy experience a greater comorbid burden, especially for cardiovascular-related conditions [42]. In the 2005 CHIS, the prevalence ratios of many comorbid conditions remained significantly higher in persons with a history of epilepsy, including type II diabetes (OR = 1.4), asthma (OR = 1.7), high cholesterol (OR = 1.3), heart disease (OR = 1.6), stroke (OR = 4.3), arthritis (OR = 1.7), and cancer (OR = 1.4) [42]. The

Centers for Disease Control and Prevention (CDC) found similar results in their analysis of 19 US states surveyed about epilepsy in 2005 [27].

Persons with epilepsy are also at greater risk for premature death when compared to the general population. Several longitudinal studies from England found newly diagnosed persons with epilepsy had a 30–42% increase in mortality when compared to age- and gender-matched controls without epilepsy [43,44]. Persons with uncontrolled epilepsy had double the expected number of deaths [45], primarily to cerebrovascular disease, cancer, and respiratory diseases such as pneumonia and chronic obstructive pulmonary disease (COPD) [43–45].

Physician–patient interactions

Clinicians are in a unique position to influence the health of persons with epilepsy. Unfortunately, time considerations and reimbursement issues are a significant barrier to their care. In general, medical literature has often reported poor communication between providers and patients [46]. The medical interview tends to be viewed as primarily a data-collection exercise, where there is typically an avoidance of psychological and social issues [47]. On average, physicians interrupt their patients within the first 18 seconds [48] of the interview and frequently overlook significant psychosocial issues [49].

A recent survey of persons with epilepsy in an outpatient setting revealed a selective gap between patients and their practitioners in understanding patients' concerns. Although there was overlap, patients were more concerned about life issues (memory and being a burden to others) and practitioners were more concerned about clinical issues (seizure activity and medication side effects). However well-meaning health care practitioners may be, attention should be spent on aligning their priorities with those of their patients [50].

Patient education has been shown to be effective in improving health outcomes such as reduction of medication needs, reduction of treatment duration and hospitals stays, improvement in risk-reducing behavior, and reduction of risk factors [51]. Doctors who express doubts about their success in patient education tend to be pessimistic about their ability to influence their patients' lifestyles [52,53].

Physicians who practice healthy personal behaviors are reported to have more credibility and ability to counsel patients effectively about improving their own health behavior. In one study, neurologists rank among the least likely to provide prevention-related counseling or screening to their patients [54]. Improved exercise and dietary habits are complementary to each other and are typically of interest to patients in the clinical setting, potentially impacting the development or progression of comorbidities common in persons with epilepsy.

Health behavior and lifestyle factors

Sleep problems
Despite concern that persons with epilepsy should avoid sleep deprivation since as far back as Claudius Galen [55], persons with epilepsy are relatively sleepy compared to controls [56]. There are several likely causes for persons with epilepsy being excessively sleepy, including seizures, alteration of circadian rhythms, and the sedating effect of antiepileptic drugs (AEDs) [57]. Persons with epilepsy have more arousals and poorer sleep architecture [58]. They are also more likely to have other comorbidities that contribute to sleep deprivation, including obstructive sleep apnea [59].

Smoking
Smoking is a significant concern, because studies have demonstrated a direct link with coronary artery disease, cancer, and stroke – the top three leading causes of death in the United States [60,61]. The 2003 and 2005 CHIS found significantly higher rates of smoking in persons with epilepsy [29,62]; these rates were confirmed in larger data from the Behavioral Risk Factor Surveillance System (BRFSS) [27].

Exercise
A lack of understanding about epilepsy among many health professionals and sports instructors led to unnecessary restriction of physical activity [63]. Less than half of patients had ever talked to their doctor about physical activity [63]. In addition, overprotection by family members, understimulation, low self-esteem, isolation, depression, and anxiety are significant barriers to a healthy lifestyle [64]. The combination of these factors has likely had an untoward effect on mortality, morbidity, and QOL for persons with epilepsy.

Exercise has been shown to improve depressive symptoms in people who admit to symptoms of depression but would not meet criteria for a diagnosis [65]. This is particularly important when considering exercise advice for persons with epilepsy, since many would not meet diagnostic criteria for depression but are thought to suffer from an interictal dysphoric disorder [66]. Population surveys from the United States have consistently found that persons with epilepsy exercise much less frequently than those without epilepsy [27,62].

Clinically based studies of exercise in persons with epilepsy suggest patients benefit from a structured exercise program. A prospective, parallel, randomized controlled study evaluating the impact of 12 weeks of exercise on clinical, behavioral, and physiological outcomes in 28 patients with epilepsy found significant improvements in the overall Quality Of Life In Epilepsy-89 (QOLIE-89) score, especially in the physical function and energy/fatigue domains, without adverse impact on clinical outcomes such as antiepileptic drug concentrations or seizure activity [67]. Mood, as measured by the Profile of Mood States (POMS), was also significantly improved in the exercise group. Cardiovascular and resistance training significantly improved strength, peak oxygen consumption, endurance time, and lipid profiles. A 12-week exercise training program resulted in positive outcomes for patients with epilepsy [68].

Exercise participation recommendations should be reviewed with regard to seizure control, medications, proper diet, and rest, and AED levels should be monitored if necessary. If these aspects are taken into account, persons with epilepsy can participate in most types of physical activity, including some contact sports [69].

Nutrition

Nutritional factors and poor diets may also contribute to the development of comorbidities in persons with epilepsy. In the United States, significant nutrient deficiencies (vitamins D, E, and K, folic acid, calcium, linoleic acid, and α-linolenic acid) were found in more than 30% of children with intractable epilepsy through a recent analysis of the National Health and Nutrition Examination Survey (NHANES) for 2001–02 [70].

An examination of the 2005 CHIS found that persons with a history of epilepsy drank more soda and consumed less salad than the non-epilepsy population [62]. However, the 2008 CDC report on epilepsy using the 2005 BRFSS data found persons with epilepsy reported consuming five servings of fruit and vegetables at the same rate as the non-epilepsy population [27].

AEDs and nutritional factors

AEDs, the basis of all therapy for persons with epilepsy, have been found to deplete vitamins B6 and B2 [71–73] and lower blood folate levels [74–79]. Enzyme-inducing AEDs are known to cause vitamin D deficiency in persons with epilepsy [80,81]. Carbamazepine reduces blood levels of omega-3 fatty acids [82]. Other AEDs, particularly valproic acid, are also known to cause weight gain and increased carbohydrate cravings [83].

The therapeutic use of nutrition and nutritional supplementation is of interest in epilepsy [84]. However, due to methodological issues and a limited number of studies, there is presently little support [85] beyond the ketogenic diet [86] for such therapies in epilepsy.

AEDs and comorbidity risk factors

Valproic acid, carbamazepine, or phenobarbital as long-term monotherapy have demonstrated atherogenic effects in children [87–89], although these effects are inconsistent [90]. Carbamazepine also increases atherogenic lipoproteins [91] and lipoprotein(a) in adult men [92]. However, carbamazepine has been found to increase high-density lipoproteins (HDL) in humans [93] and phenytoin has been found to reduce atherosclerosis by raising HDL in mice [94]. In children who complete AED treatment, lipids and lipoproteins typically return to normal 1 year after the end of treatment [95]. Additionally, carbamazepine and valproic acid can lead to significant weight gain, thereby increasing risk for metabolic syndrome and diabetes [96].

Since the 1980s, hypothyroidism has been associated with AED use. The mechanism is poorly understood but does not appear to be immune-mediated. Hypothyroidism may be more common in children and with the use of certain drugs, such as valproic acid, phenytoin, carbamazepine, and oxcarbazepine [97,98].

Conclusion

Recognizing persons with epilepsy are at risk for many other problems allows physicians to anticipate and potentially mitigate these comorbidities. These topics will be expanded in the following chapters. Since persons with epilepsy develop many comorbid medical problems as a result of their own behaviors, patients should be regularly counseled about the importance of limiting weight gain through adequate dietary and exercise habits and about other factors such as avoidance of smoking. Appropriate counseling could reduce the risk of developing other future comorbidities, such as hypertension, vascular disease, and sleep apnea. Health care workers should also be vigilant for patient concerns that may not align with their own.

References

1 Sander JW: Ultimate success in epilepsy – the patient's perspective. *Eur J Neurol* 2005; **12(Suppl. 4)**:3–11.

2 US Department of Health and Human Services: Healthy People 2010: understanding and improving health. http://www.healthypeople.gov/Document/pdf/uih/2010uih.pdf (last accessed July 15, 2014).

3 Gaitatzis A, Carroll K, Majeed A, Sander JW. The epidemiology of the comorbidity of epilepsy in the general population. *Epilepsia* 2004; **45(12)**:1613–1622.

4 Moore JL, Elliott JO, Lu B et al.: Serious psychological distress among persons with epilepsy based on the 2005 California Health Interview Survey. *Epilepsia* 2009; **50(5)**: 1077–1084.

5 Morrell MJ. Stigma and epilepsy. *Epilepsy Behav* 2002; **3(6S2)**:21–25.

6 Fisher RS, Vickrey BG, Gibson P et al.: The impact of epilepsy from the patient's perspective. II: Views about therapy and health care. *Epilepsy Res* 2000; **41(1)**:53–61.

7 Leaffer EB, Jacoby A, Benn E et al.: Associates of stigma in an incident epilepsy population from northern Manhattan, New York City. *Epilepsy Behav* 2011; **21(1)**:60–64.

8 Raty LK, Soderfeldt BA, Wilde Larsson BM: Daily life in epilepsy: patients' experiences described by emotions. *Epilepsy Behav* 2007; **10(3)**:389–396.

9 DeVillis RF, DeVellis BM, Wallston BS, Wallston KA: Epilepsy and learned helplessness. *Basic Appl Soc Psych* 1980; **1(3)**:241–253.

10 Rosenbaum M, Palmon N: Helplessness and resourcefulness in coping with epilepsy. *J Consult Clin Psychol* 1984; **52(2)**: 244–253.

11 Gehlert S: Perceptions of control in adults with epilepsy. *Epilepsia* 1994; **35(1)**:81–88.

12 DiIorio C, Shafer PO, Letz R et al.: Behavioral, social, and affective factors associated with self-efficacy for self-management among people with epilepsy. *Epilepsy Behav* 2006; **9(1)**:158–163.

13 Pramuka M, Hendrickson R, Zinski A, Van Cott AC: A psychosocial self-management program for epilepsy: a randomized pilot study in adults. *Epilepsy Behav* 2007; **11(4)**: 533–545.

14 Hermann BP: Developing a model of quality of life in epilepsy: the contribution of neuropsychology. *Epilepsia* 1993; **34(Suppl. 4)**:S14–S21.

15 Bautista RE, Glen ET, Wludyka PS, Shetty NK: Factors associated with utilization of healthcare resources among epilepsy patients. *Epilepsy Res* 2008; **79(2–3)**:120–129.

16 Amir M, Roziner I, Knoll A, Neufeld MY: Self-efficacy and social support as mediators in the relation between disease severity and quality of life in patients with epilepsy. *Epilepsia* 1999; **40(2)**:216–224.

17 Heritage Z, Wilkinson RG, Grimaud O, Pickett KE: Impact of social ties on self reported health in France: is everyone affected equally? *BMC Public Health* 2008; **8**:243.

18 Browning CR, Cagney KA, Wen M: Explaining variation in health status across space and time: implications for racial and ethnic disparities in self-rated health. *Soc Sci Med* 2003; **57(7)**:1221–1235.

19 House JS, Landis KR, Umberson D: Social relationships and health. *Science* 1988; **241(4865)**:540–545.

20 Holt-Lunstad J, Smith TB, Layton JB: Social relationships and mortality risk: a meta-analytic review. *PLoS Med* 2010; **7(7)**:e1000316.

21 Sillanpaa M, Jalava M, Kaleva O, Shinnar S: Long-term prognosis of seizures with onset in childhood. *N Engl J Med* 1998; **338(24)**:1715–1722.

22 Jalava M, Sillanpaa M, Camfield C, Camfield P: Social adjustment and competence 35 years after onset of childhood epilepsy: a prospective controlled study. *Epilepsia* 1997; **38(6)**:708–715.

23 Morgan CL, Ahmed Z, Kerr MP: Social deprivation and prevalence of epilepsy and associated health usage. *J Neurol Neurosurg Psychiatry* 2000; **69(1)**:13–17.

24 Heaney DC, MacDonald BK, Everitt A et al.: Socioeconomic variation in incidence of epilepsy: prospective community based study in south east England. *BMJ* 2002; **325(7371)**: 1013–1016.

25 Tellez-Zenteno JF, Pondal-Sordo M, Matijevic S, Wiebe S: National and regional prevalence of self-reported epilepsy in Canada. *Epilepsia* 2004; **45(12)**:1623–1629.

26 Noronha AL, Borges MA, Marques LH et al.: Prevalence and pattern of epilepsy treatment in different socioeconomic classes in Brazil. *Epilepsia* 2007; **48(5)**:880–885.

27 Kobau R, Zahran H, Thurman DJ et al.: Epilepsy surveillance among adults: 19 States, Behavioral Risk Factor Surveillance System, 2005. *MMWR Surveill Summ* 2008; **57(6)**:1–20.

28 Elliott JO, Moore JL, Lu B: Health status and behavioral risk factors among persons with epilepsy in Ohio based on the 2006 Behavioral Risk Factor Surveillance System. *Epilepsy Behav* 2008; **12(3)**:434–444.

29 Kobau R, Zahran H, Grant D et al.: Prevalence of active epilepsy and health-related quality of life among adults with self-reported epilepsy in California: California Health Interview Survey, 2003. *Epilepsia* 2007; **48(10)**:1904–1913.

30 Bautista RE, Wludyka P: Factors associated with employment in epilepsy patients. *Epilepsy Behav* 2007; **10(1)**:89–95.

31 Ross CE, Wu C: The links between education and health. *Am Sociological Rev* 1995; **60(5)**:719–745.

32 Black D, Laughlin S: Poverty and health: the old alliance needs new partners. *Benefits* 1996: **5–9**.

33 Macintyre S, Hiscock R, Kearns A, Ellaway A: Housing tenure and car access: further exploration of the nature of their relations with health in a UK setting. *J Epi Comm Health* 2001; **55**:330–331.

34 Kushel MB, Gupta R, Gee L, Haas JS: Housing instability and food insecurity as barriers to health care among low-income Americans. *J Gen Intern Med* 2006; **21(1)**:71–77.

35 Elliott JO, Lu B, Shneker BF et al.: The impact of "social determinants of health" on epilepsy prevalence and reported medication use. *Epilepsy Res* 2009; **84(2–3)**:135–145.

36 Tanumihardjo SA, Anderson C, Kaufer-Horwitz M et al.: Poverty, obesity, and malnutrition: an international perspective recognizing the paradox. *J Am Diet Assoc* 2007; **107(11)**: 1966–1972.

37 Stuff JE, Casey PH, Szeto KL et al.: Household food insecurity is associated with adult health status. *J Nutr* 2004; **134(9)**:2330–2335.

38 Fuller-Thomson E, Brennenstuhl S: The association between depression and epilepsy in a nationally representative sample. *Epilepsia* 2009; **50(5)**:1051–1058.

39 Drukker M, van Os J: Mediators of neighbourhood socioeconomic deprivation and quality of life. *Soc Psychiatry Psychiatr Epidemiol* 2003; **38(12)**:698–706.

40 Hill TD, Ross CE, Angel RJ: Neighborhood disorder, psychophysiological distress, and health. *J Health Soc Behav* 2005; **46(2)**:170–186.

41 Stimpson JP, Ju H, Raji MA, Eschbach K: Neighborhood deprivation and health risk behaviors in NHANES III. *Am J Health Behav* 2007; **31(2)**:215–222.

42 Elliott JO, Lu B, Shneker B et al.: Comorbidity, health screening, and quality of life among persons with a history of epilepsy. *Epilepsy Behav* 2009; **14(1)**:125–129.

43 Mohanraj R, Norrie J, Stephen LJ et al.: Mortality in adults with newly diagnosed and chronic epilepsy: a retrospective comparative study. *Lancet Neurology* 2006; **5(6)**:481–487.

44 Lhatoo SD, Johnson AL, Goodridge DM et al.: Mortality in epilepsy in the first 11 to 14 years after diagnosis: multivariate analysis of a long-term, prospective, population-based cohort. *Ann Neurol* 2001; **49(3)**:336–344.

45 Morgan CL, Kerr MP: Epilepsy and mortality: a record linkage study in a UK population. *Epilepsia* 2002; **43(10)**: 1251–1255.

46 Mason C, Fenton GW, Jamieson M: Teaching medical students about epilepsy. *Epilepsia* 1990; **31(1)**:95–100.

47 Brody DS: Physician recognition of behavioral, psychological, and social aspects of medical care. *Arch Intern Med* 1980; **140(10)**:1286–1289.

48 Beckman HB, Frankel RM: The effect of physician behavior on the collection of data. *Ann Intern Med* 1984; **101(5)**: 692–696.

49 Cohen-Cole SA, Boker J, Bird J, Freeman AM 3rd: Psychiatric education for primary care: a pilot study of needs of residents. *J Med Educ* 1982; **57(12)**:931–936.

50 McAuley JW, Elliott JO, Patankar S et al.: Comparing patients' and practitioners' views on epilepsy concerns: a call to address memory concerns. *Epilepsy Behav* 2010; **19(4)**: 580–583.

51 Keulers BJ, Welters CF, Spauwen PH, Houpt P: Can face-to-face patient education be replaced by computer-based patient education? A randomised trial. *Patient Educ Couns* 2007; **67(1–2)**:176–182.

52 Valente CM, Sobal J, Muncie HL Jr,: Health promotion: physicians' beliefs, attitudes, and practices. *Am J Prev Med* 1986; **2(2)**:82–88.

53 Wechsler H, Levine S, Idelson RK et al.: The physician's role in health promotion – a survey of primary-care practitioners. *N Engl J Med* 1983; **308(2)**:97–100.

54 Frank E, Breyan J, Elon L: Physician disclosure of healthy personal behaviors improves credibility and ability to motivate. *Arch Fam Med* 2000; **9(3)**:287–290.

55 Temkin O: *The Falling Sickness:* A History of Epilepsy from the Greeks to the Beginnings of Modern Neurology. Johns Hopkins University Press: Baltimore, MD, 1994.

56 De Weerd A, de Haas S, Otte A et al.: Subjective sleep disturbance in patients with partial epilepsy: a questionnaire-based study on prevalence and impact on quality of life. *Epilepsia* 2004; **45(11)**:1397–1404.

57 Kothare SV, Kaleyias J: Sleep and epilepsy in children and adolescents. *Sleep Med* 2010; **11(7)**:674–685.

58 Touchon J, Baldy-Moulinier M, Billiard M et al.: Sleep organization and epilepsy. *Epilepsy Res* 1991; **2**:73–81.

59 Malow BA, Levy K, Maturen K, Bowes R: Obstructive sleep apnea is common in medically refractory epilepsy patients. *Neurology* 2000; **55(7)**:1002–1007.

60 Rosamond W, Flegal K, Friday G et al.: Heart disease and stroke statistics – 2007 update: a report from the American Heart Association Statistics Committee and Stroke Statistics Subcommittee. *Circulation* 2007; **115(5)**:e69–171.

61 Stewart SL, Cardinez CJ, Richardson LC et al.: Surveillance for cancers associated with tobacco use – United States, 1999–2004. *MMWR Surveill Summ* 2008; **57(8)**:1–33.

62 Elliott JO, Lu B, Moore JL et al.: Exercise, diet, health behaviors, and risk factors among persons with epilepsy based on the California Health Interview Survey, 2005. *Epilepsy Behav* 2008; **13(2)**:307–315.

63 Steinhoff BJ, Neususs K, Thegeder H, Reimers CD: Leisure time activity and physical fitness in patients with epilepsy. *Epilepsia* 1996; **37(12)**:1221–1227.

64 Dubow JS, Kelly JP: Epilepsy in sports and recreation. *Sports Med* 2003; **33(7)**:499–516.

65 Brosse AL, Sheets ES, Lett HS, Blumenthal JA: Exercise and the treatment of clinical depression in adults: recent findings and future directions. *Sports Med* 2002; **32(12)**:741–760.

66 Blumer D, Montouris G, Davies K: The interictal dysphoric disorder: recognition, pathogenesis, and treatment of the major psychiatric disorder of epilepsy. *Epilepsy Behav* 2004; **5(6)**:826–840.

67 McAuley JW, Long L, Heise J et al.: A prospective evaluation of the effects of a 12-week outpatient exercise program on clinical and behavioral outcomes in patients with epilepsy. *Epilepsy Behav* 2001; **2(6)**:592–600.

68 Heise J, Buckworth J, McAuley JW et al.: Exercise training results in positive outcomes in persons with epilepsy. *Clin Exer Phys* 2002; **4(2)**:79–84.

69 Howard GM, Radloff M, Sevier TL: Epilepsy and sports participation. *Curr Sports Med Rep* 2004; **3(1)**:15–19.

70 Volpe SL, Schall JI, Gallagher PR et al.: Nutrient intake of children with intractable epilepsy compared with healthy children. *J Am Diet Assoc* 2007; **107(6)**:1014–1018.

71 Apeland T, Mansoor MA, Pentieva K et al.: Fasting and post-methionine loading concentrations of homocysteine, vitamin B2, and vitamin B6 in patients on antiepileptic drugs. *Clin Chem* 2003; **49(6 Pt 1)**:1005–1008.

72 Apeland T, Kristensen O, Strandjord RE, Mansoor MA: Thyroid function during B-vitamin supplementation of patients on antiepileptic drugs. *Clin Biochem* 2006; **39(3)**:282–286.

73 Sener U, Zorlu Y, Karaguzel O et al.: Effects of common anti-epileptic drug monotherapy on serum levels of homocysteine, vitamin B12, folic acid and vitamin B6. *Seizure* 2006; **15(2)**:79–85.

74 Schwaninger M, Ringleb P, Winter R et al.: Elevated plasma concentrations of homocysteine in antiepileptic drug treatment. *Epilepsia* 1999; **40(3)**:345–350.

75 Karabiber H, Sonmezgoz E, Ozerol E et al.: Effects of valproate and carbamazepine on serum levels of homocysteine, vitamin B12, and folic acid. *Brain Dev* 2003; **25(2)**:113–115.

76 Apeland T, Mansoor MA, Strandjord RE: Antiepileptic drugs as independent predictors of plasma total homocysteine levels. *Epilepsy Res* 2001; **47(1–2)**:27–35.

77 Apeland T, Mansoor MA, Strandjord RE, Kristensen O: Homocysteine concentrations and methionine loading in patients on antiepileptic drugs. *Acta Neurol Scand* 2000; **101(4)**:217–223.

78 Verrotti A, Pascarella R, Trotta D et al.: Hyperhomocysteinemia in children treated with sodium valproate and carbamazepine. *Epilepsy Res* 2000; **41(3)**:253–257.

79 Kishi T, Fujita N, Eguchi T, Ueda K: Mechanism for reduction of serum folate by antiepileptic drugs during prolonged therapy. *J Neurol Sci* 1997; **145(1)**:109–112.

80 Krause KH, Berlit P, Bonjour JP et al.: Vitamin status in patients on chronic anticonvulsant therapy. *Int J Vitam Nutr Res* 1982; **52(4)**:375–385.

81 Bouillon R, Reynaert J, Claes JH et al.: The effect of anticonvulsant therapy on serum levels of 25-hydroxy-vitamin D, calcium, and parathyroid hormone. *J Clin Endocrinol Metab* 1975; **41(6)**:1130–1135.

82 Yuen AW, Sander JW, Flugel D et al.: Erythrocyte and plasma fatty acid profiles in patients with epilepsy: does carbamazepine affect omega-3 fatty acid concentrations? *Epilepsy Behav* 2008; **12(2)**:317–323.

83 El-Khatib F, Rauchenzauner M, Lechleitner M et al.: Valproate, weight gain and carbohydrate craving: a gender study. *Seizure* 2007; **16(3)**:226–232.

84 Gaby AR: Natural approaches to epilepsy. *Altern Med Rev* 2007; **12(1)**:9–24.

85 Ranganathan LN, Ramaratnam S: Vitamins for epilepsy. *CDSR* 2007; **2**:DOI:10.1002/14651858.CD004304.pub2.

86 Yudkoff M, Daikhin Y, Melo TM et al.: The ketogenic diet and brain metabolism of amino acids: relationship to the anticonvulsant effect. *Ann Rev Nutr* 2007; **27**:415–430.

87 Eiris J, Novo-Rodriguez MI, Del Rio M et al.: The effects on lipid and apolipoprotein serum levels of long-term carbamazepine, valproic acid and phenobarbital therapy in children with epilepsy. *Epilepsy Res* 2000; **41(1)**:1–7.

88 Demircioglu S, Soylu A, Dirik E: Carbamazepine and valproic acid: effects on the serum lipids and liver functions in children. *Pediatr Neurol* 2000; **23(2)**:142–146.

89 Mahmoudian T, Iranpour R, Messri N: Serum lipid levels during carbamazepine therapy in epileptic children. *Epilepsy Behav* 2005; **6(2)**:257–259.

90 Tekgul H, Demir N, Gokben S: Serum lipid profile in children receiving anti-epileptic drug monotherapy: is it atherogenic? *J Pediatr Endocrinol Metab* 2006; **19(9)**:1151–1155.

91 Bramswig S, Kerksiek A, Sudhop T et al.: Carbamazepine increases atherogenic lipoproteins: mechanism of action in male adults. *Am J Physiol Heart Circ Physiol* 2002; **282(2)**:H704–H716.

92 Bramswig S, Sudhop T, Luers C et al.: Lipoprotein(a) concentration increases during treatment with carbamazepine. *Epilepsia* 2003; **44(3)**:457–460.

93 Yalcin E, Hassanzadeh A, Mawlud K: The effects of long-term anticonvulsive treatment on serum lipid profile. *Acta Paediatr Jpn* 1997; **39(3)**:342–345.

94 Trocho C, Escola-Gil JC, Ribas V et al.: Phenytoin treatment reduces atherosclerosis in mice through mechanisms independent of plasma HDL-cholesterol concentration. *Atherosclerosis* 2004; **174(2)**:275–285.

95 Verrotti A, Basciani F, Domizio S et al.: Serum lipids and lipoproteins in patients treated with antiepileptic drugs. *Pediatr Neurol* 1998; **19(5)**:364–367.

96 Jallon P, Picard F: Bodyweight gain and anticonvulsants: a comparative review. *Drug Saf* 2001; **24(13)**:969–978.

97 Cansu A, Serdaroglu A, Camurdan O et al.: The evaluation of thyroid functions, thyroid antibodies, and thyroid volumes in children with epilepsy during short-term administration of oxcarbazepine and valproate. *Epilepsia* 2006; **47(11)**:1855–1859.

98 Simko J, Horacek J: Carbamazepine and risk of hypothyroidism: a prospective study. *Acta Neurol Scand* 2007; **116(5)**: 317–321.

CHAPTER 3

Epilepsy, comorbidities, and consequences: implications for understanding and combating stigma

Rosemarie Kobau,[1] Colleen K. DiIorio,[2] Nancy J. Thompson,[2] Yvan A. Bamps,[2] and Erik K. St. Louis[3]

[1] Division of Population Health, Centers for Disease Control and Prevention, USA
[2] Department of Behavioral Sciences and Health Education, Rollins School of Public Health, Emory University, USA
[3] Department of Neurology, Mayo Clinic, USA

Disclaimer

The findings and conclusions in this report are those of the authors and do not necessarily represent the official position of the Centers for Disease Control and Prevention.

Introduction

Despite the gains made in the last 50 years in the treatment of epilepsy, for many, the diagnosis of epilepsy leads to major changes in health status and lifestyle and to profound changes in self-identity, social interactions, and life opportunities. This label of epilepsy can be attached to a "spoiled identity" with stigma at its core [1]. Early accounts of epilepsy attributed the disorder primarily to demonic or divine supernatural causes [2,3]. These beliefs are reflected in writings and art throughout history, framing social norms [4]. As a consequence, people with epilepsy were often banished from their communities or persecuted. During the 18th and 19th centuries, people with epilepsy were viewed by the public as "socially unfit" and "defective" and housed in asylums or sent to epilepsy colonies. In the United States, laws forbade people with epilepsy from marriage, reproduction, or adoption, and restricted other activities, including employment [5,6]. Although most of these restrictive laws were abolished in the 20th century and substantial social progress has been made with the passage of civil and human rights legislation,[1] this history frames the context for stigma of people with epilepsy, which persists today and can still be observed in contemporary media [6–8]. For many people with epilepsy in the United States, stigma remains among the worst things about the disorder [9]. This parallels findings from Europe, Asia, and Africa, where studies have found that about one-third to one-half of people with epilepsy report feeling stigmatized or very stigmatized by their disorder [10,11]. Individuals with epilepsy and comorbidities such as depression or anxiety face a "double stigma" associated with both an epilepsy and a mental illness diagnosis [12]. Additionally, the social disadvantages that many people with epilepsy face (e.g., unemployment, loss of income) and other health and social issues (e.g., obesity, special education, the need for caregiving in some cases) can further deflate self-esteem and marginalize people with epilepsy, compounding

[1] Section 504 of the Rehabilitation Act of 1973, The Americans with Disabilities Act, Public Law 101-336, and the 2010 Americans with Disabilities Act. The purpose of these laws is to provide uniform protection against discrimination of people with disabilities throughout the United States. Civil rights legislation in other countries and international principles on human rights prohibit discriminatory practices against people with disabilities, including those with epilepsy.

Epilepsy and the Interictal State: Co-Morbidities and Quality of Life, First Edition.
Edited by Erik K. St. Louis, David M. Ficker, and Terence J. O'Brien.
© 2015 John Wiley & Sons, Ltd. Published 2015 by John Wiley & Sons, Ltd.

the stigma. Stigma toward people with epilepsy poses a formidable burden in resource-poor regions, where more than 95% of people with epilepsy do not receive adequate treatment and where stigma interferes with basic human rights [13–18]. Thus, combating epilepsy stigma remains a public health priority worldwide [16,17].

Understanding stigma

Stigma theory

To begin to understand the causes and pervasive nature of epilepsy stigma, it is important to provide some conceptual frameworks. "Stigma" may be defined as an attribute that is perceived by others as deeply discrediting, that ultimately makes a person "of a less desirable kind" [19]. A seizure that occurs in public "discredits" a person with epilepsy, while those with better seizure control remain "discreditable" [19]. Inherent in the stigma process is the social context in which the negative characteristics are perceived and the tension between disclosure and discernment. Living among "normals," stigmatized individuals learn that they are different and come to accept the same beliefs as others about themselves. This internal devaluation, or "felt stigma," may be distinguished from "enacted stigma": overt social distancing behaviors, institutional practices (e.g., exclusion from insurance; driving and occupational restrictions), or discrimination [1,20]. For those whose stigma is not readily apparent, concealment is often used as a strategy to reduce the probability of enacted stigma. For those with visible stigmatized identities, disclosure is not an issue, but in many cases epilepsy is a "concealable stigmatized identity," where individuals must selectively weigh the pros and cons of disclosure in the context of anticipated stigma, often resulting in increased psychological distress [21].

"Courtesy stigma" is the process by which "normals" acquire some of the negative characteristics of the stigmatized, by virtue of mere association (e.g., family members, health care providers, neighbors) [19]. A recent study from China found that as much as 76% of family members of people with epilepsy felt stigmatized [22]. Observed lower employee evaluations for parents of children with epilepsy have been attributed to courtesy stigma [23]. Family members might serve as

stigma coaches, encouraging persons with epilepsy to conceal their diagnosis from others, thus perpetuating felt stigma [24]. Courtesy stigma has arguably resulted in fewer resources being allocated to patients and to professionals working on these topics, with negative implications for individuals living with these disorders [6,25].

Common dimensions of stigma may be relevant to many "marks" [26] (Table 3.1). Seizures can potentially impact social interactions, resulting in social distancing behaviors. A seizure can interrupt communication with a person with epilepsy (disruptiveness). Witnessing some types of seizures, especially for the first time, can evoke an unintended visceral response associated with aversion (esthetics) and, in some, a sense of personal threat to physical well-being (peril). In some cases, marked individuals obligate bystanders to provide help, which may be a source of distress for those unprepared to offer assistance, thus potentially evoking social distancing behaviors. While teachers report generally favorable views about the abilities of children with epilepsy, some prefer not to have them in their classrooms because of their fear of seizures and lack of knowledge about how to respond to a seizure [11,27]. In one survey, only about one-third of US adults believed they knew how to appropriately respond to a seizure, although the accuracy of their knowledge was not assessed [28]. Improving confidence and skills for seizure first aid and minimizing perceptions of harm or risk to self from seizures may minimize stigma, especially since peril (i.e., danger) is a highly salient stigma domain [26].

More contemporary views of stigma, especially in the field of mental illness stigma, focus attention on political disadvantage associated with discrimination [29–31]. Marked individuals who face discrimination are often the victims of social disadvantage, which can decrease self-esteem and lead to more dysfunction or disability, resulting in a vicious cycle of stigma (Figure 3.1) [31]. Disability, unemployment, and low income characterize the life circumstances of many people with epilepsy [16,17,32], undoubtedly contributing to the cycle [16,31].

Language and cognitive biases

Language can be a powerful weapon to demean or empower and cognitive biases can affect thinking and

Table 3.1 Dimensions of stigma and their potential implications in epilepsy. Data from Jones et al., 1984 [26].

Dimension	Characteristic	Implications/challenges
Concealability	Is the condition hidden or obvious? To what extent is its visibility controllable?	• If hidden, disclosure can become a burden, and this can be anxiety-provoking for a person with epilepsy or family members
Course	What pattern of change over time is usually shown by the condition? What is its ultimate outcome?	• Responsibility for altering the course of the condition is unclear • Treatment may be ineffective in spite of diligent self-management efforts, increasing distress in a person with epilepsy or family members • Complete remission of seizures might be a life-long concern for some, even in remission
Disruptiveness	Does the condition block or hamper interaction and communication?	• Communication interruption following a seizure may result in social distancing
Esthetic qualities	To what extent does the mark make the possessor repellent, ugly, or upsetting?	• A seizure can evoke a negative "gut reaction" that is sometimes impossible to conceal
Origin	Under what circumstances did the condition originate? Was anyone responsible for it and what was he or she trying to do?	• Blame might be assumed by those with seizures who have suffered some types of head injuries • Cultural views on epilepsy causes may dominate perceptions
Peril	What kind of danger is posed by the mark and how imminent and serious is it?	• Some might perceive a person's seizure as an immediate threat to their physical well-being • Some might resent feeling an obligation to provide help and/or lack the confidence to provide assistance, resulting in social distancing behaviors

Source: Data from Jones et al. (1984) [26]. Adapted with permission of WH Freeman.

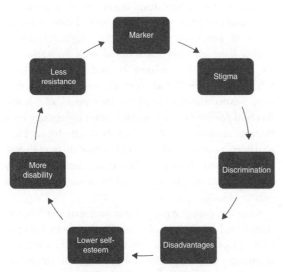

Figure 3.1 Cycles of stigma. Source: Smith [31]. Reproduced with permission from the Royal College of Psychiatrists.

decision-making skills [33]. Cognitive biases are the mental shortcuts that people engage in when making decisions. These shortcuts are influenced by anticipated emotions, framing effects, tradeoffs, and other psychological processes [33]. People may be subject to an "availability bias." When asked their opinions about epilepsy or when encountering a person with epilepsy, persons without epilepsy might be more likely to retrieve the preponderance of negative views about epilepsy, because such information is readily available, and anchor their judgment negatively [34]. In the absence of clear contrary evidence, "normals" may be biased toward attuning to behaviors that confirm negative expectations or rigid beliefs that can validate stigma [26]. "Familiarity bias" occurs when familiar false statements are accepted as true [35]. Denying myths often requires repeating false information, which may paradoxically reinforce and perpetuate mythic falsehoods [36]. The persistence of the common myth that people with epilepsy may swallow their tongue during a seizure (often refuted in educational material on epilepsy) demonstrates the pervasiveness of some "familiarity biases." Prospect theory suggests that most decisions are grounded in perceptions of gains or losses and that people are risk-averse when faced with uncertainty [37]. Losses hurt more than gains feel good, so people are risk-averse, even in relatively benign situations [37]. Whether cognitive biases or decision theory could influence efforts to combat stigma requires further study.

Person-centered language (PCL) can affect cognitive biases. The characteristics and abilities of "people with epilepsy" are viewed significantly more favorably when contrasted with "epileptics" [38]. PCL is a more empowering way to recognize persons who need services or supports because of disabilities or chronic illness [39]. The use of PCL challenges myths and stereotypes associated with stigmatizing labels that connote disability or dysfunction [39]. The reductionist term "epileptic" pejoratively connotes a person characterized primarily by seizures and may imply the additional presence of aberrant personality traits [40]. Even though worldwide epilepsy patient advocacy organizations discourage labeling people with epilepsy as "epileptics," this term and other stigmatizing language is unfortunately still commonly used [7,41]. We recommend refraining from use of this language when referring to a person and instead using PCL to help minimize epilepsy stigma [38,39].

The burden of epilepsy stigma

In people with epilepsy

People with epilepsy across cultures generally report feeling embarrassed or ashamed by the condition and associate epilepsy with fear, losses, difficulties, personal devaluation, and stigma [9,10,20,42–45]. Stigma appears to affect women and men equally, but younger people are more likely to report feelings of stigma than older people [46,47]. However, different stigma patterns by age have been found (e.g., low perceived stigma among adolescents, but the youngest (12–16-year-olds) reporting more stigma

than older adolescents (17–20-year-olds)) [48], perhaps related to small study samples, sample characteristics, nuances in how investigators operationalized stigma, or confounding uncontrolled covariates [48,49].

Employment, income, and social support may serve to buffer stigma independently or synergistically [50,51]. People who are not employed or who are unemployed and disabled tend to report higher levels of stigma [52,53]. Likewise, persons who believe that their employment status is related to their epilepsy are more likely to perceive stigma [52]. Working and earning income demonstrates social participation and integration, and confers a number of physical and mental resources (self-esteem) that may buffer stigma [53,54]. The complex associations between employment and stigma might be due in part to the nature of seizures, as people with frequent seizures are less likely to be employed [53] and are more likely to express feelings of stigma [46,52,55,56].

Seizure frequency and type play a role in the perception of stigma. Feelings of stigma are greater for those recently diagnosed with epilepsy, those still having seizures compared to those who are seizure-free, and those with more frequent seizures [10,46,50]. Likewise, people with tonic–clonic seizures tend to report higher levels of stigma [55], as do people with a combination of seizure types [57]. Individuals with simple and complex partial seizures may be able to better hide their seizure symptoms from others, resulting in less felt stigma.

Nonadherence behaviors have been linked to higher levels of perceived stigma [50,58]. Higher levels of stigma have also been associated with greater activity limitations, less seizure control, lower levels of self-efficacy for self-management, more negative outcome expectations related to treatment, and lower levels of patient satisfaction [50]. After controlling for a number of covariates, higher levels of self-efficacy have also been associated with lower levels of stigma [49,50]. Improving self-efficacy for the management of epilepsy and its effects may be warranted to minimize perceived stigma [49,50].

However, people with epilepsy do not universally feel stigmatized by the disorder, so there is room for optimism [45,59,60]. Public educational and promotional campaigns that share the stories of people (including professional athletes, musicians, and the general public) successfully living with epilepsy could help counter epilepsy stigma [6].[2]

In the public

Through the efforts of multiple organizations and campaigns over the last 50 years and following break-throughs in civil rights legislation and declarations on human rights, public awareness of epilepsy and some attitudes toward epilepsy have generally improved in regions such as North America, Europe, and some parts of Africa and Asia, but they still remain suboptimal [61–66]. The US public's attitudes regarding social-ization with and employment of people with epilepsy have improved; 57% of survey respondents in 1949 indicated that they would not object to their children playing with a child with epilepsy; this increased to 89% by 1979 [67]. In 2006, generally more than 80% of US community-dwelling adults disagreed with negative stereotypes about people with epilepsy [68],[3] but substantial proportions of the general population expressed risk and safety concerns related to seizures [68]. A majority of Spanish-speaking adults living in metropolitan areas believed that a person with epilepsy needs total supervision, while about 8% believed that an evil spirit causes epilepsy [69].

In resource-poor countries, stigma is still widespread, with as many as 51% objecting to associating with a person with epilepsy [70]. Beliefs about epilepsy having supernatural causes [71–74], fear of conta-gion [75,76], and general opposition to marriage or employment of a person with epilepsy [70,74,75,77,78] persist. Cross-cultural research on epilepsy stigma has differed, with emphasis on perceived or felt stigma in resource-rich countries (North America, Europe) and on enacted stigma or discrimination in resource-poor countries, suggesting the need for more consistency in theoretical approaches in the future [44].

Epilepsy comorbidities and stigma

Epilepsy can be complicated by neurobehavioral comor-bidities, which include psychiatric disorders, cognitive impairment, and other psychosocial and lifestyle prob-lems [79,80]. These comorbidities carry their own qual-ity of life (QOL) burden associated with impaired health status, activity limitations, disability, and stigma. Men-tal illness alone carries substantial stigma and prejudice, and others have pointed out that this is an especially damaging combination for people with epilepsy [81].

Psychiatric disorders

Psychiatric disorders such as depression and anxi-ety disorders are identified in up to half of patients with epilepsy, with higher prevalence among patients with poorly controlled seizures [82]. The relationship between psychiatric disorders and epilepsy is com-plex, related potentially to shared disease pathways, functional impairment, maladaptive coping styles, attributional style, treatment effects (medication or surgical), and other psychosocial and sociodemographic factors known to be associated with depression (e.g., sex) [42,79,81,83–86].

The lifetime prevalence of mood disorders is almost two times higher in patients with epilepsy than in those with chronic conditions such as diabetes and asthma [87]. Depression is one of the most important factors associated with patients' QOL, more powerful as a predictor than seizure frequency and severity [88,89]. In spite of its importance, depression is often unrecog-nized among people with epilepsy. Lack of recognition and treatment have been attributed to difficulty in diagnosing atypical clinical presentations of depressive disorders in epilepsy (e.g., interictal or periictal mood disorders); the myth on the part of patients, family members, and clinicians that depression is a normal

---

[2]Spokespersons with epilepsy who have participated in activities to raise public awareness about epilepsy include Tony Coelho, former US congressman and past board chair of the US Epilepsy Foundation; Chanda Gunn, US Olympic women's hockey team Olympic bronze medalist and goalie; and Jason Snelling and Alan Faneca, National Football League players. These and other individuals' stories have appeared in national press outlets (http://www.cnn.com/2006/HEALTH/02/07/profile.gunn/index.html?iref=newssearch; last accessed July 15, 2014), on YouTube (http://www.youtube.com/watch?v=zDGkYwDJsgA; last accessed July 15, 2014), and in *Epilepsy Advocate* (www.epilepsyadvocate.com; last accessed July 15, 2014).

[3]Examples of statements on the negative stereotypes subscale are: "I believe people with epilepsy should not marry," "I believe people with epilepsy are unreliable," "I believe people with epilepsy should not have biological children"; examples of statements on the risk and safety concerns subscale are: "I would ride in a car if the driver has epilepsy," "I would hire someone with epilepsy to babysit for my infant child," "I believe people with epilepsy should not drive, even if the state allows them to get a driver's license."

reaction to a condition such as epilepsy; and concern about added pharmacologic treatment [84,90].

Anxiety disorders have received less attention than depression as a comorbid psychiatric disorder in epilepsy. However, anxiety is perhaps even more common than depression and just as disabling [91,92]. Reduced health-related quality of life (HRQOL) in patients with epilepsy is strongly associated with anxiety, possibly trumping both depression and seizure frequency [93]. Elevated rates of panic attacks, panic disorder, obsessive–compulsive disorder (OCD), and generalized anxiety have been reported in adult epilepsy patients when compared with the general population [91]. Unpredictability of seizures and the resulting helplessness patients feel may contribute to high rates of anxiety, and generalized anxiety disorder is frequently associated with excessive fears of future seizures [91].

In addition to depression and anxiety, people with epilepsy suffer higher rates of attention deficit/hyperactivity disorder (ADHD), autism, and psychotic disorders [94]. Psychiatric disorders often go unrecognized and untreated in people with epilepsy, despite their high prevalence [79,84,86], which may be the direct result of stigma: patients with epilepsy might minimize their psychiatric symptoms for fear of being further stigmatized [90], while professional prejudice against people with epilepsy might impact willingness to treat those with epilepsy and comorbid psychiatric disorders [12].

Cognitive impairment

Although many people with epilepsy have normal or above normal intelligence, as a group people with epilepsy have more cognitive dysfunction than controls matched for age and education [95]. Cognitive problems can stem from seizures themselves, with loss of consciousness and postictal dysfunction, such as dysphasia; from psychological factors, such as depression; and from side effects of anti-seizure drugs, such as memory impairment.

For individuals with epilepsy and comorbid cognitive impairment, engaging in daily activities may be especially challenging. Loss of independence and withdrawal and other avoidance behaviors can reinforce self-criticism and social isolation, which may contribute to the cycle of stigma [31]. Thus, providing prompt and appropriately aggressive care for people with epilepsy and comorbid psychiatric disorders or cognitive impairment is a priority.

Along with cognitive impairment, problems with attention are common among people with epilepsy. Reports indicate that those with generalized epilepsies have attentional difficulties more frequently than do patients suffering from partial seizures [96]. Problems with attention are also stigmatized, especially among youth, who may be placed in special-education classes. Furthermore, like ADHD, frontal-lobe epilepsy can result in behaviors such as disinhibition, impulsivity, and irritability [96]. These behaviors cause people with epilepsy to behave in socially inappropriate ways, further contributing to their stigmatization. In children with epilepsy, problems with behavior are more frequent than expected in the 6 months before their first seizure is recognized [97].

Lifestyle factors

Comorbid lifestyle factors can also contribute to stigmatization of, or in, people with epilepsy. Overweight body habitus and obesity occur at elevated rates [32,98], which has been attributed to their medication regimens and reduced rates of physical activity [99]. In addition, smoking is more frequent among people with epilepsy [32,98,100]. Both of these behaviors are highly stigmatized in today's society [101,102].

Impact on QOL

The cumulative effects of living with epilepsy and associated social disadvantages (e.g., unemployment) are reflected in the substantially lower levels of QOL and life satisfaction among people with epilepsy [32,103–109]. Those with more frequent or severe seizures tend to report lower levels of QOL compared to those with well-controlled seizures [103,104,106–114]. Mental health issues, including depression and stigma, have been found to contribute to diminished feelings of well-being. In adults with epilepsy, the perception of stigma is a strongly negative predictor of lower QOL [115]. Depression, seizures within the past year, and activity restrictions are also important predictors of QOL. In adults living with epilepsy in the Netherlands, sociopsychological variables including stigma, psychological distress, coping, and loneliness were the most important predictors of QOL, contributing about twice as much as did "medical variables," including seizure frequency [51]. Stigma limits a person's social interactions, educational attainment, and employment opportunities, ultimately limiting independence. Activity restrictions and loneliness impact feelings of well-being. Moreover, people who feel uncomfortable in social situations tend to report less satisfaction with their lives [51].

The relationship between stigma and QOL is evident among adolescents, as well. Higher perceived levels of stigma have been associated with poorer self-esteem among adolescents [48]. Moreover, adolescents from lower socioeconomic households and those requiring special-education classes report higher perceived stigma and lower overall QOL [116]. A general lack of knowledge about epilepsy and perceptions reflecting stigma contribute to a peer social environment that

is especially stressful for youths with epilepsy [66]. Society also suffers without the contributions of people with epilepsy to the larger social fabric.

Combating stigma

Stigma-mitigating strategies often require multiple approaches, including disease prevention, public information to improve understanding and correct perceptions of risk or danger, the provision of counseling services for those affected by a disorder, and social policies and regulatory action that promote integration [60,117]. Many of these anti-stigma strategies have been

Table 3.2 Select examples of epilepsy stigma-reduction initiatives, resources, and toolkits.

Source	Toolkit/campaign	Web site	Population targeted
International League Against Epilepsy, International Bureau for Epilepsy, and World Health Organization	Global Campaign Against Epilepsy: Out of the Shadows	http://globalcampaignagainstepilepsy.org	General public, health care professionals, and policy makers
National Epilepsy Foundation and US Centers for Disease Control and Prevention		http://www.epilepsyfoundation.org/	General public
	Talk About It	http://www.talkaboutit.org/	General public
	La Epilepsia es Mas Comun de lo Que Piensas	http://209.66.116.43/epilepsia/	Hispanics
	Take Charge of the Facts	http://www.epilepsy.com/make-difference/public-awareness/take-charge-facts	Adolescents (14–17 years)
	Take Charge of the Storm	http://www.epilepsy.com/make-difference/public-awareness/take-charge-storm	Adolescents (11–14 years)
	Managing Students with Seizures	http://www.epilepsy.com/get-help/services-and-support/training-programs/managing-students-seizures-school-nurse-training	School nurses
	You Are Not Alone	http://www.cdc.gov/epilepsy/toolkit/index.htm	Parents of teens with epilepsy
	Epilepsy Training for First Responders	http://www.epilepsy.com/get-help/services-and-support/training-programs/first-responder-training	First responders
	1 in 26 Campaign	http://www.epilepsy.com/make-difference/public-awareness/1-26	General public and targeted subgroups (e.g., Asian-Americans)

implemented over the past few decades by worldwide government agencies and nongovernmental epilepsy and general health organizations. Extensive educational information about epilepsy, community-based stigma reduction toolkits for targeted groups (e.g., students, first responders, parents of children with epilepsy), community-based anti-stigma campaign material for special populations, and guidance documents are publicly available (Table 3.2). Readers are encouraged to access these resources and to check for updated materials as they become available, and ultimately to use and disseminate these materials in their local communities.

New communication approaches that consider cognitive biases and make use of social media innovations to combat epilepsy stigma require research. PCL should be used when communicating about people with epilepsy. Professional educational programs with general health care providers aimed at improving epilepsy knowledge and effective treatment strategies might help ease any apprehension in treating people with epilepsy. Continued public education about epilepsy, in addition to enhancing individuals' skills and reducing their anxiety over administering seizure first aid, may help minimize discomfort concerning seizures and improve attitudes toward people with epilepsy.

References

1 Scambler G, Hopkins A: Generating a model of epileptic stigma: the role of qualitative analysis. *Soc Sci Med* 1990; **30(11)**:1187–1194.

2 Masia SL, Dovinsky O: Epilepsy and behavior: a brief history. *Epilepsy Behav* 2000; **1(1)**:27–36.

3 Baxendale S. The intriguing case of Christina the Astonishing. *Neurology* 2008;**70(21)**:2004–2007.

4 Wolf P: Epilepsy in contemporary fiction: fates of patients. *Can J Neurol Sci* 2000; **27**:166–172.

5 Hermann B: 100 years of *Epilepsia*: landmark papers and their influence in neuropsychology and neuropsychiatry. *Epilepsia* 2010; **51(7)**:1107–1119.

6 Jacoby A: Stigma, epilepsy, and quality of life. *Epilepsy Behav* 2002; **3**:S10–S20.

7 Krauss GL, Gondek S, Krumholz A et al.: The scarlet E: the presentation of epilepsy in the English language print media. *Neurology* 2000; **54(10)**:1894–1898.

8 Morrell MJ, Pedley TA: "The scarlet E": epilepsy is still a burden. *Neurology* 2000; **54**:1882–1883.

9 Fisher RS: Epilepsy from the patient's perspective: review of results of a community-based survey. *Epilepsy Behav* 2000; **1**:S9–S14.

10 Baker GA: People with epilepsy: what do they know and understand, and how does this contribute to their perceived level of stigma? *Epilepsy Behav* 2002: S26–S32.

11 Lee SA, Yoo HJ, Lee BI: Korean QoL in Epilepsy Study Group – factors contributing to the stigma of epilepsy. *Seizure* 2005; **14(3)**:157–163.

12 Marchetti RL, Werneck de Castro AP, Salles Daltio C et al.: Attitudes of Brazilian psychiatrists toward people with epilepsy. *Epilepsy Behav* 2004: **999–1004**.

13 Onwuekwe IO, Onodugo OD, Ezeala-Adikaibe B et al.: Pattern and presentation of epilepsy in Nigerian Africans: a study of trends in the southeast. *Trans R Soc Trop Med Hyg* 2009; **103(8)**:785–789.

14 Rafael F, Houinato D, Nubukpo P et al.: Sociocultural and psychological features of perceived stigma reported by people with epilepsy in Benin. *Epilepsia* 2010; **51(6)**: 1061–1068.

15 Shafiq M, Tanwir M, Tariq A et al.: Myths and fallacies about epilepsy among residents of a Karachi slum area. *Trop Doct* 2008; **38(1)**:32–33.

16 World Health Organization: Neurological disorders: public health challenges. http://www.who.int/mental_health/neurology/neurodiso/en/index.html (last accessed July 15, 2014).

17 World Health Organization: Mental health and development: targeting people with mental health conditions as a vulnerable group. http://www.who.int/mental_health/policy/mhtargeting/en/index.html (last accessed July 15, 2014).

18 deBoer HM, Mula M, Sander JW: The global burden of stigma. *Epilepsy Behav* 2008; **12(4)**:540–546.

19 Goffman E: *Stigma: Notes on the Management of Spoiled Identify*. Penguin: London, 1963.

20 Jacoby A: Felt versus enacted stigma: a concept revisited. *Soc Sci Med* 1994; **38(2)**:269–274.

21 Quinn DM, Chaudoir SR: Living with a concealable stigmatized identity: the impact of anticipated stigma, centrality, salience and cultural stigma on psychological distress and health. *J Pers Soc Psychol* 2009; **97(4)**:634–651.

22 Li S, Wu J, Wang W et al.: Stigma and epilepsy: the Chinese perspective. *Epilepsy Behav* 2010; **17(2)**:242–245.

23 Parfene C, Stewart TL, King TZ: Epilepsy stigma and stigma by association in the workplace. *Epilepsy Behav* 2009; **15(4)**:461–466.

24 Schneider JW, Conrad P: Medical and sociological typologies: the case of epilepsy. *Soc Sci Med* 1981; **15A**:212–219.

25 Weiss MG, Ramakrishna J: Interventions: research on reducing stigma. Paper presented at US *NIH Conference on Stigma and Global Health: Developing a Research Agenda*. Bethesda, MD, September 2001.

26 Jones EE, Farina A, Hastorf AH et al.: *The Dimensions of Stigma: The Psychology of Marked Relationships*. WH Freeman & Company: New York, 1984.

27 Prpic I, Korotaj Z, Vlasic-Cicvaric I et al.: Teachers' opinions about capabilities and behavior of children with epilepsy. *Epilepsy Behav* 2003; **4**:142–145.

28 Kobau R, Price PH: Knowledge of epilepsy and familiarity with this disorder in the U.S. population: results from the 2002 Health Styles Survey. *Epilepsia* 2003; **44(11)**: 1449–1454.

29 Sayce L: Stigma, discrimination and social exclusion: what's in a word? *J Ment Health* 1998; **7(4)**:331–343.

30 Link BG, Phelan JC: Stigma and its public health implications. *Lancet* 2006; **367**:528–529.

31 Smith M: Stigma. *Adv Psych Treat* 2002; **8**:317–325.

32 CDC: Epilepsy surveillance among adults – 19 states, Behavioral Risk Factor Surveillance System, 2005. *MMWR* 2008; **57(SS-6)**:1–20.

33 Kahneman D, Slovic P, Tversky A: *Judgment Under Uncertainty: Heuristics and Biases*. Cambridge University Press: New York, 1982.

34 Taylor S: The availability bias in social perception and interaction. In: Kahneman D, Slovic P, Tversky A (eds): *Judgment Under Uncertainty: Heuristics and Biases*. Cambridge University Press: New York, 1982, pp. 190–208.

35 Skurnik I, Yoon C, Park DC, Schwarz N: How warnings about false claims become recommendations. *J Consumer Res* 2005; **31**:713–723.

36 Vedantam S, Washington Post: Persistence of myths could alter public policy approach. http://freedom-school.com/reading-room/persistence-of-myths-could-alter-public-policy-approach.pdf (last accessed July 15, 2014).

37 Kahneman D: A perspective on judgment and choice. *Am Psychol* 2003; **58**:697–720

38 Fernandes PT, deBarros NF, Li LM: Stop saying epileptic. *Epilepsia* 2009; **50(5)**:1280–1283.

39 National Center on Birth Defects and Developmental Disabilities: Communication with and about people with disabilities. No. CS214598-A, CDC. Atlanta, GA. http://www.cdc.gov/ncbddd/disabilityandhealth/pdf/disabilityposter_photos.pdf (last accessed July 15, 2014).

40 Ritaccio AL, Devinsky O: Personality disorders in epilepsy. In: Ettinger AB, Kanner AM (eds.): *Psychiatric Issues in Epilepsy*. Lippincott Williams & Wilkins: Philadelphia, 2001, pp. 147–161.

41 Caspermeyer JJ, Sylvester EJ, Drazkowski JF et al.: Evaluation of stigmatizing language and medical errors in neurology coverage by US newspapers. *Mayo Clin Proc* 2006; **81(3)**:300–306.

42 De Souza EAP, Salgado PCB: A psychosocial view of anxiety and depression in epilepsy. *Epilepsy Behav* 2006; **8**: 232–238.

43 Kilinc S, Campbell C: "It shouldn't be something that's evil, it should be talked about": a phenomenological approach to epilepsy and stigma. *Seizure* 2009; **18(10)**:665–671.

44 Reis R, Meinardi H: ILAE/WHO "Out of the Shadows Campaign": Stigma: does the flag identify the cargo? *Epilepsy Behav* 2002; **3**:S33–S37.

45 Ryan R, Kempner K, Emlen AC: The stigma of epilepsy as a self-concept. *Epilepsia* 1980; **21**:433–444.

46 Jacoby A, Baker GA, Steen N et al.: The clinical course of epilepsy and its psychosocial correlates: findings from a U.K. community study. *Epilepsia* 1996; **37(2)**:148–161.

47 Ridsdale L, Robins D, Fitzgerald A et al.: Epilepsy in general practice: patients' psychological symptoms and their perception of stigma. *Br J Gen Pract* 1996; **46**:365–366.

48 Westbrook LE, Bauman LJ, Shinnar S: Applying stigma theory to epilepsy: a test of a conceptual model. *J Pediatr Psychol* 1992; **17(5)**:633–649.

49 Smith G, Ferguson PL, Saunders LL et al.: Psychosocial factors associated with stigma in adults with epilepsy. *Epilepsy Behav* 2009; **16**:484–490.

50 DiIorio C, Osborne Shafer P, Letz R et al. and the Project EASE Study Group: The association of stigma with self-management and perceptions of health care among adults with epilepsy. *Epilepsy Behav* 2003; **4**:259–267.

51 Suurmeijer TPBM, Reuvekamp MF, Aldenkamp BP: Social functioning, psychological functioning, and quality of life in epilepsy. *Epilepsia* 2001; **42(9)**:1160–1168.

52 Chaplin JE, Wester A, Tomson T: Factors associated with the employment problems of people with established epilepsy. *Seizure* 1998; **7(4)**:299–303.

53 Smeets VMJ, van Lierop BAG, Vanhoutvin JPG et al.: Epilepsy and employment: literature review. *Epilepsy Behav* 2007; **10**:354–362.

54 Schachter SC, Shafer PI, Murphy W: The personal impact of seizures: correlations with seizure frequency, employment, cost of medical care, and satisfaction with physician care. *J Epilepsy* 1993; **6**:224–227.

55 Baker GA, Brooks J, Buck D, Jacoby A: The stigma of epilepsy: a European perspective. *Epilepsia* 1999; **41**: 98–104.

56 Baker GA, Jacoby A, Chadwick DW: The associations of psychopathology in epilepsy: a community study. *Epilepsy Res* 1996; **25(1)**:29–39.

57 Ratsepp M, Oun A, Haldre S, Kaasik A: Felt stigma and impact of epilepsy on employment status among Estonian people: exploratory study. *Seizure* 2000; **9**:394–401.

58 Buck D, Jacoby A, Baker GA, Chadwick DW: Factors influencing compliance with antiepileptic drug regimes. *Seizure* 1997; **6**:87–93.

59 MacLeod JS, Austin JK. Stigma in the lives of adolescents with epilepsy: a review of the literature. *Epilepsy Behav* 2003; **4**:112–117.

60 Morrell MJ. Stigma and epilepsy. *Epilepsy Behav* 2002: S21–S25.

61 Doughty J, Baker GA, Jacoby A, Lavaud V: Cross-cultural differences in levels of knowledge about epilepsy. *Epilepsia* 2003; **44(1)**:115–123.

62 Hasan SS, Alen YK, Wayne WG et al.: Understanding of and attitudes toward epilepsy among the urban Chinese population in Malaysia. *Epilepsy Behav* 2010; **51(4)**:290–299.

63 Jacoby A, Gorry J, Gamble C, Baker GA: Public knowledge, private grief: a study of public attitudes to epilepsy in the United Kingdom and implications for stigma. *Epilepsia* 2004; **45(11)**;1405–1415.

64 Mirnics Z, Czikor G, Zavecz T, Halasz P: Changes in public attitudes toward epilepsy in Hungary: results of surveys conducted in 1994 and 2000. *Epilepsia* 2001; **42(1)**:86–93.

65 Shibre T, Alem A, Takle-Haimanot R et al.: Community attitudes towards epilepsy in a rural Ethiopian setting: a re-visit after 15 years. *Ethiop Med J* 2008; **46(3)**:251–259.

66 Austin JK, Shafer PO, Deering JB: Epilepsy familiarity, knowledge, and perceptions of stigma: report from a survey of adolescents in the general population. *Epilepsy Behav* 2002; **3(4)**:368–375.

67 Caveness WF, Gallup GH Jr: A survey of public attitudes toward epilepsy in 1979 with an indication of trends over the past thirty years. *Epilepsia* 1980; **21(5)**:509–518.

68 Kobau R, DiIorio CA, Anderson LA, Price PH: Further validation and reliability testing of the Attitudes and Beliefs about Living with Epilepsy (ABLE) components of the CDC Epilepsy Program Instrument on Stigma. *Epilepsy Behav* 2006; **8(3)**:552–559.

69 Sirven JI, Lopez RA, Vazquez B, Van Haverbeke P: Qué es la Epilepsia? Attitudes and knowledge of epilepsy by Spanish-speaking adults in the United States. *Epilepsy Behav* 2005; **7**:259–265.

70 Njamnshi AK, Yepnjio FN, Bissek AC et al.: A survey of public knowledge, attitudes, and practices with respect to epilepsy in Badissa village, centre region of Cameroon. *Epilepsy Behav* 2009; **16(2)**:254–259.

71 Birbeck GL, Chomba E, Atadzhanov M et al.: Zambian teachers: what do they know about epilepsy and how can we work with them to decrease stigma? *Epilepsy Behav* 2006; **9(2)**:275–280.

72 Sanya EO, Salami TA, Goodman OO et al.: Perception and attitude to epilepsy among teachers in primary, secondary and tertiary educational institutions in middle belt Nigeria. *Trop Doc* 2005; **35(3)**:153–156.

73 Shafiq M, Tanwir M, Tariz A et al.: Myths and fallacies about epilepsy among residents of a Karachi slum area. *Trop Doct* 2008; **38(1)**:32–33.

74 Tran DS, Odermatt P, Singphuoangphet S et al.: Epilepsy in Laos: knowledge, attitudes, and practices in the community. *Epilepsy Behav* 2007; **10(4)**:565–570.

75 Awad A, Sarkhoo F: Public knowledge and attitudes toward epilepsy in Kuwait. *Epilepsia* 2008; **49(4)**:564–572.

76 Millogo A, Siranyan AS: Knowledge of epilepsy and attitudes towards the condition among schoolteachers in Bob-Dioulasso (Burkina Faso). *Epileptic Disord* 2004; **6(1)**: 21–26.

77 Choi-Kwon S, Park KA, Lee HJ et al.: Familiarity with, knowledge of, and attitudes toward epilepsy in residents of Seoul, South Korea. *Aca Neurol Scand* 2004; **110(1)**:39–45.

78 Nuhu FT, Fawole JO, Babalola OJ et al.: Social consequences of epilepsy: a study of 231 Nigerian patients. *Ann Afr Med* 2010; **9(3)**:170–175.

79 Devinsky O: Psychiatric comorbidity in patients with epilepsy: implications for diagnosis and treatment. *Epilepsy Behav* 2003: S2–S10.

80 Hermann BP, Seidenberg M, Jones J: The neurobehavioral comorbidities of epilepsy: can a natural history be developed? *Lancet Neurol* 2008; **7(2)**:151–160.

81 Krishnamoorthy ES. Treatment of depression in patients with epilepsy: problems, pitfalls, and some solutions. *Epilepsy Behav* 2003: S46–S54.

82 LaFrance WC Jr, Kanner AM, Hermann B: Psychiatric comorbidities in epilepsy. *Int Rev Neurobiol* 2008; **83**: 347–383.

83 Amann B, Grunze, H: Neurochemical underpinnings in bipolar disorder and epilepsy. *Epilepsia* 2005; **46(S4)**: 26–30.

84 Barry JJ. The recognition and management of mood disorders as a comorbidity of epilepsy. *Epilepsia* 2003; **44(S4)**:30–40.

85 Hermann BP, Trenerry MR, Colligan RC: Learned helplessness, attributional style, and depression in epilepsy. *Bozeman Epilepsy Surgery Consortium. Epilepsia* 1996; **37(7)**: 680–686.

86 Kanner AM. Depression in epilepsy: a frequently neglected multifaceted disorder. *Epilepsy Behav* 2003: S11–S19.

87 Blum D, Reed M, Metz A: Prevalence of major affective disorders and manic/ hypomanic symptoms in persons with epilepsy: a community survey. *Neurology* 2002; **Suppl. 3**:A175.

88 Johnson EK, Jones JE, Seidenberg M, Hermann BP: The relative impact of anxiety, depression, and clinical seizure features on health-related quality of life in epilepsy. *Epilepsia* 2004; **45**:544–550.

89 Tracy JI, Dechant V, Sperling MR et al.: The association of mood and quality of life ratings in epilepsy. *Neurology* 2007; **68(14)**:1101–1107.

90 Kanner AM, Balabov A: Depression and epilepsy: how closely related are they? *Neurology* 2002; **58(8 Suppl. 5)**: S27–S39.

91 Beyenburg S, Mitchell AJ, Schmidt D et al.: Anxiety in patients with epilepsy: systematic review and suggestions for clinical management. *Epilepsy Behav* 2005; **7**:161–171.

92 Vazquez B, Devinsky O: Epilepsy and anxiety. *Epilepsy Behav* 2003; **4(Suppl. 4)**:S20–S25.

93 Choi-Kwon S, Chung C, Kim H et al.: Factors affecting the quality of life in patients with epilepsy in Seoul, South Korea. *Acta Neurologica Scandinavica* 2003; **108**:428–434.

94 Ekinci O, Titus JB, Rodopman AA et al.: Depression and anxiety in children and adolescents with epilepsy: Prevalence, risk factors, and treatment. *Epilepsy Behav* 2009; **14**:8–18.

95 Meador KJ: Cognitive outcomes and predictive factors in epilepsy. *Neurology* 2002; **58(8)**:S21–S26.

96 Parisi P, Moavero R, Verrotti A, Curatolo P: Attention deficit hyperactivity disorder in children with epilepsy. *Brain Dev* 2010; **32**:10–16.

97 Austin JK, Harezlak J, Dunn DW et al.: Behavior problems in children before first recognized seizures. *Pediatrics* 2001; **107(1)**:115–122.

98 Hinnell C, Williams J, Metcalfe A et al.: Health status and health-related behaviors in epilepsy compared to other chronic conditions: a national population-based study. *Epilepsia* 2010; **51(5)**:853–861.

99 Kobau R, DiIorio C, Price PH et al.: Prevalence of epilepsy and health status of adults with epilepsy in Georgia and Tennessee: Behavioral Risk Factor Surveillance System, 2002. *Epilepsy Behav* 2004; **5(3)**:358–366.

100 Ben-Menachem E: Weight issues for people with epilepsy – a review. *Epilepsia* 2007; **38(Suppl. 9)**:42–45.

101 Puhl RM, Heuer CA: Obesity stigma: important consider-ations for public health. *Am J Public Health* 2010; **100(6)**:1019–1028.

102 Ritchie D, Amos A, Martin C: "But it just has that sort of feel about it, a leper": stigma, smoke-free legislation, and public health. *Nicotine & Tobacco Research* 2010; **12(6)**:622–629.

103 Berto P: Quality of life in patients with epilepsy and impact of treatments. *Pharmacoeconomics* 2002; **20(15)**:1039–1059.

104 Bishop M, Berven NL, Hermann BP, Chan F: Quality of life among adults with epilepsy: an exploratory model. *Rehabil Couns Bull* 2002; **45**:87–95.

105 Hermann BP: The evolution of health-related quality-of-life assessment in epilepsy. *Qual Life Res* 1995; **4(2)**:87–100.

106 Leidy NK, Elixhauser A, Vickrey B et al.: Seizure frequency and the health-related quality of life of adults with epilepsy, 1999. *Neurology* 2001; **57(11 Suppl 4)**:S69–S73.

107 Mrabet H, Mrabet A, Zouari B, Ghachem R: Health-related quality of life of people with epilepsy compared with a general reference population: a Tunisian study. *Epilepsia* 2004; **45(7)**:838–843.

108 Raty L, Hamrin E, Soderfeldt B: Quality of life in newly-debuted epilepsy – an empirical study. *Acta Neurol Scand* 1999; **100(4)**:221–226.

109 Wagner JL, Sample PL, Ferguson PL et al.: Impact of pediatric epilepsy: voices from a focus group and implica-tions for public policy change. *Epilepsy Behav* 2009; **16(1)**:161–165.

110 Argyriou AA, Papapetropoulos S, Polychronopoulos P et al.: Psychosocial effects and evaluation of the health-related quality of life in patients suffering from well-controlled epilepsy. *J Neurol* 2004; **251(3)**:310–313.

111 Collings JA: Psychosocial well-being and epilepsy – an empirical-study. *Epilepsia* 1990; **31(4)**:418–426.

112 Kugoh T: Quality of life in adult patients with epilepsy. *Epilepsia* 1996; **37**:37–40.

113 Leppik IE: Quality of life of people with epilepsy in the United States. *Clin Therapeutics* 1998; **20(Suppl. A)**:A13–A18, disc. A58–A60.

114 Sillanpaa M, Haataja L, Shinnar S: Perceived impact of childhood-onset epilepsy on quality of life as an adult. *Epilepsia* 2004; **45(8)**:971–977.

115 Whatley AD, DiIorio CK, Yeager K: Examining the relation-ships of depressive symptoms, stigma, social support and regimen-specific support on quality of life in adult patients with epilepsy. *Health Educ Res* 2010; **25(4)**:575–584.

116 Devinsky O, Westbrook L, Cramer J et al.: Risk factors for poor health-related quality of life in adolescents with epilepsy. *Epilepsia* 1999; **40(12)**:1715–1720.

117 Weiss MG, Ramakrishna J, Somma D: Health-related stigma: rethinking concepts and interventions. *Psychol Health Med* 2006; **11(3)**:277–287.

SECTION II
Cognition and epilepsy

CHAPTER 4

Causes and types of cognitive domain impairments in epilepsy

Sections

Impairment of consciousness in epilepsy

Luigi Maccotta,[1] Clemente Vega,[2] and R. Edward Hogan[1]

[1] *Comprehensive Epilepsy Center, Barnes Jewish Hospital and Washington University, USA*

[2] *Division of Epilepsy and Clinical Neurophysiology, Children's Hospital Boston and Harvard University, USA*

Ictal cognitive impairments due to nonconvulsive status epilepticus

Elizabeth Waterhouse[3]

[3] *Department of Neurology, Virginia Commonwealth University School of Medicine, USA*

Memory and dysexecutive impairments in epilepsy

Erik K. St. Louis[4] and Ashley M. Enke[5]

[4] *Department of Neurology, Mayo Clinic, USA*

[5] *Creighton University, USA*

Attention deficit/hyperactivity disorder, disordered attention, and epilepsy

David W. Dunn[6] and William G. Kronenberger[6]

[6] *Department of Psychiatry and Neurology, Indiana University School of Medicine, USA*

Behavioral and developmental disorders in epilepsy

Michael Smith[7] and Esmeralda L. Park[7]

[7] *Rush Epilepsy Center, Rush University Medical Center, USA*

Introduction

Cognition is a key domain impacting the quality of life (QOL) of patients with epilepsy and cognitive impairments are a common problem affecting many epilepsy patients. Several cognitive domains may be impaired in epilepsy, including memory and executive functioning, language, and attention. Furthermore, complex cognitive disorders such as attention deficit disorder, psychomotor maldevelopment accompanying cortical malformations or static encephalopathies resulting from antenatal, perinatal, or postnatal cerebral brain

Epilepsy and the Interictal State: Co-Morbidities and Quality of Life, First Edition.
Edited by Erik K. St. Louis, David M. Ficker, and Terence J. O'Brien.
© 2015 John Wiley & Sons, Ltd. Published 2015 by John Wiley & Sons, Ltd.

injuries, and autism are frequent comorbid cognitive disorders in children, adolescents, and younger adults with epilepsy, while dementia is an increasingly recognized condition associated with epilepsy in the elderly. Causes of cognitive impairments are complex, multiple, and overlapping, and include structural brain lesions underlying epilepsy, nociferous epileptic cortex causing cognitive dysfunction, type and frequency of seizures, duration of epilepsy, interictal spiking, ictal or lingering postictal consciousness and other cognitive impairments, and cognitive problems due to adverse effects of antiepileptic drugs (AEDs), neurostimulation therapies, and surgical lesions. Determining the causes of cognitive impairments that impact QOL for epilepsy patients is often difficult and given the general lack of direct treatments, therapeutic approaches for cognitive impairments in epilepsy are necessarily multipronged, including optimizing treatment for the epilepsy itself through medication, surgery, or neurostimulation therapy, restructuring AED polytherapy regimens, and, increasingly, cognitive rehabilitation strategies.

Impairment of consciousness in epilepsy

Introduction

From the beginnings of modern concepts of the pathophysiology of epileptic seizures, consciousness has played a central role in the proposed etiology and classification of epilepsy [1]. In modern classification systems [2], consciousness continues to be a major criterion in definitions; for example, partial (or focal) seizures are defined as either simple (with retained consciousness) or complex (with loss of consciousness). The continued inclusion of consciousness in the definition of seizures and epilepsy is related to the concerning clinical morbidity associated with global encephalopathy and altered perception during the ictal and periictal states. Typical ictal and postictal complex partial seizures are stereotyped within individual patients and can involve either arrested activity or actions that are simple, unsustained, and not supported by a consecutive series of purposeful movements [3]. Clinical periictal semiological concomitants can include: 1) continuation of actions ongoing before the seizure (although often in an imperfect way); 2) disorientation and mild delirium, sometimes associated with wandering; and rarely 3) more dramatic symptoms of struggling, shouting, kicking, and "hysteria" [4]. With repeated episodes of disruption of consciousness in subjects with intractable epilepsy, associated problems range from social stigmatization to trauma (especially in the context of operating an automobile or machinery), severe burns, and drowning. Clinical semiology in the periictal state is the manifestation of differential dysfunction of specific brain regions. Often there is a relative delay in the recovery of higher perceptive and motor functions, causing patients to "misperceive" their environment and therefore react inappropriately [3,5]. Illustrative of this concept is the phenomenon of "resistive violence," associated with periictal aggressive behavior, in which attempts to restrain patients in a postictal confusional state produce violent reactive automatisms [6]. Patients misperceive the restraining attempts as threatening and "fight back" during the encounter. Most investigators emphasize that the clinical situation, and specifically the reaction of bystanders during the periictal state, is one of the most important factors in provoking aggressive behavior [3,6].

Despite longstanding interest in consciousness and epilepsy and the importance of deficits of consciousness in clinical epileptology, defining consciousness and establishing objective relationships between conscious states and epileptic seizures remains difficult [5,7]. Neurobiological research can inform this definition with the study of aspects of conscious experience, such as perception, attention, memory, language, and voluntary movement [8]. Yet using a complex neurobiological definition of consciousness ultimately yields too broad a construct to provide a useful basis for the purposes of clinical epilepsy. The semiology of epileptic seizures can provide objective observations on how initial signs and symptoms can progress to global neurological dysfunction, potentially linking seizure pathophysiology with basic neurobiological mechanisms of brain function. To illustrate recent advances in the understanding of epilepsy and consciousness, we will review recent findings in two epilepsy syndromes, focusing on ictal SPECT findings in temporal-lobe epilepsy (TLE) and functional magnetic resonance imaging (fMRI) findings in absence epilepsy. Additionally, we will examine the concept of functional neurologic networks in epilepsy, focusing on resting-state networks.

Temporal-lobe epilepsy

In his landmark clinical observations on TLE and consciousness [9,10], John Hughlings-Jackson noted the clinical association of the mesial TLE aura of fear and epigastric sensation with loss of consciousness, stating that "it seems strange that these sensations should, as is most common, occur in those cases of epilepsy in which loss of consciousness is, next to such warning, the first event in the paroxysm" [11]. Using the equivalent of the modern concept of focal epileptic seizures, defined as "a seizure whose initial semiology indicates, or is consistent with, initial activation of only part of one cerebral hemisphere" [12], Hughlings-Jackson postulated that seizures arising from the "uncinate" region (contemporarily defined as mesial TLE) were closely functionally related to mechanisms controlling global brain functions. Additionally, he observed that the semiology of temporal-lobe seizures often included both positive and negative components. Using the clinical example of the aura of déjà vu, he described a positive component of a feeling of familiarity and a negative component of misperception of reality and a "clouded" recollection of events. Importantly, behaviors observed after seizures often begin during the epileptic discharge and persist into the postictal period [5]. From these clinical observations in TLE, one can speculate that 1) mesial temporal structures may be functionally related to global brain functions, including those supporting the conscious state; 2) positive and negative periictal symptoms may represent the manifestation of the activation or inhibition of specific brain regions, often occurring simultaneously; and 3) the region of initial brain activation (the "epileptogenic" mesial temporal region) secondarily affects other brain structures, which, in turn, at least in part, produce changes in consciousness, with symptoms that often continue into the postictal period.

Ictal single-photon emission computed tomography (SPECT), which enables measurement of ictal blood perfusion changes over the entire brain, has enabled measurement of global brain changes during TLE seizures. Ictal SPECT studies in TLE show broad regions of hyperperfusion (activation) and hypoperfusion (inhibition) during temporal-lobe seizures, with primary activation of contiguous structures of the the ipsilateral anteromedial temporal region, corpus striatum, and insula [13–17]. In addition, there are broad regions of inhibition in distant brain regions, with perfusion decreases in the frontoparietal association cortex, precuneus, and cingulate gyrus during and following seizures, similar in distribution to the "default-mode" network (see subsequent discussion) [18]. Interestingly, regions of SPECT hypoperfusion during TLE seizures are larger than in extratemporal epileptic seizures [19], implying that TLE seizures preferentially inhibit broad brain regions, which likely contributes to loss of consciousness [15]. SPECT findings provide interesting correlations with Jacksonian theories derived from clinical observations of TLE seizures, confirming simultaneous excitatory and inhibitory periictal brain changes and secondary involvement of broad brain regions beyond the temporal lobe during the periictal state. How activation and inhibition of brain regions produce clinical symptoms remains an important question in the basic pathophysiology of TLE seizures. The "network inhibition hypothesis" addresses this issue by proposing that temporal-lobe seizures spread to midline subcortical structures, leading in turn to bilateral cortical inhibition [20]. This hypothesis incorporates the idea of interactions between neuronal networks to explain how focal-onset seizures cause global changes in brain function and consciousness.

Childhood absence epilepsy

Studying childhood absence epilepsy (CAE) provides a reliable model for examining brain changes responsible for alterations in consciousness. Typical episodes are associated with a brief period of unresponsiveness, usually lasting 5–10 seconds, without additional clinical correlates such as tonic–clonic movements or automatisms [21]. The typical electrical pattern in absence seizures involves 3–4 Hz bilateral spike-and-wave discharges and normal background activity [22], described early in the history of the EEG [23].

In order to increase our understanding of periictal changes in cognition observed in absence epilepsy, we must explore the neural pathways involved in alteration of consciousness. Abnormalities in thalamico-cortical pathways have been suggested as likely to be responsible for the generation of spike-and-wave discharges based on thalamic stimulation in animal models and in human subjects [24] and, as with other epilepsies, disruption of thalamic function is believed to play a central role in the alteration of consciousness observed in absence [25]. However, thalamic dysfunction alone does not account for the variability in cognitive changes reported in the literature; disruption of normal communication between specific bilateral anterior neocortical areas and subcortical structures (e.g., thalamus) during the ictal period creates specific cognitive changes associated with that neocortical region, mediating the type of impairment [21].

Decades of literature investigating ictal changes in consciousness in absence epilepsy reveal variability in degree of impairment based on a number of variables. For example, simple tasks such as repetitive fine-motor movements have been found to be relatively unaffected during seizures, while tasks requiring more complex actions involving attention, memory, and language comprehension are most vulnerable [26,27]. The timing of the onset of alteration in consciousness also varies. Researchers have identified greater vulnerability toward brief cognitive impairments in the middle stage of a seizure, with relatively intact performance during the few seconds at the beginning and end of the episode, while preictal changes in cognition, described as retrograde amnesia, have also been reported [26]. Notably, painful or loud stimuli have been found to suddenly stop seizures, suggesting some ability to respond to the external environment [28]. A more extensive recent review of the medical literature describing consciousness in absence epilepsy is available for the interested reader [21].

Arguably the most arduous challenge we face when studying neural activity in absence epilepsy is related to inaccuracies in the temporal and spatial resolution of neurodiagnostic procedures [29]. This problem is exacerbated by the relatively short duration of the ictal period in absence seizures and the difficulties in assessment of young patients [30]. As a result, it has been proposed that simultaneous recording of scalp EEG and fMRI provides the most accurate method for measuring ictal changes in neural activity during seizures [29]. Furthermore, by engaging patients in different behavioral tasks while employing these methods, we can ultimately provide a real-time course for alterations in consciousness and associated changes in brain mechanisms [31].

During absence seizures, overactivation of the bilateral thalamic, superior temporal gyrus, and superior rolandic, occipital, and lateral frontal regions and deactivation of the parietal region, cingulate gyrus, and basal ganglia are evident during simultaneous recording of EEG, fMRI, and various behavioral tasks [30]. Behaviorally, subjects exhibited an ictal error rate of 81% on a behavioral task measuring attentional vigilance and reaction time; ictal errors were less than half as likely (39%) on a repetitive finger-tapping task. Variable cognitive changes observed in absence may occur as a result of concurrent abnormal activity in thalamic and frontoparietal neocortical regions that mediate attention *and* aberrant involvement of primary auditory, visual, somatosensory, and motor processing areas [30]. Interestingly, greater fMRI activation in the orbital, medial frontal, and parietal cortices occurs more than 5 seconds prior to onset of spike-and-wave activity on EEG, followed by deactivation in these same regions and generalized brain deactivation up to 20 seconds postictally [31]. Based on time-course analysis, disruption in cognition was only observed in the presence of spike-and-wave discharges, despite clear evidence of preictal hemodynamic changes.

Finally, it is important to mention that absence epilepsy is also associated with interictal changes in cognition. Despite the traditional understanding of this disease as having minimal impact in normal functioning, recent work has identified a number of attention-related deficits in everyday activities compared to healthy peers [32]. Permanent disruption of mechanisms involved in sustained attention is conceivable given the proposed mechanism of epileptogenesis just described, involving thalamico-cortical pathways that mediate attention.

In summary, many challenges remain in studying mechanisms of absence seizures during periictal periods and development of better paradigms that include simultaneous EEG, functional imaging, and behavioral tasks will shed light on the specific neuroanatomical substrates responsible for changes observed in cognition. Research suggests intact ability to perform simple tasks and compromised complex processing of motor, visual, and auditory information. Recent advances have shed light on the possible brain networks involved in ictal cognitive impairments associated with absence epilepsy, focusing on concurrent dysfunction of thalamico-cortical (frontoparietal regions) pathways and primary sensory processing areas. Further, changes in blood oxygenation levels precede measurable alterations in consciousness and cognitive changes are likely dependent on the presence of spike-and-wave activity.

Resting-state brain networks, consciousness, and epilepsy

The question of what is responsible for the awake, conscious state of the human brain is one of the most fundamental issues in the field of neuroscience. In the second half of the 20th century, noninvasive techniques such as fMRI, EEG, magnetoencephalography (MEG), and positron emission tomography (PET) have focused on tracking regional changes in brain activity and metabolism that index the brain as it engages in different aspects of a cognitive task. More recently, however, significant attention has been directed to what happens in the brain "at baseline"; that is, when one is awake but not actively engaged in a cognitive task. Low-frequency fluctuations in the MRI-BOLD (blood oxygenation level-dependent) signal in such a resting state have been shown to form reproducible networks of distinct brain regions [33–35]. Such networks emerge when one calculates the *functional connectivity* between brain regions; that is, how well the activity of one region predicts that of another over time.

The nature of some of the resting-state networks in the healthy adult brain remains speculative. Some of the resting-state networks mirror the sets of regions active during specific cognitive tasks (such as performance of a motor act), implying that the activity detected at rest has functional validity and indexes and reflects the network of connections used during a given cognitive function [33,36–38]. An example is the tight coupling of activity observed at rest, in the absence of movement, between ipsilateral and contralateral primary motor cortices [39]. The resting-state crosstalk between the two regions presumably reflects the underlying functional connections between the regions that allow their coordination during performance of a motor task.

A different set of resting-state networks that do not correspond to known networks of regions engaged by specific cognitive functions has also been described. In these networks, activity is more pronounced in the *absence* of a cognitive task and typically decreases during performance of *any* cognitive task. This generic behavior has led some to suggest that these regions are not networks *per se* but rather reflect core baseline brain physiology independent of neuronal activity or anatomical or functional connections [40–42]. Others have instead speculated that they indeed reflect specific neuronal networks that are engaged when goal-directed action and external input are absent; that is, a *default network* [36,38,43–45]. Some researchers have even speculated that such default networks may be at the heart of what underlies the awake, conscious state of the human brain [46].

The ability to study functional networks noninvasively, of particular value in a patient population, has made the study of resting-state networks very appealing for epilepsy research. The classical notion of epileptic seizures being caused by a single, localized, ictal focus is now often complemented by a more distributed view, whereby epileptic seizures, including focal or partial seizures, arise from and reflect abnormalities in an epileptogenic *network* of regions [47]. Indeed, as examined in previous sections, epilepsy appears to have a widespread and yet targeted effect on the human brain, with localized structural and/or metabolic abnormalities observed in multiple, nonlimbic brain regions, most prominently in lateral temporal and frontal regions

[48–54]. Furthermore, there is evidence, primarily from animal models, that ictal onset is distributed and that seizures arise from specific cortico-cortical and cortico-subcortical networks and can have stereotyped clinical appearance despite onset from different cortical foci [47,55–59]. This suggests that the foci of seizure onset may belong to a functional network, activation of which leads to a stereotyped clinical manifestation. This manifestation can include alteration of consciousness, leading to the speculation that some of the disruptions of the conscious state produced by epileptic seizures may be due to abnormal interactions with specific functional brain networks, including the resting-state networks.

A few studies have examined resting-state networks in epilepsy patients. The majority focused on TLE, often with the additional goal of attempting to localize the ictal focus by using abnormalities in network connectivity [60–66]. Nearly all studies discovered abnormalities in functional connectivity, but findings were not always concordant. Several groups noted *decreases* in functional connectivity that were often localized near the region of an ictal focus [61,62,66], potentially arguing that the pathological changes brought on by the disease also result in functional network disruption. However, decreased connectivity was not a universal finding. Using techniques from graph theory to examine functional connectivity in a broad set of brain regions in patients with TLE, significantly *increased* connectivity has been reported within the medial temporal lobes, but decreased connectivity within frontal and parietal regions [63]. Increased interictal connectivity within the ictal zone was identified using surface EEG in a smaller group of TLE patients [60]. Such apparent discrepancies reflect in part the nascent nature of the techniques used to analyze resting-state activity, including how one defines regions of interest to then use as "seeds" to calculate functional connectivity with other brain regions.

Default-mode networks also appear to be affected by epilepsy, but preliminary findings thus far do not definitively prove this one way or the other. Several previously mentioned studies of TLE showed findings of decreased functional connectivity or decreased activity in default-mode networks. Fewer studies have focused on primary generalized epilepsy. In a study of patients with idiopathic generalized epilepsy, examples of both decreased and increased connectivity in typical default-mode networks were shown [67]. In a similar group of patients with analysis restricted to interictal discharges, decreased *activity* in default-mode networks occurred during interictal discharges but functional connectivity was unaffected [68]. This latter study illustrates another potential outcome of this line of research: functional brain networks defined using resting-state activity may be affected by epilepsy in terms of overall activity as a network but the functional connectivity between regions within the network may be unimpaired.

In conclusion, new techniques have allowed the study of functional networks of brain regions by examining the coupling of their resting-state activity with fMRI. Some of these networks reflect known anatomical and functional connections between brain regions involved in specific cognitive functions. Others, termed "default-mode networks," show greater activity in the absence of an active cognitive task and may underlie a default mode of consciousness. Resting-state brain networks are under initial exploration in epilepsy. Preliminary studies hint at the disruption of functional connectivity both in regions directly affected by the disease and in more remote ones. Default-mode networks seem also to be affected but the complex interplay between default-mode networks, consciousness, and epilepsy is only beginning to be unraveled.

References

1 Temkin O: *The Falling Sickness: A History of Epilepsy from the Greeks to the Beginning of Modern Neurology*. Johns Hopkins University Press, Baltimore, MD, 1971, pp. 328–346.
2 Anon: Proposal for revised clinical and electroencephalographic classification of epileptic seizures. From the Commission on Classification and Terminology of the International League Against Epilepsy. *Epilepsia* 1981; **22**: 489–501.
3 Treiman DM: Epilepsy and violence: medical and legal issues. *Epilepsia* 1986; **27(Suppl. 2)**:S77–S104.
4 Hughlings-Jackson J: Lectures on the diagnosis of epilepsy (Harveian Society). In: Taylor J (ed.): *The Selected Writings of John Hughlings Jackson*. Basic Books, New York, NY, 1958, pp. 276–307.
5 Hogan RE, Kaiboriboon K: The "dreamy state": John Hughlings-Jackson's ideas of epilepsy and consciousness. *Am J Psychiatry* 2003; **160**:1740–1747.
6 Fenwick P: The nature and management of aggression in epilepsy. *J Neuropsychiatry* 1989; **1**:418–424.
7 Blumenfeld H, Taylor J: Why do seizures cause loss of consciousness? *Neuroscientist* 2003; **9**:301–310.
8 Gloor P: Consciousness as a neurological concept in epileptology: a critical review. *Epilepsia* 1986; **27(Suppl. 2)**: S14–S26.
9 Hughlings-Jackson J: On a particular variety of epilepsy ("intellectual aura"), one case with symptoms of organic brain disease. *Brain* 1888; **11**:179–207.
10 Hughlings-Jackson J: Intellectual warnings of epileptic seizures. In: Taylor J (ed.): *The Selected Writings of John Hughlings Jackson*. Basic Books, New York, NY, 1958, pp. 274–275.
11 Hughlings-Jackson J: Remarks on systemic sensations in epilepsies. In: Taylor J (ed.): *The Selected Writings of John Hughlings Jackson*. Basic Books, New York, NY, 1958, p.118.
12 Blume WT, Luders HO, Mizrahi E et al.: Glossary of descriptive terminology for ictal semiology: report of the ILAE Task Force on Classification and Terminology. *Epilepsia* 2001; **42**:1212–1218.
13 Hogan RE, Kaiboriboon K, Bertrand ME et al.: Composite SISCOM perfusion patterns in right and left temporal seizures. *Arch Neurol* 2006; **63**:1419–1426.
14 Van Paesschen W, Dupont P, Van Driel G et al.: SPECT perfusion changes during complex partial seizures in patients with hippocampal sclerosis. *Brain* 2003; **126**:1103–1111.
15 Blumenfeld H, McNally KA, Vanderhill SD et al.: Positive and negative network correlations in temporal lobe epilepsy. *Cereb Cortex* 2004; **14**:892–902.
16 Hogan RE, Kaiboriboon K, Osman M: Composite SISCOM images in mesial temporal lobe epilepsy: technique and illustration of regions of hyperperfusion. *Nucl Med Commun* 2004; **25**:539–545.
17 Tae WS, Joo EY, Kim JH et al.: Cerebral perfusion changes in mesial temporal lobe epilepsy: SPM analysis of ictal and interictal SPECT. *Neuroimage* 2005; **24**:101–110.
18 Blumenfeld H, Varghese GI, Purcaro MJ et al.: Cortical and subcortical networks in human secondarily generalized tonic-clonic seizures. *Brain* 2009; **132**:999–1012.
19 Newton MR, Berkovic SF, Austin MC et al.: SPECT in the localisation of extratemporal and temporal seizure foci. *J Neurol Neurosurg Psychiatry* 1995; **59**:26–30.
20 Norden AD, Blumenfeld H: The role of subcortical structures in human epilepsy. *Epilepsy Behav* 2002; **3**:219–231.
21 Blumenfeld H: Consciousness and epilepsy: why are patients with absence seizure absent? *Prog Brain Res* 2005; **150**: 271–286.
22 Commission on Classification and Terminology of the International League Against Epilepsy: Proposal for revised classification of epilepsies and epileptic syndromes. *Epilepsia* 1989; **30**:389–399.
23 Gibbs FA, Davis H, Lennox WG: The electro-encephalogram in epilepsy and in conditions of impaired consciousness. *Arch Neurol Psychiatr* 1935; **34**:1133–1148.
24 Blumenfeld H: From molecules to networks: cortical/subcortical interactions in the pathophysiology of idiopathic generalized epilepsy. *Epilepsia* 2003; **44(2)**:7–15.

25 Englot D, Blumenfeld H: Consciousness and epilepsy: why are complex-partial seizures complex? *Prog Brain Res* 2009; **177**:147–170.

26 Mirsky AF, Buren JMV: On the nature of the "absence" in centrencephalic epilepsy: a study of some behavioral, electroencephalographic, and autonomic factors. *Electroen Clin Neuro* 1965; **18**:334–348.

27 Courtois GA, Ingvar DH, Jasper HH: Nervous and mental defects during petit mal attacks. *Electroen Clin Neuro* 1953; **Suppl. 3**:87.

28 Boudin G, Barbizet J, Masson S: Etude de la dissolution de la conscience dans 3 cas de petit mal avec crises prolongees. *Rev Neurol* 1958; **99**:483–487.

29 Motelow JE, Blumenfeld H: Functional imaging of spike-wave seizures. *Methods Mol Biol* 2009; **489**:189–209.

30 Berman R, Negishi M, Vestal M et al.: Simultaneous EEG, fMRI, and behavior in typical childhood absence seizures. *Epilepsia* 2010; **50(10)**:2011–2022.

31 Bai X, Vestal M, Berman R et al.: Dynamic time course of typical absence seizures: EEG, behavior, and functional magnetic resonance imaging. *J Neurosci* 2010; **30(17)**: 5884–5893.

32 Vega C, Vestal M, DeSalvo M et al.: Differentiation of attention-related problems in childhood absence epilepsy. *Epilepsy Behav* 2010; **19(1)**:82–85.

33 Lowe MJ, Dzemidzic M, Lurito JT et al.: Correlations in low-frequency BOLD fluctuations reflect cortico-cortical connections. *Neuroimage* 2000; **12(5)**:582–587.

34 Cordes D, Haughton VM, Arfanakis K et al.: Frequencies contributing to functional connectivity in the cerebral cortex in "resting-state" data. *AJNR* 2001; **22(7)**:1326–1333.

35 Achard S, Salvador R, Whitcher B et al.: A resilient, low-frequency, small-world human brain functional network with highly connected association cortical hubs. *J Neurosci* 2006; **26(1)**:63–72.

36 Gusnard D, Raichle ME, Raichle ME: Searching for a baseline: functional imaging and the resting human brain. *Nat Rev Neurosci* 2001; **2(10)**:685–694.

37 Lewis CM, Baldassarre A, Committeri G et al.: Learning sculpts the spontaneous activity of the resting human brain. *Proc Natl Acad Sci USA* 2009; **106(41)**:17558–17563.

38 Peltier S, Noll D: T2* dependence of low frequency functional connectivity. *Neuroimage* 2002; **16(4)**:985–992.

39 Biswal B, Yetkin FZ, Haughton VM, Hyde JS: Functional connectivity in the motor cortex of resting human brain using echo-planar MRI. *Magn Reson Med* 1995; **34**:537–541.

40 Obrig H, Neufang M, Wenzel R et al.: Spontaneous low frequency oscillations of cerebral hemodynamics and metabolism in human adults. *Neuroimage* 2000; **12**:623–639.

41 Wise RG, Ide K, Poulin MJ, Tracey I: Resting fluctuations in arterial carbon dioxide induce significant low frequency variations in BOLD signal. *Neuroimage* 2004; **21**:1652–1664.

42 Birn RM, Diamond JB, Smith MA, Bandettini PA: Separating respiratory-variation-related fluctuations from neuronal-activity-related fluctuations in fMRI. *Neuroimage* 2006; **31**:1536–1548.

43 Raichle ME, MacLeod AM, Snyder AZ et al.: A default mode of brain function. *Proc Natl Acad Sci USA* 2001; **98**:676–682.

44 Damoiseaux JS, Rombouts ARB, Barkhof F et al.: Consistent resting-state networks across healthy subjects. *Proc Natl Acad Sci USA* 2006; **103**:13848–13853.

45 De Luca M, Beckmann CF, De Stefano N et al.: fMRI resting state networks define distinct modes of long-distance interactions in the human brain. *Neuroimage* 2006; **29**: 1359–1367.

46 He B, Raichle ME: The fMRI signal, slow cortical potential and consciousness. *Trends Cogn Sci* 2009; **13**:302–309.

47 Spencer SS: Neural networks in human epilepsy: evidence of and implications for treatment. *Epilepsia* 2002; **43(3)**:219–227.

48 Arnold S, Schlaug G, Niemann H et al.: Topography of interictal glucose hypometabolism in unilateral mesiotemporal epilepsy. *Neurology* 1996; **46(5)**:1422–1430.

49 Bernhardt BC, Bernasconi N, Concha L, Bernasconi A: Cortical thickness analysis in temporal lobe epilepsy: reproducibility and relation to outcome. *Neurology* 2010; **74(22)**: 1776–1784.

50 Henry TR, Mazziotta JC, Engel J: Interictal metabolic anatomy of mesial temporal lobe epilepsy. *Arch Neurol* 1993; **50(6)**:582–589.

51 Margerison JH, Corsellis JA: Epilepsy and the temporal lobes: a clinical, electroencephalographic and neuropathological study of the brain in epilepsy, with particular reference to the temporal lobes. *Brain* 1966; **89(3)**:499–530.

52 Spanaki MV, Kopylev L, DeCarli C et al.: Postoperative changes in cerebral metabolism in temporal lobe epilepsy. *Arch Neurol* 2000; **57(10)**:1447–1452.

53 Theodore WH, Sato S, Kufta C et al.: Temporal lobectomy for uncontrolled seizures: the role of positron emission tomography. *Ann Neurol* 1992; **32(6)**:789–794.

54 Maccotta L, Buckner RL, Gilliam FG, Ojemann JG: Changing frontal contributions to memory before and after medial temporal lobectomy. *Cereb Cortex* 2007; **17(2)**:443–456.

55 Bear J, Fountain NB, Lothman EW: Responses of the superficial entorhinal cortex in vitro in slices from naive and chronically epileptic rats. *J Neurophysiol* 1996; **76(5)**: 2928–2940.

56 Bertram EH: Functional anatomy of spontaneous seizures in a rat model of limbic epilepsy. *Epilepsia* 1997; **38(1)**: 95–105.

57 Paré D, Decurtis M, Llinas R: Role of the hippocampal-entorhinal loop in temporal lobe epilepsy: extra-and intracellular study in the isolated guinea pig brain in vitro. *J Neurosci* 1992; **12(5)**:1867–1881.

58 Rafiq A, DeLorenzo RJ, Coulter DA: Generation and propagation of epileptiform discharges in a combined entorhinal cortex/hippocampal slice. *J Neurophysiol* 1993; **70(5)**: 1962–1974.

59 White L, Price J: The functional anatomy of limbic status epilepticus in the rat. II: The effects of focal deactivation. *J Neurosci* 1993; **13(11)**:4810–4830.

60 Bettus G, Wendling F, Guye M et al.: Enhanced EEG functional connectivity in mesial temporal lobe epilepsy. *Epilepsy Res* 2008; **81(1)**:58–68.

61 Bettus G, Guedj E, Joyeux F et al.: Decreased basal fMRI functional connectivity in epileptogenic networks and contralateral compensatory mechanisms. *Hum Brain Mapp* 2009; **30(5)**:1580–1591.

62 Bettus G, Bartolomei F, Confort-Gouny S et al.: Role of resting state functional connectivity MRI in presurgical investigation of mesial temporal lobe epilepsy. *J Neurol Neurosurg Psychiatry* 2010; **81(10)**:1147–1154.

63 Liao W, Zhang Z, Pan Z et al.: Altered functional connectivity and small-world in mesial temporal lobe epilepsy. *PloS One* 2010; **5(1)**:e8525.

64 Morgan VL, Gore JC, Abou-Khalil B: Functional epileptic network in left mesial temporal lobe epilepsy detected using resting fMRI. *Epilepsy Res* 2010; **88**:168–178.

65 Waites AB, Briellmann RS, Saling MM et al.: Functional connectivity networks are disrupted in left temporal lobe epilepsy. *Ann Neurol* 2010; **59(2)**:335–343.

66 Zhang Z, Lu G, Zhong Y et al.: Altered spontaneous neuronal activity of the default-mode network in mesial temporal lobe epilepsy. *Brain Res* 2010; **1323**:152–160.

67 Wang Z, Lu G, Zhang Z et al.: Altered resting state networks in epileptic patients with generalized tonic-clonic seizures. *Brain Res* 2010; **1374**:134–141.

68 Moeller F, Maneshi M, Pittau F et al.: Functional connectivity in patients with idiopathic generalized epilepsy. *Epilepsia* 2011; **52(3)**:515–522.

Ictal cognitive impairments due to nonconvulsive status epilepticus

Introduction

Altered mental status is one of the most common reasons for a neurological consultation in the hospital or emergency department. Nonconvulsive status epilepticus (NCSE) is not one of the most common causes of altered mentation but is eminently treatable, often with immediate and dramatic improvement. NCSE is an easily missed diagnosis. The savvy clinician should maintain a high index of suspicion for NCSE when evaluating the confused or encephalopathic patient and should request an EEG for further investigation.

Continuous or intermittent seizure activity lasting at least 30 minutes without recovery of consciousness is a widely accepted definition for status epilepticus [1]. NCSE refers to prolonged electrographic seizure activity unassociated with clinical convulsions. NCSE type is determined by the underlying EEG findings and the underlying clinical syndrome. Absence status epilepticus, complex partial status epilepticus, electrographic status epilepticus during slow-wave sleep, NCSE in coma, and "subtle" NCSE following convulsive status epilepticus are all forms of NCSE and have varied effects on cognition. An EEG is required to make the diagnosis of NCSE and typically demonstrates continuous, almost continuous, or waxing and waning electrographic ictal activity.

Clinical setting

NCSE should be considered in the differential diagnosis of all cases of altered mental status, ranging from subtle cognitive slowing and mild confusion to obtundation. NCSE may be precipitated by a variety of acute medical conditions, including metabolic derangement, infection, acute or chronic brain lesion, intoxication, and withdrawal. NCSE frequently occurs in the setting of epilepsy and may occur as the initial presentation of epilepsy or be precipitated by medication noncompliance in patients with known seizure disorders. There should be a particularly high index of suspicion for NCSE in a patient with altered mental status and a known history of epilepsy or a recent convulsive seizure. NCSE occurs in approximately 20% of patients with complex partial seizure disorders. NCSE frequently follows convulsive seizure activity, so obtaining an EEG to assess patients who remain confused or stuporous following a convulsive seizure is important; up to 14% of such patients have ongoing electrographic status epilepticus [2].

Because many other medical and psychiatric conditions give rise to similar clinical manifestations, the diagnosis of NCSE is easily missed or delayed. Table 4.1 lists a variety of clinical signs and symptoms that can occur in NCSE. Table 4.2 lists psychiatric and neurologic disorders that mimic NCSE [3]. Diagnosis of NCSE is made by EEG, which shows ongoing electrographic ictal activity. Brain MRI may be helpful in demonstrating underlying structural epileptogenic cortical neuropathology in patients with *de novo* NCSE with an unexplained mechanism. Single-photon emission computed tomography (SPECT) and positron emission tomography (PET) scans can be helpful in localizing ictal activity. When feasible, neuropsychological testing provides details of the cognitive domains involved.

Table 4.1 Symptoms and signs of nonconvulsive status epilepticus (NCSE).

Physical	Cognitive
Ataxia and falling	Absentmindedness
Change in heart rate	Agitation
Diaphoresis	Alteration of speech
Eye blinking	Altered level of consciousness
Gesticulations	Aphasia
Head nodding	Apraxia
Increased salivation	Attitudinal change
Oral automatisms	Atypical behavior
Picking	Change in affect
Posturing	Disorientation
Shivering	Euphoria
Smiling/laughing	Experiential
Staring	Hallucinations
Twitching	Impaired memory
Wandering	Inattentiveness
	Perseveration
	Somnolence
	Slow speech
	Unresponsiveness

Table 4.2 Disorders that can mimic nonconvulsive status epilepticus (NCSE).

Psychiatric disorders	Medical and neurological disorders
Acute psychotic reactions	Apraxia
Akinetic mutism	Amnesia
Attention deficit disorder	Aphasia
Catatonia	Coma
Conversion disorder	Creutzfeldt–Jakob disease
Dissociative fugue state	Delirium
Delusions	Dementia
Depression	Drug toxicity
Hallucinations	Drug withdrawal
Major depression	Encephalitis
Malingering	Locked-in state
Paranoia	Medication toxicity
Schizophrenia	Metabolic encephalopathy
	Minimally conscious state
	Periodic paralysis
	Persistent vegetative state
	Postictal state
	Sleep disorders
	Stroke
	Transient global amnesia

Absence status epilepticus

Typical absence status epilepticus begins abruptly, with onset of a variable degree of alteration of consciousness, and lasts hours to days, terminating either spontaneously, following treatment, or following a convulsive seizure. The hallmark of absence status epilepticus is clouding of consciousness. Typically, the patient is ambulatory but slow, with staring, a blank expression, and fluctuating confusion. States of severe somnolence or stupor are less common. Responses are slow and speech is sparse. About half of the time, there are associated motor signs, such as rapid blinking or facial myoclonia. Depending on the epilepsy syndrome, there may be a history of prior convulsive, absence, or myoclonic seizures. Precipitating factors for absence status epilepticus include medication withdrawal, inappropriate narrow-spectrum medications (carbamazepine, tiagabine, and others), metabolic abnormalities, alcohol, sleep deprivation, menstruation, hyperventilation, and strobe lights [4,5].

The first detailed characterization of absence status epilepticus was published in 1941 [6], describing 10 cases with diagnostic clinical and EEG features that remain relevant today. Most patients had a history of convulsive seizures and absence seizures with intervals of absence status epilepticus lasting hours to several days. During absence status epilepticus, symptoms included dullness and mental slowing, difficulty with comprehension and calculation, confusion, disorientation, dysarthria, forgetfulness, grogginess, subjective ataxia, apathy, and poor school performance. The authors distinguished absence status epilepticus from neurological deterioration or psychological states by the qualities of intermittence, lack of severe affective disturbance, correlation with generalized spike-and-wave activity on EEG, and improvement or elimination when treated with a nonsedative anticonvulsant. Most patients were aware of their prolonged absences and described mental slowing and other features.

New onset of NCSE in later life

While most absence status epilepticus occurs in the setting of epilepsy, *de novo* NCSE in later life has been described [7,8], with features distinct from typical or childhood-onset absence status. Psychiatric symptoms and bizarre behavior are common, leading to frequent misdiagnosis. The EEG typically shows continuous or almost continuous runs of generalized spike-and-wave discharges of 1.0–2.5 Hz. Onset is usually abrupt, with duration of symptoms ranging from 1 day to 2 months. A common precipitant of late-onset absence status epilepticus is benzodiazepine withdrawal [7,8]. Other provoking factors include excessive use of psychotropic drugs, electrolyte abnormalities, and alcoholism.

In older patients, the degree of alteration in mental status ranges from mild disorientation to confusion and psychiatric symptoms may include hallucinations, thought broadcasting, paranoia, fear, and flight of ideas. Additional symptoms, including memory disturbance, agitation, irritability, euphoria, apraxia, slow speech or speech arrest, and intermittent unresponsiveness have also been described. Intermittent lucid intervals may be helpful in diagnosing seizure activity but may also lead to the erroneous conclusion of a psychogenic disturbance or malingering.

Examples of bizarre behavior exhibited by older patients with confusion and generalized EEG ictal activity include the following [7]:

- A 64-year-old man sat in his car in the garage, trying to navigate it as if it were an airplane and claiming that he had been to the airport twice that day.
- In the middle of a psychiatric interview, a patient stood up suddenly, sang "thank you, Jesus," and started dancing.
- A man took a gun up on to the roof to "patch a hole" and asked his daughter to drive their (nonexistent) dump truck. He telephoned several community members and spoke bizarrely or said nothing.
- A man said that he could read minds and was in direct communication with God.

NCSE of focal onset

By definition, there is no alteration of awareness with simple partial status epilepticus. While the most commonly recognized type of simple partial status epilepticus involves persistent motor twitching of the face or limb, as in *epilepsia partialis continua*, diverse cognitive changes may occur, depending on the localization of the ictal discharge. Cases of *aura continua*, lasting hours to days, have been reported, associated with a wide range of symptoms, including gustatory hallucinations, repetitive musical hallucinations, vertigo, epigastric sensations, focal pain, and autonomic phenomena [9].

The symptoms and signs of simple partial status epilepticus are determined by the brain region involved in the seizure activity. Focal temporal ictal activity may result in behavioral changes, depression, fear, or other emotions [10,11]. Patients have also described auditory hallucinations and thought intrusion, déjà vu, and various distortions of perception or experience. Left frontal or left temporal ictal activity can cause speech arrest due to ictal aphasia, with preserved awareness. Parietal status epilepticus is rare but alien-hand syndrome due to spread from a frontotemporal focus has been described [12]. Occipital status epilepticus may cause complex visual hallucinations, ictal amaurosis, cortical blindness, hemianopsia, or the erroneous interpretation of visual phenomena, including misperception of an object's size [13–15].

Complex partial status epilepticus

Clinically, complex partial status epilepticus may be difficult to distinguish from absence status epilepticus because both include impaired executive functioning. EEG differentiates the two entities, with complex partial status epilepticus demonstrating a rhythmic focal ictal pattern or a generalized pattern with focal features [16]. Complex partial status epilepticus has a more variable presentation than absence status epilepticus, with clinical manifestations depending on the localization of the electrographic discharge. The cognitive changes in complex partial status epilepticus typically fluctuate, in contrast to the steadily persistent clouded consciousness of absence status epilepticus.

Ictal cognitive impairment is most commonly associated with complex partial status epilepticus arising from either the frontal or the temporal lobe. In a series of 52 NCSE patients, one-third had frontal NCSE and many had an underlying focal brain lesion [17]. Altered awareness occurred in 57% of patients with complex partial status epilepticus of frontal onset – less often than with absence status epilepticus (100%) or temporal status epilepticus (66%). Mood changes were common in frontal-lobe NCSE. Some patients had a flat or slow affect, while others were euphoric, with smiling and laughter. Although psychomotor slowing was also described in some patients with absence status epilepticus, jocularity, when present, was unique to the frontal NCSE group [17].

A series of 10 cases of frontal NCSE identified two distinct types [18]. The first was associated with mild cognitive dysfunction, mood disturbance, and a normal level of alertness without postictal amnesia. Mood disturbance ranged from emotional disinhibition and talkativeness to indifference and psychomotor slowing. Neurological findings included perseveration, confabulation, and impaired performance of complex bimanual tasks, serial subtractions, and pattern drawing. At the onset of ictal EEG activity, motor manifestations included head turning, subtle perioral myoclonia, and loss of postural tone. Because of the subtlety of the clinical findings, the authors proposed an alternative classification as simple partial status epilepticus with affective or cognitive features. The second type of frontal NCSE had markedly altered awareness, with postictal stupor and amnesia, cyclic spatiotemporal disorientation, behavior disturbance, and motor and verbal perseveration. The EEG typically showed abnormal background activity with bilateral frontotemporal or frontocentral ictal activity [18].

Differentiating frontal NCSE from temporal status epilepticus on the basis of clinical manifestations is often challenging. Complex partial status epilepticus of the temporal lobe, known in the past as "psychomotor status" or "twilight state," is suggested by perceptual hallucinations, memory disturbance (déjà vu, jamais vu, flashbacks), emotional states (fear, sadness, pleasure, anger), or experiential distortions (feelings of unreality, dreamlike states, out-of-body experiences). Typical mesial temporal status epilepticus presents with fluctuating confusion and emotional overtones and with automatisms such as lip smacking, picking, or fumbling hand movements. The mental state associated with temporal status epilepticus varies widely between patients, ranging from mild confusion to catatonia or stupor and postictal amnesia. Speech arrest, perseverative gesticulations, and vocalizations may occur. The presence of visual hallucinations, gaze deviation, nystagmus, or posturing suggests spread of the ictal discharge, with extratemporal involvement.

A small case series of six patients who had neuropsychological testing during focal NCSE found impaired executive functioning in all, including lack of self-initiated directed behavior, slowed responses, perseveration, and limited working memory [19]. These patients had either a right-brain focus on ictal EEG or bilateral generalized ictal activity with focal features. Impairments of high-order function were present in all subjects, including apraxia, receptive/expressive dysphasia, transcortical aphasia, dyscalculia, dyslexia, and agnosia.

NCSE in coma

Nonconvulsive seizures are common in comatose individuals with serious medical conditions and have been found in 8–48% of ICU patients monitored with continuous EEG [20]. A significant proportion of these patients have prolonged or waxing and waning ictal activity consistent with NCSE. The EEG patterns of NCSE may be partial or generalized and the background is usually slow or suppressed. The mental status of ICU patients with NCSE ranges from mildly encephalopathic to comatose. NCSE should be evaluated in patients with a fluctuating level of consciousness, an acute brain injury, a recent convulsive seizure, or subtle rhythmic limb or eye movements.

The etiology of NCSE in this setting is more often related to acute or ongoing medical problems than to a diagnosis of epilepsy, making it difficult to determine the extent to which NCSE *per se* contributes to the patient's alteration in consciousness. Structural brain abnormalities that precipitate NCSE – such as stroke, edema, hemorrhage, and neurosurgical postoperative changes – impair mental functions even when epileptiform discharges are absent. In these complex ICU cases, NCSE may be just one of several factors that alter mental status, since organ failure, metabolic abnormalities, and anesthetic or sedative medication effects contribute to encephalopathy.

EEG and the diagnosis of NCSE

EEG is the most important test for evaluation of NCSE. Various EEG patterns are associated with NCSE at different stages of life and with a range of syndromes [21]. Electrographic criteria for NCSE depend upon the frequency of epileptiform discharges. If discharges occur with a frequency exceeding 2.5 Hz, no additional criteria are required. If the frequency is less than 2.5 Hz, one of the following must also apply: clinical and electrographic improvement after an intravenous AED, subtle associated clinical ictal signs, or typical spatiotemporal evolution of discharges [22].

Typical absence status epilepticus demonstrates a continuous or nearly continuous EEG pattern of generalized ≥3 Hz spike-and-wave or polyspike-and-wave discharges, with a normal interictal background. Onset and termination of absence status epilepticus are usually abrupt. The frequency of discharges in atypical absence status epilepticus is less than 3 Hz and the interictal background is diffusely slow. Absence status epilepticus with onset in later life demonstrates spike-and-wave or polyspike-and-wave discharges with a frequency of 1–4 Hz, often with a mild or moderately slow interictal background.

The EEG diagnosis of NCSE remains somewhat controversial. Difficulties arise when a diffuse EEG pattern arises from a discrete focus, which may not be evident if the seizure onset is not recorded. In the past, this has led to the erroneous grouping of complex partial status epilepticus cases with cases of primary generalized status epilepticus, compounding the difficulty in characterizing and differentiating these entities. Focal NCSE with secondary involvement of both hemispheres is now considered a form of complex partial status epilepticus. Prolonged continuous EEG monitoring is helpful in differentiating complex partial status epilepticus from absence status epilepticus. While both complex partial status epilepticus and absence status epilepticus have similar clinical phenomentology of staring, unresponsiveness, and variable oral and manual automatisms, complex partial status epilepticus demonstrates waxing and waning electrographic epileptiform activity, either focal or sometimes generalized, evolving in morphological or spatiotemporal characteristics such as amplitude, frequency, waveform, and electrical field distribution – as distinct from absence status epilepticus, which typically maintains a generalized and relatively stereotypic, monomorphic appearance of repetitive generalized spike-and-wave complexes.

Simple partial status epilepticus presents a diagnostic challenge, as routine EEG may be nondiagnostic. In order to record epileptic activity with scalp electrodes, an estimated cortical volume of at least $10\,cm^2$ must be involved in a synchronous discharge [23]. Electrographic seizure activity from a distant focus, or from a population of neurons oriented parallel to the scalp, may generate minimal – or no – scalp discharges. The diagnosis of simple partial status epilepticus should be considered based on recurrent episodes of stereotyped symptoms or signs and response to antiepileptic medication.

Additional challenges arise in determining whether ongoing rhythmic EEG patterns are ictal or encephalopathic in patients with altered mental status. Resolution of EEG discharges and improvement in the patient's mental status in response to an intravenous benzodiazepine are diagnostic of nonconvulsive seizure activity. However, in the ICU setting, benzodiazepine administration may improve the EEG but not the patient's mental status, resulting in a diagnostic impasse.

Another "gray zone" in EEG interpretation of NCSE involves identifying the beginning and end of seizure activity, especially when other causes of encephalopathy (such as metabolic changes or structural lesions)

cause altered mentation and an abnormal baseline EEG. Clinical and EEG improvement may not occur for hours to several days after treatment. EEG is recommended to monitor the response of NCSE to treatment but it is often difficult to determine when a seizure pattern stops and the postictal state begins. Seizures usually stop abruptly and are followed by postictal suppression or slowing but in some cases of complex partial status epilepticus the transition to the postictal state is more ambiguous [24].

Treatment

Aggressive emergency treatment is warranted for convulsive status epilepticus but is not indicated for patients with absence status epilepticus. Patients that are stable from a cardiac and respiratory standpoint are at low risk for neuronal damage. Intravenous lorazepam, 0.5 mg intravenously, is an appropriate initial dose for most adults; additional doses may be administered several minutes apart if there is partial or no response. Large doses or continuous infusions of AEDs that could cause sedation or respiratory compromise should be avoided. Intravenous valproate, 20–40 mg/kg, is an alternative when a benzodiazepine cannot be used. If medications are identified as having precipitated absence status epilepticus (such as a narrow-spectrum drug like carbamazepine), they should be discontinued.

Provoked *de novo* absence status epilepticus may not require chronic antiepileptic medication if the provoking factor is removed [8]. However, those with idiopathic generalized epilepsy do require ongoing treatment, as well as a prescription for a benzodiazepine to have on hand at home, because there is a risk of recurrent absence status epilepticus episodes [5]. Benzodiazepines should not be given intravenously to patients with Lennox–Gastaut syndrome (LGS) and atypical absence status epilepticus, however, as they can precipitate tonic status epilepticus in these patients [25].

The treatment of complex partial status epilepticus is controversial because its sequellae are not well understood. Complex partial status epilepticus causes neuronal damage in animal models but human case series have reported contradictory outcomes [26–30]. The management of focal NCSE involves treating the seizure activity and its cause. Patients with complex partial status epilepticus due to epilepsy have a better prognosis than those who develop complex partial status epilepticus in the setting of an acute medical condition [31].

In an awake patient with status epilepticus, large doses of sedating medications should be avoided because these may lead to central nervous system (CNS) depression and respiratory depression requiring ventilatory support. In this setting, intravenous lorazepam, 0.5–1.0 mg, can be administered, and repeated several minutes later if there is no response. If necessary, a loading dose of a nonsedating AED, such as fosphenytoin, valproate, or levetiracetam, should also be given. EEG should be obtained to monitor the response to treatment. Because some intravenous antiepileptic medications may cause hypotension, respiratory depression, and other adverse effects, they should be used with caution. In general, anesthetic coma induction is reserved for refractory cases of convulsive status epilepticus. In cases of NCSE in an unconscious patient, intubation may be needed for airway protection, and risks of seizure activity must be balanced against risks associated with aggressive treatment and the prognosis of the underlying condition.

The cause of complex partial status epilepticus must be rapidly investigated and treated. Status epilepticus may not resolve until metabolic disturbances are corrected and rapid treatment of toxic, infectious, or autoimmune etiologies has been initiated. Patients with known epilepsy may also have additional precipitating causes of NCSE. If epilepsy is found to be the sole cause of NCSE then the patient's AED regimen should be optimized and compliance should be assessed at regular intervals.

Conclusion

NCSE is an increasingly recognized acute cause of cognitive impairment, with a variety of clinical manifestations depending on the region of the brain that is involved. NCSE may be provoked by acute medical illnesses or may occur as a manifestation of epilepsy. Given the protean manifestations of NCSE and the frequent presence of comorbidities that also alter mental status, the diagnosis may be missed, so a high index of suspicion for NCSE is necessary. The diagnosis is confirmed by correlating cognitive and behavioral changes with ictal EEG activity. Clinical signs and EEG seizures usually resolve in response to treatment with one or more antiepileptic medication. Management of

NCSE involves treating both the seizure activity and its underlying cause.

References

1 Epilepsy Foundation of America's Working Group on Status Epilepticus: The treatment of convulsive status epilepticus. *JAMA* 1993; **270**:854–859.
2 DeLorenzo RJ, Waterhouse E, Towne AR et al.: Persistent non-convulsive status epilepticus following the control of convulsive status epilepticus. *Epilepsia* 1998; **39(3)**: 833–840.
3 Kaplan PW: Behavioral manifestations of nonconvulsive status epilepticus. *Epilepsy Behav* 2002; **3**:122–139.
4 Agathonikou A, Panayiotopoulos CP, Giannakodimos S, Koutroumanidis K: Typical absence status in adults: diagnostic and syndromic considerations. *Epilepsia* 1998; **39(12)**: 1265–1276.
5 Shorvon S, Walker M: Status epilepticus in idiopathic generalized epilepsy. *Epilepsia* 2005; **46(Suppl. 9)**:73–79.
6 Putnam TJ, Merrit HH: Dullness as an epileptic equivalent. *Arch Neurol Psychiatry* 1941; **45**:797–813.
7 Lee SI: Nonvconvulsive status epiletpicus: ictal confusion in later life. *Arch Neurol* 1985; **42**:778–781.
8 Thomas P, Beaumanoir A, Genton P et al.: "De novo" absence status of late onset: report of 11 cases. *Neurology* 1992; **42**:104–110.
9 Wieser HG, Fischer M: Temporal lobe nonconvulsive status epilepticus. In: Kaplan PW, Drislane FW (eds): *Nonconvulsive Status Epilepticus*. Demos Medical, New York, NY, 2009, pp. 119–137.
10 Henriksen GF: Status epilepticus partialis with fear as clinical expression: report of a case and ictal EEG findings. *Epilepsia* 1973; **14**:39–46.
11 McLachlan RS, Blume WT: Isolated fear in complex partial status epilepticus. *Ann Neurol* 1980; **8**:639–641.
12 Feinberg TE, Roane DM, Cohen J: Parital status epilepticus associated with asomatognosia and alien hand-like behaviors. *Arch Neurol* 1998; **55**:1574–1576.
13 Jobst BC, Roberts DW, Williamson PD: Occipital lobe nonconvulsive status epilepticus. In: Kaplan PW, Drislane FW (eds): *Nonconvulsive Status Epilepticus*. Demos Medical, New York, NY, 2009, pp. 139–150.
14 Thomas P, Barrès P, Chatel M: Complex partial status epilepticus of extratemporal origin: report of a case. *Neurology* 1991; **41(7)**:1147–1149.
15 Walker MC, Smith SJ, Sisodiya SM, Shorvon SD: Case of simple partial status epilepticus in occipital lobe epilepsy misdiagnosed as migraine: clinical, electrophysiological, and magnetic resonance imaging characteristics. *Epilepsia* 1995; **36(12)**:1233–1236.
16 Granner MA, Lee SI: Nonconvulsive status epilepticus : EEG analysis in a large series. *Epilepsia* 1994; **35**:42–47.

17 Rohr-Le Floch J, Gauthier G, Beaumanoir A: Confusional states of epileptic origin: value of emergency EEG. *Rev Neurol (Paris)* 1988; **144(6–7)**:425–436.

18 Thomas P, Zifkin B: Frontal lobe status epilepticus. In: Kaplan PW, Drislane FW (eds): *Nonconvulsive Status Epilepticus*. Demos Medical, New York, NY, 2009, pp. 97–107.

19 Profitlich T, Hoppe C, Reuber M et al.: Ictal neuropsychological findings in focal nonconvulsive status epilepticus. *Epilepsy Behav* 2008; **12**:269–275.

20 Friedman D, Claassen J, Hirsch LJ: Continuous electroencephalogram monitoring in the intensive care unit. *Anesth Analg* 2009; **109(2)**:506–523.

21 Sutter R, Kaplan PW: Electroencephalographic criteria for nonconvulsive status epilepticus: synopsis and comprehensive survey. *Epilepsia* 2012; **53(Suppl. 3)**:1–51.

22 Beniczky S, Hirsch LJ, Kaplan PW et al.: Unified EEG terminology and criteria for nonconvulsive status epilepticus. *Epilepsia* 2013; **54(Suppl. 6)**:28–29.

23 Tao JX, Ray A, Hawes-Ebersole S, Ebersole JS: Intracranial EEG substrates of scalp EEG interictal spikes. *Epilepsia* 2005; **46(5)**:669–676.

24 Fisher RS, Engel JJ Jr,: Definition of the postictal state: when does it start and end? *Epilepsy Behav* 2010; **19**:100–104.

25 Tassinari CA, Dravet C, Roger J et al.: Tonic status epilepticus precipitated by intravenous benzodiazepine in five patients with Lennox-Gastaut syndrome. *Epilepsia* 1972; **13**:421–435.

26 Cockerell OC, Walker MC, Sander JW, Shorvon SD: Complex partial status epilepticus: a recurrent problem. *J Neurol Neurosurg Psychiatry* 1994; **5**:835–837.

27 Drislane FW: Evidence against permanent neurologic damage from nonconvulsive status epilepticus. *J Clin Neurophysiol* 1999; **16(4)**:323–331.

28 Kaplan PW: Assessing the outcomes in patients with nonconvulsive status epilepticus: nonconvulsive status epilepticus is underdiagnosed, potentially overtreated, and confounded by comorbidity. *J Clin Neurophysiol* 1999; **16(4)**:341–352.

29 Krumholz A: Epidemiology and evidence for morbidity of nonconvulsive status epilepticus. *J Clin Neurophysiol* 1999; **16(4)**:314–322.

30 Krumholz A, Sung GY, Fisher RS et al.: Complex partial status epilepticus accompanied by serious morbidity and mortality. *Neurology* 1995; **45**:1499–1504.

31 Shneker BF, Fountain NB: Assessment of acute morbidity and mortality in nonconvulsive status epilepticus. *Neurology* 2003; **61**:1066–1073.

Memory and dysexecutive impairments in epilepsy

Introduction

Memory, executive function, and language impairments are common in both focal and primary generalized epilepsy patients and significantly impact their QOL, as well as practical daily school and work role functioning. Assessment and treatment of cognitive impairments is thus a crucial consideration in epilepsy care. This section reviews some potential underlying causes of memory, executive function, and language cognitive domain impairments in epilepsy and briefly examines some possible indirect and direct therapeutic strategies for improving these cognitive difficulties in epilepsy patients.

Epilepsy is associated with several comorbidities, including problems with emotional and behavioral control, socialization, and cognition [1]. Cognitive impairment is a major concern among people with epilepsy: it was the most significant concern reported in a large survey involving over 1000 epilepsy patients [2]. Problems with memory difficulties affect approximately 20–50% of persons with epilepsy, representing the most commonly reported cognitive problem [3], and are among the most significant factors that may lead to poorer QOL in epilepsy patients [4]. In this section, we will review memory, executive function, language, and other related cognitive impairments, as well as possible treatment approaches to problems in these cognitive domains in epilepsy patients. We will begin with a brief overview of cognitive domains and then look at cognitive impairments noted in newly diagnosed and chronic epilepsies. We will then progress to an overview of the range, types, and severities of cognitive dysfunction seen in different common epilepsy syndromes. The impact of transient cognitive impairments (TCIs) accompanying epileptiform EEG activity are considered next, followed by a discussion of the peculiar and unique syndrome of transient epileptic forgetting. We then highlight the frequent lack of patient awareness of memory and cognitive impairments and the frequent lack of provider assessment of memory and cognitive problems in people with epilepsy and offer a practical overview of potentially useful measures for assessing problems

with memory and cognition in epilepsy patients. We conclude with a brief summary of possible future direct treatment approaches toward memory and related cognitive impairments in people with epilepsy. Detailed reviews of the scope and impact of epilepsy comorbidities, the influence of mood-state problems and AED adverse effects, and strategies for diagnostic and treatment approaches to these problems are given elsewhere in this book (see Chapters 1, 2, 5, 7, 10, and 13).

Background and introduction to memory, executive function, and language in epilepsy

While deficits in several aspects of memory functioning occur in epilepsy patients (working memory, semantic memory, autobiographical memory including "flashbulb" emotionally charged memories, implicit memory, recognition memory, and others), our use of the terms "memory" and "memory impairment" throughout this section refers principally to the types of deficits tested in neuropsychological examinations, which concentrate on the evaluation of declarative memory (demonstrated by what the tested patient says, versus procedural memory, which is evaluated by what the tested patient does during a procedure), especially explicit, episodic, anterograde memory (related to a specific, previously learned episode). Episodic memory is thought to be largely dependent on the hippocampus and parahippocampal gyrus structures, including the entorhinal and perirhinal cortices. Declarative, material-specific memories depend on the ability of the patient to learn and recall new episodic information and are typically evaluated as either verbal or nonverbal/visuospatial information. Episodic memories are generally expected to have differential, lateralized representation in most right-handed individuals with traditional functional neuroanatomy, with verbal memory functioning relatively lateralized to the left and visual memory lateralized to the right mesial temporal regions. Dysfunction in these regions thus predominantly causes either verbal or nonverbal memory impairments, and unilateral structural lesions (hippocampal sclerosis (HS), low-grade neoplasms, malformations of cortical development) may cause relatively lateralized impairments ipsilateral to the side of the lesion. When brain lesions are acquired early in life, cerebral plasticity may lead to rerouting of some functional abilities to either the ipsilateral posterior temporal or frontoparietal brain regions or the contralateral, healthy (or relatively spared) mesial temporal region. The modifying influence of education is perhaps an even more significant influence on the degree of cognitive reserve and subsequent capacity for resilience toward additional injury to memory function beyond the epileptogenic focus, frequent seizure, or brain lesion itself, such as may occur following temporal-lobe resection. Research using fMRI has rapidly expanded our understanding of memory functioning in TLE and other epilepsy syndromes, however, particularly with regard to the interdependence between the mesial temporal region and broader network connectivity related to specific tasks.

Executive function involves working memory and several higher-order and integrative cognitive abilities, such as reasoning, abstract thinking, organization, planning, judgment, impulse control, problem-solving, decision-making, motivated behavior, and motor execution. The cognitive control of executive functioning is thought to principally involve the frontal lobe, although integrative functioning of other brain regions from widely distributed brainstem, subcortical, and posterior cortical regions is also involved. Frontal-lobe structures that are especially integral to executive function include the dorsolateral prefrontal cortex, the anterior cingulate cortex, and the orbitofrontal cortex.

Language abilities involve both expressive and receptive capacities for spoken and written communication, which depend especially on the dominant left frontotemporoparietal regions. Language development is impacted by epilepsy in children and language disruption may result in the postictal state in adults and is an integral consideration in patients being considered for epilepsy surgery.

For a detailed review of neuropsychological functioning and evaluation, the reader is referred to other detailed authoritative sources, especially concerning typical neuropsychological test battery measures utilized in assessing epilepsy patients and the roles of neuropsychological testing in localization and preoperative evaluation, including applications in functional cortical mapping and the intracarotid amobarbital procedure (IAP, a.k.a. "Wada") [5–8].

Epilepsy-related factors impacting cognitive functioning

Several epilepsy-related factors may affect cognitive functioning in people with epilepsy, including: the duration of epilepsy (newly diagnosed or chronic); the type of epilepsy syndrome (generalized or focal); the location of focal epileptogenic foci (temporal or extratemporal); the type and frequency of seizures (focal or generalized tonic–clonic); any underlying brain lesions associated with epilepsy; the frequency and distribution of interictal epileptiform discharges (IEDs), which may induce TCIs; and the peculiar and poorly understood syndrome of transient epileptic amnesia (TEA) [4]. Epilepsy comorbidities such as mood and anxiety disorders, AED therapies, neurostimulation, and surgical therapies are additional influences on cognition that must be considered. Cognitive impairments in epilepsy are addressed indirectly by effective seizure control, careful selection and adjustment of AED doses, polytherapy reduction, and treatment of comorbid depression [9]. Additionally, indirect approaches of neurostimulaton and epilepsy surgery, which target improvement in seizure control, may also in some cases have favorable impact on cognitive functioning, particularly memory, executive functioning, and language. Unfortunately, direct approaches to memory impairments are limited; these include neurocognitive rehabilitation approaches and pharmacologic treatments, although the evidence base for both remains limited currently.

Duration of epilepsy: cognitive impairments in newly diagnosed and chronic epilepsies

Problems with memory and cognition appear to begin quite early in the course of newly diagnosed epilepsy. Cognitive impairments in memory and executive function have been found with objective neurocognitive assessments in approximately 72% of those with newly diagnosed epilepsy, with memory problems occurring particularly in those with generalized tonic–clonic seizures and executive dysfunction in those with lower education or structural brain lesions [10]. Recent evidence suggests that verbal memory dysfunction may be present in 60% of patients following presentation with a first seizure and that depressive symptoms are present in 21% of these patients prior to first seizure occurrence [11]. Many children with newly diagnosed epilepsy show evidence for neurocognitive impairments even before initiation of treatment and, in a subset of patients, academic underachievement and cognitive impairment may antedate seizure onset [12]. Prior to treatment initiation, newly diagnosed adult patients in the VA Cooperative study demonstrated impaired motor speed, cognitive attention, and mood state compared to controls [13]; in another recent large prospective sample of epilepsy patients drawn from the SANAD cohort, 53.5% of patients with newly diagnosed epilepsy demonstrated poorer neuropsychological task performance in at least a single domain before AED therapy, in comparison to 20.7% of controls who demonstrated a similar level of dysfunction, especially in the domains of memory and processing speed [14]. One year following initiation of AED treatment, a subset of the SANAD cohort demonstrated persisting dysfunction in several cognitive domains relative to controls, including memory, executive functioning, and psychomotor processing speed, with poorer performance associated with receiving topiramate, generalized seizures, and achieving immediate 12-month remission [15]; after 5-year follow-up, 38% of SANAD patients demonstrated further subtle decline in these domains [16].

In a large cohort of children and adolescents aged 8–18 years with newly diagnosed or recent-onset epilepsy, there was also evidence for significant cognitive impairment in both broad-band (including 41 idiopathic generalized epilepsy (IGE) and 53 idiopathic localization-related epilepsy patients) and narrow-band syndromes (childhood/juvenile absence, juvenile myoclonic, benign epilepsy with centrotemporal spikes, and focal (temporal/frontal/not otherwise specified) syndromes). Cognitive dysfunction was similar to that in adult cohorts, with deficits in psychomotor slowing across syndromes, as well as epilepsy syndrome-specific impairments in memory and language in focal syndromes and executive dysfunction in IGE, when compared to age- and gender-matched controls [17]. Notably, approximately 50% had academic difficulties, even in epilepsy syndromes typically thought of as benign. In a smaller study, children with complex partial seizures (CPS) had more prominent cognitive dysfunction than those with CAE or controls, although both epilepsy groups (CPS and CAE) had more verbal memory dysfunction than controls [18].

Interestingly, neuropsychiatric deficits have also recently been found to be predictive of AED treatment response. An Australian study cohort of 138 evaluable patients who completed the A-B Neuropsychological Assessment Scale (ABNAS) before initiation of AED therapy and were followed for 12 months showed that higher pretreatment ABNAS score was independently predictive of failure to respond to AED treatment, along with brain lesion on MRI imaging and a genomic classifier [19]. Thus, neuropsychological deficits at presentation appear likely to be an important determinant of the likelihood of developing medically refractory seizures.

Chronic epilepsy syndromes and cognitive impairment: temporal-lobe, extratemporal, and primary generalized epilepsies

Chronic epilepsy effects on cognition have predominantly been analyzed in specific epilepsy syndromes, with most studies focused on TLE. In this section we will also discuss extratemporal focal epilepsies and juvenile myoclonic epilepsy (JME), the most widely studied primary generalized epilepsy type.

Temporal-lobe epilepsy

Memory and cognitive impairments are a major feature in the clinical presentation of TLE, due both to lesional and nonlesional impairments of function in the mesial temporal lobe and temporal neocortex, as well as to more widely distributed network alterations in structure and function in subcortical and extratemporal structures [20]. Memory impairment may affect up to 37% of TLE patients and is predominantly related to problems in declarative, episodic memory, with relative sparing of semantic memory [21]. In one large, single-center, 20-year longitudinal German cohort study of 1156 TLE patients aged 6–68 years, memory problems appeared to occur due to both inadequate learning achievement and premature decline in memory functioning at older ages; since TLE patients achieve lower levels of memory in early life, despite losses of memory functioning with age paralleling controls, TLE patients reached impaired memory levels earlier in life than did controls [22]. Patients with left TLE and with HS had the greatest degree of memory loss [22]. A retrospective study of childhood-onset mesial TLE associated with unilateral HS found that deficits in memory, learning, and cognition occurred in early life and remained stable throughout adulthood and that patients of female gender and those with left lateralized HS had more frequent generalized cognitive impairments [23]. Another longitudinal study of medical and surgically treated TLE patients from the same German center suggested that seizure control was the most important variable in arresting or improving memory impairments [24].

Among patients with TLE in a large American series, 20–25% demonstrated cognitive impairments on detailed neuropsychological testing, especially in memory and executive functioning, which correlated with lower baseline IQ scores, more baseline quantitative MRI volumetric abnormalities, a longer duration of epilepsy, and older chronological age [25]. In chronic refractory TLE, seizure frequency has been associated with progressive hippocampal atrophy [26], which probably underlies progressive memory loss. Longer-duration epilepsy has been associated with lower IQ in one large cross-sectional study of chronic refractory TLE [27], while in a different longitudinal study of refractory TLE, about 38% of all patients treated either surgically or medically showed progression in memory and executive function impairments unless seizures were controlled [28]. Chronic epilepsy duration and earlier age of TLE onset have been independently associated with verbal memory, working memory, and executive function impairments in chronic refractory TLE [29,30].

Most memory dysfunction in TLE is material-specific. Lateralized material-specific memory deficits in TLE are relatively specific but infrequent. In one large series of unilateral mesial temporal sclerosis (MTS) TLE patients, selective verbal memory impairment was noted in 25.6% of left MTS cases (82.2% specificity) and nonverbal memory impairments in 26.2% of right MTS cases (92% specificity), while 52.9% of patients had intact memory functions and 13.8% had global memory impairments [31].

The nature of declarative memory dysfunction may relate to age of onset and to the locations of mesial and/or lateral temporal pathology and epileptogenic pathophysiology. In one study of children and adolescents with TLE tested with both semantic and episodic memory tasks, a subset of patients demonstrated a "double dissociation" of impaired memory functioning, whereby some children were impaired on episodic

but not semantic memory and others had intact episodic but impaired semantic memory, implying that patients with more mesial functioning deficits may have episodic memory problems, while more lateral, neocortical-based pathology may contribute to semantic memory dysfunction [32]. Studies that have correlated associative and recognition memory task performance with structural and functional neuroimaging have found that lesions involving the anterior parahippocampal gyrus structures (entorhinal and perirhinal cortices) are more likely to have problems with recognition and associative memory for objects and faces [33,34]. The extent of lateral temporal lobe involvement may also determine whether TLE patients have semantic memory deficits, impairing neocortical memory storage and retrieval [35].

An increasing body of structural and functional neuroimaging research has also confirmed that TLE patients have more broadly distributed connectivity, dysfunction, and structural pathology that likely underlies both seizure generation and cognitive dysfunction. Cognitive phenotypes in TLE have recently been eloquently correlated with either relatively more restricted or more diffuse alterations in temporal and extratemporal cortical thickness, with corresponding gray-matter volume changes to subcortical structures, the corpus callosum, and the cerebellum [36]. The investigators found that anatomical MRI was relatively intact in a minimally impaired TLE group, while increasingly more severe and extensive corresponding anatomical loss was evident in TLE patients with impaired memory, executive function, and processing speed, suggesting a direct correspondence between the severity of TLE cognitive impairments and the distribution of anatomical abnormalities on structural volumetric MRI in widely distributed cortical, subcortical, callosal, and cerebellar networks [36]. Several studies have shown evidence for diffuse extratemporal cerebral function network alterations in both task-specific and resting-state (default-mode network) connectivity on fMRI studies [37–43]. Functional-connectivity (FC) fMRI analyzes blood oxygen level-dependent (BOLD) signal correlation between brain regions, which show reproducible functional networks both during the resting state and linked to the performance of specific tasks. During the resting state of relaxed conscious wakefulness, when the subject is not focused on any specific outward task, the active resting-state network is termed the "default-mode network," which chiefly involves the medial temporal lobes, including the hippocampus, the ventromedial prefrontal cortex, the posterior cingulate cortex (PCC), the precuneus, and the medial, lateral, and inferior parietal cortices. One default-mode network study in unilateral TLE patients showed decreased FC between the amygdala and hippocampus on the affected side of the epileptic focus, as well as altered FC on the temporal lobe contralateral to the focus [37]. Another study instead showed nonlateralized altered FC between the anterior and posterior default-mode network in both right and left TLE subjects [38], while a third showed that FC between the PCC and hippocampal formation was associated with better memory performance and that higher preoperative connectivity with an epileptic focus is correlated with a higher risk for postoperative memory loss. Alternatively, greater preoperative and postoperative FC with the contralateral healthy hippocampal region is associated with better postoperative memory functioning [39]. A similar finding during a verbal memory task-specific fMRI experiment also suggests that abnormal left hippocampal–PCC FC may be responsible for impaired verbal memory [40]. Such default-mode network alterations have been hypothesized to potentially explain cognitive and psychiatric impairments in TLE patients and may be useful in localizing likely deficits and functional memory reserve when considering epilepsy surgery [37–40].

Studies using fMRI to analyze FC in unilateral TLE patients while performing working memory tasks have also shown disrupted connectivity in frontoparietal networks and abnormalities in both gray and white matter in widespread functionally relevant areas [41,42]. In another memory task-specific experiment, extratemporal activations in the anterior cingulate and insula correlated with better verbal and visual memory performance in both left and right TLE patients, which were thought to be evidence for effective compensatory extratemporal recruitment [43].

Temporal and extratemporal network dysfunction likely explains executive dysfunction and language impairments in TLE. Several neuropsychological, imaging, and intracerebral neurophysiologic studies have shown evidence for executive dysfunction in chronic TLE patients arising from the lateral temporal and frontal cortices, with impaired performance on measures of working memory, attention, mental flexibility, categorical verbal fluency, set-shifting ability, categorization, initiation, planning, decision-making, and motor control [44–49].

While most individuals have left hemispheric dominance for language abilities, those with left hemispheric focal epilepsies in the temporal or frontal lobes may have atypical language localization and, more frequently, nontraditional right or mixed language lateralization [50]. Several epilepsy-related variables may account for the development of nontraditional language anatomy with right or mixed language dominance or for the reorganization of language centers within the same hemisphere, including seizure focus localization, age at seizure onset, and the distribution and frequency of IEDs [51]. The IAP has been the traditional standard for language and memory function lateralization [52], although invasive cortical stimulation studies are usually needed to adequately localize nontraditional language anatomy, especially in the setting of nonlesional or cortical malformation focal epilepsy surgical cases [53].

TLE surgery may either impair or improve cognition. Deteriorations in memory, language, and other cognitive functions may result from the removal of functionally normal tissue, while improvements may result from resultant seizure control, removal of nociferous epileptogenic cortex, and reduction of AEDs. The most common functions to be lost postoperatively include verbal and nonverbal, visual memory, naming, and face-recognition functions. Factors that may lead to cognitive decline following TLE surgery include surgery on the language/memory dominant temporal lobe, older age at seizure onset or at the time of temporal lobectomy, high preoperative memory functioning, nonlesional brain MRI study or lack of memory dysfunction ipsilateral to the epileptic focus, and lack of postoperative seizure control [54–59]. When the preoperative intracarotid amobarbital study or PET study is normal on the side of surgery, this may also portend postoperative memory impairment [53,57]. A recent functional neuroimaging study suggested that better postoperative verbal memory outcomes occurred in those patients who demonstrated more activation during a verbal task in the posterior medial temporal lobe prior to surgical resection, suggesting evidence for preoperative functional reorganization of the ipsilateral left posterior hippocampus as the mechanism for better postoperative memory outcome, rather than contralateral hippocampal functional reserve [60]. Considerable research has been devoted to identifying accurate preoperative methods for lateralization of language and memory functions before temporal lobectomy, but at many epilepsy centers the IAP remains the "gold standard" preoperative test [53,61]. Current evidence suggests that fMRI may have sufficient sensitivity and specificity for accurate preoperative language lateralization, with two recent meta-analyses each concluding that fMRI sensitivity was 83.5% (95% CI 80.2 and 86.7%) and specificity 88.1% (95% CI 87.0 and 89.2%) for correctly lateralizing language dominance [62,63]. Unfortunately, fMRI paradigms such as scene-encoding tasks currently remain much less effective at predicting post-operative naming and verbal memory outcomes related to material-specific memory, which appears to be better estimated by preoperative language lateralization [64]. Future development of multivoxel pattern analysis via fMRI may show promise in demonstrating hippocampal functional reserve in individual patients [65].

Favorable cognitive effects following anterior temporal lobectomy surgery can include verbal fluency following left-sided temporal surgery and naming outcomes following more conservative resection [56,59]. Typically, executive function, IQ, and nonverbal memory functions are not significantly impacted by temporal-lobe surgery [56]. Cognitive outcomes following alternative surgical or temporal-lobe ablative strategies such as selective hippocampectomy and gamma knife irradiation have also been reported and appear to have either relatively comparable cognitive risks to standard surgery [59] or, in the case of gamma knife, a neutral cognitive risk profile [66].

Extratemporal and cryptogenic (nonlesional) epilepsies

We will now discuss memory and executive function in extratemporal epilepsies, benign epilepsy of childhood with centrotemporal spikes (BECTS or benign rolandic epilepsy, BRE), and cryptogenic nonlesional focal epilepsies (NFLE).

Frontal-lobe epilepsy

In contrast to TLE, patients with frontal-lobe epilepsy (FLE) have not been found to have a characteristic neuropsychological profile of deficits, having highly variable cognitive impairments, but like in TLE, they do frequently show executive dysfunction, attentional, and memory problems [67–70]. However, executive dysfunction is the most prominent impairment in FLE, unlike in TLE, with problems in set shifting, motor coordination, and planning; reduced attention span; and difficulties with complex behaviors such as planning, selecting goals, anticipating outcomes, initiating action, and inhibiting response [67,69–72]. When trying to distinguish FLE from TLE via neuropsychological deficits, more specific executive measures such as set shifting appear to be more discriminative, especially for patients with nonlesional FLE or dominant lateralization of the frontal epileptogenic focus [71,72]. Resting frontal-lobe PET hypometabolism also appears to be linked to cognitive impairment in FLE patients but there may also be parietal and limbic cortical hypometabolism, suggesting that executive dysfunction is mediated by a broad frontotemporoparietal network [73]. A more recent fMRI study of FC in a cohort of children with FLE and cognitive impairment has also shown decreased frontal-lobe connectivity both within the frontal lobe and to widespread cortical and subcortical structures, including the parietal and temporal lobes, cerebellum, and basal ganglia, suggesting a mechanism for executive dysfunction and other cognitive problems seen in FLE [74]. Several neuropsychological studies have shown impaired memory function in FLE patients [75] and another recent fMRI imaging study showed that FLE patients with sufficient memory functioning had wide frontal-lobe activation contralateral to the side of the frontal-lobe seizure focus, while FLE patients with impaired memory function showed decreased hippocampal activation [76]. The major risk factor for occurrence of cognitive impairment in FLE appears to be young age at seizure onset, and behavioral disorders, especially attention deficit/hyperactivity disorder (ADHD), which is frequently seen in children with FLE [67].

In the absence of a structural lesion, specific neuropsychological deficits may be difficult to identify in FLE [69]. Following dominant frontal lobectomy, children have shown decreased verbal fluency, variable verbal IQ decrement, and problems with confrontation naming and conceptual reasoning, while adults have shown decreased verbal fluency after dominant dorsolateral frontal lesions and reduced nonverbal fluency following nondominant dorsolateral frontal lesions [69].

However, the role of mood disturbance may be a major issue in the occurrence and severity of executive dysfunction in FLE. In one recent large surgical series of FLE patients, preoperative depression was the major factor associated with presence of postoperative executive function impairment, possibly due in part to widespread damage mediated by FLE and/or surgery to the frontal-lobe structures involved in emotion regulation, including the ventral lateral and medial prefrontal cortices, as well as to structures mediating cognitive control such as the dorsolateral prefrontal cortex and medial frontal circuits neighboring the anterior cingulate cortex [77].

Occipital-lobe epilepsy

A few papers on occipital-lobe epilepsy (OLE) suggest that cognitive impairments are quite similar to those seen in FLE. One study of 20 nonsymptomatic adult OLE patients found impairments in complex visuospatial skills and executive function, which were more prominent in cryptogenic than idiopathic OLE patients, although these subgroup differences were not statistically significant [78]. In another study of 21 children aged 6–14 years with idiopathic OLE, significantly poorer attention, memory, and intellectual functioning was noted when compared to age- and gender-matched controls [79]. A study of children with benign childhood occipital epilepsy (Panayotopulos syndrome) demonstrated significant impairment of visual attentional ability, verbal and visuospatial memory, manual dexterity, language, and abilities in reading, writing, and arithmetic [80]. There are few specific published data on cognitive aspects of parietal-lobe epilepsies.

Cryptogenic/nonlesional focal epilepsies

Patients with NFLE have also been found to have similar cognitive impairments. Several recent studies that correlated structural and functional neuroimaging tests with neuropsychological functioning are of particular interest, as they provide insight into probable diffuse network dysfunction underlying cognitive impairments in patients with NFLE. One study of 36 patients found that relative to controls, NLFE patients had lower IQ, impaired information processing, and decreased working memory performance [81]. Short-term memory deficits were unrelated to hippocampal volumetry and the only group differences during a memory task were decreased activations within a prefrontal network, suggesting that working memory deficits in NLFE patients may result from impairments in prefrontal network functioning [81]. In another study of 21

NLFE patients with worse intelligence, language, and executive functioning than controls, reduced white matter measures of fractional anisotropy in multifocal bilateral frontal, temporal, and parietal regions correlated with several neuropsychological deficits, possibly underlying disturbances in diffuse cortical processing networks [82]. An fMRI study of FC in 36 NLFE patients showed they had lower IQ and verbal fluency and significantly lower prefrontal network FC during word fluency and generation tasks and lower frontotemporal network FC during text reading than controls, and that the reduced performance was correlated with these reduced FC activations [83].

Benign epilepsy of childhood with centrotemporal spikes/benign rolandic epilepsy

Children with BECTS frequently outgrow their seizures but often have a less benign neurocognitive profile of impairments identified at the time of presentation with seizures [84]. Enduring neurocognitive problems are especially common in language [85,86] and attention [87], leading to learning disabilities and developmental cognitive sequelae that may outlast their seizures. Cognitive problems are especially prominent in language, reading, attention, and memory, and general intelligence has been found to be reduced in patients with bilateral interictal epileptiform spikes compared to those with unilateral spikes [84–94]. Language problems include difficulties in reading, spelling, auditory verbal learning, auditory discrimination, and expressive grammar [85,86]. Recent functional neuroimaging studies have demonstrated compensatory reorganization of language representation in BECTS patients, with evidence for reorganization in bilateral or right hemispheric language networks [87]. While many cognitive functions improve over serial tests, particularly when seizures resolve, some deficits in language, phonologic awareness, and visual memory remain and some patients demonstrate specific learning disabilities, behavioral problems, and language delay or regression [93,95,96], while others may show resolution of language impairments when seizures remit [97]. A very small subset of patients with BECTS may follow an atypical course, with cognitive and language deterioration and evolution of electrical status epilepticus during slow-wave sleep (ESES) and Landau–Kleffner syndrome (LKS), which is thought to represent an epileptic encephalopathy. In one large single-center series of 196 BECTS cases from Israel, ESES was seen in 4.6% of patients, LKS in 2%, and other atypical presentations with cognitive or motor sequelae in another 2%. Frequent neuropsychiatric comorbidities were also seen in these patients, including ADHD in 31%, cognitive deficits in 21.9%, and neurobehavioral abnormalities including aggression, anxiety, depression, and pervasive developmental disorder in 11.7% [98]. A detailed discussion of the epileptic encephalopathies is beyond the scope of this section but practical aspects of the striking of a balance between the goals of effective seizure treatment and idiosyncratic toxicities are discussed in Chapter 11.

Serial testing for borderline or deficient neurocognitive and language abilities is recommended for all children with BECTS, to allow early intervention, timely speech and neurorehabilitation therapies, and academic accommodation where appropriate, in order to optimize development and school life. Recent evidence has also pointed to a familial BECTS neurocognitive endophenotype, with similar memory and language problems frequently being found in siblings of children with BECTS, suggesting that siblings of BECTS patients should also be screened for neurocognitive problems and possible learning disabilities [99,100]. A recent study demonstrated that striatal hypertrophy was seen in a small sample of patients with newly diagnosed BECTS and that greater hypertrophy, especially in the putamen, appeared adaptive toward better cognitive performance, suggesting that if the mechanisms for this compensatory alteration in subcortical structure and function were better understood, this could represent a future targetable pathway for improving cognitive functioning in children with BECTS [101].

Primary generalized epilepsies and cognitive impairments: juvenile myoclonic and childhood absence epilepsy

Compared to the focal epilepsies, there has until recently been considerably less research concerning cognitive aspects of the generalized epilepsies. Most data concern the common syndromes of JME and CAE.

JME is thought to be an IGE syndrome, although recent neuroimaging research has shown subtle findings suggesting that frontothalamic network dysfunction underlies both seizures and cognitive abnormalities in JME [102]. Several neuropsychological studies have confirmed widespread dysfunction in JME patients

relative to controls, particularly involving prominent dysexecutive impairments consistent with frontal-lobe dysfunction [103–109]. Specifically, impaired neuropsychological domain scores in JME patients relative to healthy controls have included attention, immediate verbal memory, mental flexibility, control of inhibition, working memory, processing speed, verbal and visual memory, naming and verbal fluency, and visuospatial skills, with deficits found to be correlated with epilepsy duration, younger age, family history, and absence seizures, although in one study impairments were partially modified by higher education [103,104]. Another study utilizing detailed executive function measures found evidence for dysexecutive impairments in 83% of JME patients, with higher seizure frequency, longer epilepsy duration, and psychiatric comorbidity [105]. Two recent studies of JME patients found that executive dysfunction may relate to poor planning ability, as represented in prospective memory impairments in JME, and that JME patients with continued seizures are prone to disadvantageous decision-making during the Iowa Gambling Task, which is associated with increased fMRI activation in the dorsolateral prefrontal cortex [107,108]. Recent imaging data have also shown evidence for hippocampal formation atrophy in JME patients with memory deficits, demonstrating a basis for structural abnormalities in addition to functional abnormalities beyond the frontothalamic network in JME patients [109]. Very recent functional neuroimaging analyses of JME network FC have shown increased FC between the prefrontal and motor cortices and abnormal coactivation of the motor and supplementary motor area cortices during cognitive tasks in JME patients, providing evidence for possible mechanistic explanations for cognitive triggering of seizures and executive cognitive dysfunction in JME patients [110,111].

CAE has been associated with a twofold greater chance of neuropsychological impairment than other seizure types in a large prospective community cohort study of 282 children with newly diagnosed seizures [112]. Of patients with idiopathic generalized epilepsies undergoing neuropsychological testing, both those with CAE and those with primary generalized tonic seizures had attentional deficits but only CAE patients had global cognitive dysfunction in attention, verbal memory, learning, fluency, visuospatial skills, and fine-motor responses, with worse function seen in CAE patients with a longer epilepsy duration [113,114]. In a recently published study of neurocognitive functioning in participants in the pivotal randomized prospective clinical trial conducted by the NIH-NINDS Childhood Absence Study Group, 36% of patients with CAE had attention deficits at baseline prior to treatment initiation, which persisted in a subset despite effective seizure control at 4–5-month follow-up, more frequently in patients treated with valproate (49%) than either ethosuximide (32%) or lamotrigine (24%) [115]. Attention deficits on a continuous performance task were also seen to occur more frequently in CAE patients with absence seizures that lasted longer than 20 seconds [116].

Attentional and cognitive problems may also create vulnerability to frequent neuropsychiatric comorbidity in CAE. In one CAE cohort, 25% of children had subtle cognitive dysfunction, 43% had language problems, and 61% were found to have a psychiatric diagnosis (most commonly either ADHD or an anxiety disorder); epilepsy duration, seizure frequency, and AED treatment were associated with severity of these comorbidities. Alarmingly, only 23% of patients were found to have appropriate interventions for these comorbid problems, suggesting a substantial unmet need to recognize and treat neuropsychiatric deficits and comorbidities in children with CAE [117]. Another study found evidence for higher frequency of hyperactivity and inattentiveness in children with CAE. These children required more classroom supervision, those who were actively seizing were more impatient, and those with longer epilepsy duration were less able to finish homework [118]. On formal measures of alertness, divided and selective attention, and impulsivity, CAE patients are impaired relative to controls [119]. Effective recognition and timely treatment of neuropsychiatric comorbidities in CAE patients is crucial, since recent evidence suggests that comorbidities often influence an epilepsy patient's overall longitudinal cognitive trajectory, leading to worsened cognitive functioning over time [120].

Diffuse neurocognitive and neuropsychiatric problems in CAE appear to be related to a diffuse brain disorder, given that CAE patients have been found to have significantly reduced gray-matter volumes in crucial structures subserving emotional and memory functioning, including the orbitofrontal cortex and bilateral temporal lobes [121].

Transient cognitive impairments associated with interictal epileptiform discharges in epilepsy

Both focal and generalized ictal seizure events frequently disturb consciousness or higher cognitive functions, causing temporary language disturbance and amnesia. However, until recently, there has been comparatively little study of cognitive impairments associated with IEDs on EEG. Early descriptions of TCI caused by IEDs began in the 1980s, when either brief generalized or focal IEDs were found to cause impairments in short-term memory tasks, particularly when IEDs occurred during the time of stimulus presentation [122,123]. Generalized IEDs of 3-second duration were generally found to cause TCIs, but briefer generalized and focal IEDs have also been found to produce TCI performance deficits, with focal left IEDs impacting verbal short-term memory task performance and right IEDs negatively affecting nonverbal short-term memory task performance, and TCIs have been recognized to impact real-world performance of educational functions in children and driving abilities in adults [123]. More recent studies of children and adults have found that when IEDs exceed 10% of continuous EEG recording time, processing speed, verbal memory, and visual–motor integration are impaired, with greater deficits seen for daytime than nocturnal IEDs, at least in children [124–126]. Recent elegant studies in rat and human hippocampus showed that IED occurrence during memory retrieval or maintenance had a prominent negative effect on performance but that IED during memory encoding did not a have substantial impact [127,128]. In humans, IEDs bilateral or contralateral to seizure focus, especially longer-duration IEDs, were most deleterious [128]. Fascinatingly, the relationship between memory processing and epileptiform activity may be bidirectional in nature. A recent human intracranial electrode study demonstrated reduction in IED frequency during successful memory encoding in the amygdala, hippocampus, and temporal cortex, suggesting that physiologic local mesial temporal network activity related to memory encoding may modulate IED occurrence [129]. Additional animal and human studies of the interplay between memory processing and IEDs are necessary to further clarify the influence of epileptiform activity on cognition, and vice versa, and to determine whether normal human cognitive processing could be applied toward a potential therapeutic purpose in epilepsy and whether treatment of IEDs could in turn improve cognitive impairments accompanying epilepsy.

Transient epileptic amnesia and accelerated long-term forgetting: a controversial epileptic syndrome

TEA is a controversial but established unique clinical syndrome characterized by recurrent witnessed transient amnesia in isolation of other cognitive deficits that has an apparent epileptic cause [130–133]. TEA tends to affect elderly individuals but may also occur in middle-aged people, especially men [131–133]. Attacks are brief (typically under 1 hour in duration), often occur upon awaking, and recur up to 12 times per year [131]. While TEA is frequently confused with incipient dementia or cerebrovascular disease and epilepsy is often not suspected initially, a workup for causes other than epilepsy is unrevealing. TEA also resembles transient global amnesia in that patients ask the same questions repeatedly, having variable and usually incomplete anterograde and variable retrograde amnesia, but attacks are more frequent and briefer in duration [130,131]. "Accelerated long-term forgetting," a form of accelerated amnesia for successfully learned memories that are then forgotten over subsequent days or weeks, is also typical [131,132,134]. Other focal seizures typical of TLE, often complex partial (or, in the new terminology, focal dysmnesic) in type, are frequent and a good response of the episodes to AEDs is seen in the majority of cases [130–133]. Persistent retrograde autobiographical amnesia for important personal or other details from past experience, either facts or events, over periods as long as decades is also usual and has been postulated to reflect the impact of epilepsy on long-term memory consolidation [130,131,134]. Further research into this intriguing entity will hopefully clarify its clinical characteristics and pathophysiology, potentially providing novel insights into the mechanisms of cognitive impairments in focal epileptic disorders.

Awareness and assessment of memory and cognitive problems in epilepsy

In a recent study of epilepsy outpatients and their providers, the top three concerns identified by patients were unexpected seizures, driving issues, and memory problems. Providers were more focused on clinical seizure management. A gap was identified between patient's and provider's prioritization of memory concerns, implying that providers need to focus more on addressing memory problems in their epilepsy patients [135]. Another recent study of patient self-reports of cognitive abilities found that patient-reported everyday memory functioning correlated better with academic performance than objective neuropsychological test scores, suggesting that patients who possess insight into their own memory abilities can provide valid and reliable information concerning their real-world academic abilities [136]. However, cognitive deficits are frequently underestimated by as many as 61% of people with epilepsy [8,137], especially those with comorbid depression or frequent seizures; those with comorbid mood or anxiety disorders also have subjective memory complaints that lack clear correlation with objective neuropsychological deficits [138–140], suggesting that objective cognitive assessments should be considered at initial presentation and sequentially over time so that perceived cognitive functioning, objective neurocognitive deficits, and mood disorders can all be identified and effectively treated to improve well-being and functioning [8,137–140].

A standard full neuropsychological testing battery remains the "gold standard" for formal assessment of cognitive functioning in patients with epilepsy, especially those with refractory epilepsy, who may be candidates for surgery or invasive neurostimulation procedures [141]. However, in newly diagnosed patients and for serial follow-up assessments, a full battery of neuropsychological testing is usually impractical and unfeasible given its expense, frequent inaccessibility, and resource intensiveness. A screening method that is quicker, easier, and highly reproducible between sessions is called for. Fortunately, a developing body of research now suggests that the use of a variety of neurocognitive assessment measures may provide valid and reliable assessments of memory and cognitive functioning in epilepsy patients [142–148].

The most familiar, inexpensive, and simplest method of assessing neurocognitive functioning is a bedside mental status examination. Recent evidence suggests that the Montreal Cognitive Assessment (MoCA) is superior to the Folstein Mini-Mental State Examination (MMSE) for evaluation of epilepsy patients, as it enables identification of subtle neurocognitive impairment (which correlates frequently with AED polytherapy) in 60% of patients who have normal scores on the MMSE [142]. The MoCA – or a similar comprehensive measure that provides a comprehensive assessment of attention, visuospatial, and language functioning, such as the Kokmen Short Test of Mental Status (STMS) – is best for the evaluation of neurological patient populations, especially in epilepsy. Another advantage of the MoCA and STMS is that they are freely available for clinical and research use, whereas the MMSE is a proprietary test, requiring royalty payments for use and intended publication.

When time permits, a longer and more comprehensive battery that also provides quantifiable measures of psychomotor processing speed is desirable and can provide detailed information on the key neurocognitive domains of memory, executive function, attention, and visuospatial abilities. There are now several well-validated and extensively normed comprehensive computerized neurocognitive batteries available [143–145], as well as more focused tests for attention and a domain-specific assessment tool for executive function [146–148]. These computerized and bedside measures have recently been analyzed in a variety of epilepsy patient populations [143–148]. While such tools are inadequate for purposes of confident localization or preoperative evaluation, they may be sufficient for initial neurocognitive screening [144,145] or serial longitudinal evaluation for change in neurocognitive functioning [145]. Computerized neurocognitive measures can also assist in tailoring AED therapy [145–147], identifying patients who may require more detailed neuropsychological testing for academic or workplace accommodation, and enabling early intervention for learning disabilities in children and adolescents with epilepsy.

Direct therapeutic approaches for memory and cognitive problems in epilepsy

While there are no currently well-established therapies that directly target the improvement of memory and cognitive problems in epilepsy, commonly employed indirect approaches that may also improve cognition include interventions to improve seizure frequency, reduce AED polytherapy, and treat mood and anxiety comorbidities. These topics will be discussed extensively in later chapters but this section will briefly discuss the rationale and preliminary research findings concerning direct pharmacologic, neurostimulation, and neurocognitive rehabilitation therapies for memory and cognitive problems in epilepsy patients.

Primary pharmacologic strategies targeting memory improvement in epilepsy patients have been very limited thus far. Donepezil, a selective, reversible acetylcholinesterase inhibitor, is an effective, highly evidence-based treatment for improving cognitive impairment in several other neurological conditions, especially Alzheimer's disease [149], in which epilepsy has been recently found to be a significant comorbidity [150]. Two studies examined donepezil therapy for memory impairment in epilepsy. One, a pilot study, found that donepezil appeared to improve some aspects of memory, especially verbal learning [151], but the other, a randomized, placebo-controlled crossover study of donepezil targeting neuropsychological memory domain performance was negative [152]. Similarly, galantamine, another selective inhibitor of acetylcholinesterase, underwent a small randomized controlled trial in patients with epilepsy and, although it was well tolerated, no improvement of memory was observed [153].

Most neurostimulation therapies have either neutral or slightly favorable effects on alertness, cognition, and memory. The most extensively studied neurostimulation therapy is vagus nerve stimulation (VNS), which has shown variable effects on memory. Some studies have shown that VNS may enhance memory or executive functions [154–157], while others show a neutral or negative impact [158–160]. Similarly, short-term VNS in treatment-resistant depression showed a variety of cognitive improvements in executive functions, language, and processing speed [161]. Invasive neurostimulation techniques, including responsive neurostimulation, deep-brain stimulation targeting the anterior nucleus of the thalamus, bilateral hippocampal stimulation, and low-frequency stimulation of the fornix, have shown neutral or mildly favorable cognitive effects [162–167]. Interestingly, stimulation of the entorhinal cortex improved spatial memory and navigation in a virtual environment [168] and stimulation of the temporal neocortex in a single case reproduced specific long-term autobiographical memories with a reproducible neural activity signature [168]. Repetitive transcranial magnetic stimulation (rTMS) improved some aspects of cognition, including Stroop performance [169].

Chapter 7 provides a detailed summary of the rationale, approaches, and efficacy of neurocognitive rehabilitation in epilepsy. Generally, compensation for deficits, rather than restoration, is the primary aim of cognitive rehabilitation [170]. Compensatory strategies are either external or internal, with external memory strategies including methods for storing information externally and reminding oneself to complete a certain activity, such as the use of an electronic agenda [171]. Internal memory strategies focus on the elaboration and visualization of information, presumably facilitating later retrieval [170]. Several studies have demonstrated the effectiveness of cognitive rehabilitation programs for the treatment of epilepsy-related memory problems [172–174]. However, methodologies and program characteristics varied significantly from study to study. A randomized controlled study of two cognitive rehabilitation programs, the retraining method and the compensation method, found both treatment strategies to be effective in improving self-reported cognitive outcomes and QOL in people with epilepsy [175].

Conclusion

Memory and cognitive problems are one of the chief concerns of patients with epilepsy and physicians tend to underestimate the importance of patient cognitive concerns. Use of objective screening tools to identify memory and cognitive impairments in people with epilepsy is suggested both on the initial visit and at regular intervals during the course of epilepsy follow-up to identify newly emerging subjective or objective cognitive difficulties that may pose risks for adverse neurodevelopmental outcomes and learning disability in children and adolescents and impact work and social role functioning and QOL in adult patients with epilepsy. There are now a variety of well-validated bedside and computerized neurocognitive assessment tools to aid clinicians in patient evaluation and in triaging patients for more intensive neuropsychological testing, which remains the "gold standard" for cognitive assessment, particularly when aiding localization or as part of a comprehensive presurgical evaluation. Both focal and generalized epilepsy syndromes feature prominent neurocognitive impairments in memory, language, and executive functioning that often correspond to underlying unique structural gray- and white-matter alterations and disturbances in FC within epileptogenic, resting-state, and task-specific networks. TCIs result from either generalized or focal interictal epileptiform activity. TEA is a controversial but well-delineated clinical entity accompanying some middle-aged and elderly men with temporal-lobe focal epilepsies. Ongoing research correlating neuropsychological, neurophysiological, and neuroimaging techniques will be necessary to better understand the complex interrelationships between memory and cognitive functioning and epilepsy.

References

1 Bell B, Lin JJ, Seidenberg M, Hermann B: The neurobiology of cognitive disorders in temporal lobe epilepsy. *Nat Rev Neurol* 2011; **7**:154–164.

2 Fisher RS, Vickrey BG, Gibson P et al.: The impact of epilepsy from the patient's perspective. I: Descriptions and subjective perceptions. *Epilepsy Res* 2000; **41**:39–51.

3 Hendriks MPH, Aldenkamp AP, Vlugt H et al.: Memory complaints in medically refractory epilepsy: relationship to epilepsy-related factors. *Epilepsy Behav* 2002; **3**:165–172.

4 Hall KE, Isaac CL, Harris P: Memory complaints in epilepsy: an accurate reflection of memory impairment or an indicator of poor adjustment? A review of the literature. *Clin Psychol Rev* 2009; **29**:354–367.

5 Trenerry MR: Neuropsychologic assessment in surgical treatment of epilepsy. *Mayo Clin Proc* 1996; **71(12)**: 1196–1200.

6 Lezak MD, Howieson DB, Loring DW: *Neuropsychological Assessment*, 4 edn. Oxford University Press, New York, NY, 2004.

7 Alvarez JA, Emory E, Julie A, Emory E: Executive function and the frontal lobes: a meta-analytic review. *Neuropsychol Rev* 2006; **16(1)**:17–42.

8 Jones-Gotman M, Smith ML, Risse GL et al.: The contribution of neuropsychology to diagnostic assessment in epilepsy. *Epilepsy Behav* 2010; **18(1–2)**:3–12.

9 Shulman MB, Barr W: Treatment of memory disorders in epilepsy. *Epilepsy Behav* 2002; **3**:S30–S34.

10 Witt JA, Helmstaedter C: Should cognition be screened in new-onset epilepsies? A study in 247 untreated patients. *J Neurol* 2012; **259(8)**:1727–1731.

11 Rühle N, Schley A, Pohley I et al.: Neuropsychological deficits after a first unprovoked seizure and depressive symptoms in the week before. *Epilepsy Behav* 2014; **31**: 334–338.

12 Hermann B, Jones J, Sheth R et al.: Children with new-onset epilepsy: neuropsychological status and brain structure. *Brain* 2006; **129**:2609–2619.

13 Smith DB, Craft BR, Collins J et al.: Behavioral characteristics of epilepsy patients compared with normal controls. *Epilepsia* 1986; **27(6)**:760–768.

14 Taylor J, Kolamunnage-Dona R, Marson AG et al.: Patients with epilepsy: cognitively compromised before the start of antiepileptic drug treatment? *Epilepsia* 2010; **51(1)**: 48–56.

15 Baker GA, Taylor J, Aldenkamp AP, SANAD group: Newly diagnosed epilepsy: cognitive outcome after 12 months. *Epilepsia* 2011; **52(6)**:1084–1091.

16 Taylor J, Baker GA: Newly diagnosed epilepsy: cognitive outcome at 5 years. *Epilepsy Behav* 2010; **18(4)**:397–403.

17 Jackson DC, Dabbs K, Walker NM et al.: The neuropsychological and academic substrate of new/recent-onset epilepsies. *J Pediatr* 2013; **162(5)**:1047–1053.

18 Kernan CL, Asarnow R, Siddarth P et al.: Neurocognitive profiles in children with epilepsy. *Epilepsia* 2012; **53(12)**: 2156–2163.

19 Petrovski S, Szoeke CE, Jones NC et al.: Neuropsychiatric symptomatology predicts seizure recurrence in newly treated patients. *Neurology* 2010; **75(11)**:1015–1021.

20 Bell B, Lin JJ, Seidenberg M, Hermann B: The neurobiology of cognitive disorders in temporal lobe epilepsy. *Nat Rev Neurol* 2011; **7(3)**:154–164.

21 Helmstaedter C: Effects of chronic epilepsy on declarative memory systems. *Prog Brain Res* 2002; **135**:439–453.

22 Helmstaedter C, Elger CE: Chronic temporal lobe epilepsy: a neurodevelopmental or progressively dementing disease? *Brain* 2009; **132(Pt 10)**:2822–2830.

23 Baxendale S, Heaney D, Thompson PJ, Duncan JS: Cognitive consequences of childhood-onset temporal lobe epilepsy across the adult lifespan. *Neurology* 2010; **75(8)**: 705–711.

24 Helmstaedter C, Kurthen M, Lux S et al.: Chronic epilepsy and cognition: a longitudinal study in temporal lobe epilepsy. *Ann Neurol* 2003; **54(4)**:425–432.

25 Hermann BP, Seidenberg M, Dow C et al.: Cognitive prognosis in chronic temporal lobe epilepsy. *Ann Neurol* 2006; **60**:80–87.

26 Fuerst D, Shah J, Shah A, Watson C: Hippocampal sclerosis is a progressive disorder: a longitudinal volumetric MRI study. *Ann Neurol* 2003; **53**:413–416.

27 Jokeit H, Ebner A: Long term effects of refractory temporal lobe epilepsy on cognitive abilities: a cross sectional study. *J Neurol Neurosurg Psychiatry* 1999; **67**:44–50.

28 Helmstaedter C, Kurthen M, Lux S et al.: Chronic epilepsy and cognition: a longitudinal study in temporal lobe epilepsy. *Ann Neurol* 2003; **54**:425–432.

29 Kent GP, Schefft BK, Howe SR et al.: The effects of duration of intractable epilepsy on memory function. *Epilepsy Behav* 2006; **9(3)**:469–477.

30 Black LC, Schefft BK, Howe SR et al.: The effect of seizures on working memory and executive functioning performance. *Epilepsy Behav* 2010; **17(3)**:412–419.

31 Castro LH, Silva LC, Adda CC et al.: Low prevalence but high specificity of material-specific memory impairment in epilepsy associated with hippocampal sclerosis. *Epilepsia* 2013; **54(10)**:1735–1742.

32 Smith ML, Lah S: One declarative memory system or two? The relationship between episodic and semantic memory in children with temporal lobe epilepsy. *Neuropsychology* 2011; **25(5)**:634–644.

33 Weniger G, Boucsein K, Irle E: Impaired associative memory in temporal lobe epilepsy subjects after lesions of hippocampus, parahippocampal gyrus, and amygdala. *Hippocampus* 2004; **14(6)**:785–796.

34 Guedj E, Barbeau EJ, Liégeois-Chauvel C et al.: Performance in recognition memory is correlated with entorhinal/perirhinal interictal metabolism in temporal lobe epilepsy. *Epilepsy Behav* 2010; **19(4)**:612–617.

35 Giovagnoli AR, Erbetta A, Villani F, Avanzini G: Semantic memory in partial epilepsy: verbal and non-verbal deficits and neuroanatomical relationships. *Neuropsychologia* 2005; **43(10)**:1482–1492.

36 Dabbs K, Jones J, Seidenberg M, Hermann B: Neuroanatomical correlates of cognitive phenotypes in temporal lobe epilepsy. *Epilepsy Behav* 2009; **15(4)**: 445–451.

37 Pittau F, Grova C, Moeller F et al.: Patterns of altered functional connectivity in mesial temporal lobe epilepsy. *Epilepsia* 2012; **53(6)**:1013–1023.

38 Haneef Z, Lenartowicz A, Yeh HJ et al.: Effect of lateralized temporal lobe epilepsy on the default mode network. *Epilepsy Behav* 2012; **25(3)**:350–357.

39 McCormick C, Quraan M, Cohn M et al.: Default mode network connectivity indicates episodic memory capacity in mesial temporal lobe epilepsy. *Epilepsia* 2013; **54(5)**: 809–818.

40 Doucet G, Osipowicz K, Sharan A et al.: Extratemporal functional connectivity impairments at rest are related to memory performance in mesial temporal epilepsy. *Hum Brain Mapp* 2013; **34(9)**:2202–2216.

41 Doucet G, Osipowicz K, Sharan A et al.: Hippocampal functional connectivity patterns during spatial working

memory differ in right versus left temporal lobe epilepsy. *Brain Connect* 2013; **3(4)**:398–406.

42 Winston GP, Stretton J, Sidhu MK et al.: Structural correlates of impaired working memory in hippocampal sclerosis. *Epilepsia* 2013; **54(7)**:1143–1153.

43 Sidhu MK, Stretton J, Winston GP et al.: A functional magnetic resonance imaging study mapping the episodic memory encoding network in temporal lobe epilepsy. *Brain* 2013; **136(Pt 6)**:1868–1888.

44 Zamarian L, Trinka E, Bonatti E et al.: Executive functions in chronic mesial temporal lobe epilepsy. *Epilepsy Res Treat* 2011, art. no. 596174.

45 Stretton J, Thompson PJ: Frontal lobe function in temporal lobe epilepsy. *Epilepsy Res* 2012; **98(1)**:1–13.

46 Longo CA, Kerr EN, Smith ML: Executive functioning in children with intractable frontal lobe or temporal lobe epilepsy. *Epilepsy Behav* 2013; **26(1)**:102–108.

47 Yamano M, Akamatsu N, Tsuji S et al.: Decision-making in temporal lobe epilepsy examined with the Iowa gambling task. *Epilepsy Res* 2011; **93(1)**:33–38.

48 Rusnáková S, Daniel P, Chládek J et al.: The executive functions in frontal and temporal lobes: a flanker task intracerebral recording study. *J Clin Neurophysiol* 2011; **28(1)**:30–35.

49 Bocková M, Chládek J, Jurák P et al.: Executive functions processed in the frontal and lateral temporal cortices: intracerebral study. *Clin Neurophysiol* 2007; **118(12)**: 2625–2636.

50 Berl MM, Balsamo LM, Xu B et al.: Seizure focus affects regional language networks assessed by fMRI. *Neurology* 2005; **65(10)**:1604–1611.

51 Hamberger MJ, Cole J: Language organization and reorganization in epilepsy. *Neuropsychol Rev* 2011; **21(3)**: 240–251.

52 Hamberger MJ: Cortical language mapping in epilepsy: a critical review. *Neuropsychol Rev* 2007; **17(4)**:477–489.

53 Sharan A, Ooi YC, Langfitt J, Sperling MR: Intracarotid amobarbital procedure for epilepsy surgery. *Epilepsy Behav* 2011; **20(2)**:209–213.

54 Helmstaedter C. Neuropsychological aspects of epilepsy surgery. *Epilepsy Behav* 2004; **5(Suppl. 1)**:S45–S55.

55 Helmstaedter C, Petzold I, Bien CG: The cognitive consequence of resecting nonlesional tissues in epilepsy surgery: results from MRI- and histopathology-negative patients with temporal lobe epilepsy. *Epilepsia* 2011; **52**: 1402–1408.

56 Sherman EM, Wiebe S, Fay-McClymont TB et al.: Neuropsychological outcomes after epilepsy surgery: systematic review and pooled estimates. *Epilepsia* 2011; **52(5)**: 857–869.

57 Henry TR, Roman DD: Presurgical epilepsy localization with interictal cerebral dysfunction. *Epilepsy Behav* 2011; **20(2)**:194–208.

58 Baxendale S, Thompson PJ, Sander JW: Neuropsychological outcomes in epilepsy surgery patients with unilateral hippocampal sclerosis and good preoperative memory function. *Epilepsia* 2013; **54(9)**:e131–e134.

59 Tanriverdi T, Dudley RW, Hasan A et al.: Memory outcome after temporal lobe epilepsy surgery: corticoamygdalohippocampectomy versus selective amygdalohippocampectomy. *J Neurosurg* 2010; **113(6)**:1164–1175.

60 Bonelli SB, Thompson PJ, Yogarajah M et al.: Memory reorganization following anterior temporal lobe resection: a longitudinal functional MRI study. *Brain* 2013; **136(Pt 6)**:1889–1900.

61 Loring DW, Bowden SC, Lee GP, Meador KJ: Diagnostic utility of Wada Memory Asymmetries: sensitivity, specificity, and likelihood ratio characterization. *Neuropsychology* 2009; **23(6)**:687–693.

62 Spritzer SD, Hoerth MT, Zimmerman RS et al.: Determination of hemispheric language dominance in the surgical epilepsy patient: diagnostic properties of functional magnetic resonance imaging. *Neurologist* 2012; **18(5)**:329–331.

63 Dym RJ, Burns J, Freeman K, Lipton ML: Is functional MR imaging assessment of hemispheric language dominance as good as the Wada test? *A meta-analysis. Radiology* 2011; **261(2)**:446–455.

64 Binder JR, Swanson SJ, Sabsevitz DS et al.: A comparison of two fMRI methods for predicting verbal memory decline after left temporal lobectomy: language lateralization versus hippocampal activation asymmetry. *Epilepsia* 2010; **51(4)**:618–626.

65 Bonnici HM, Sidhu M, Chadwick MJ et al.: Assessing hippocampal functional reserve in temporal lobe epilepsy: a multi-voxel pattern analysis of fMRI data. *Epilepsy Res* 2013; **105(1–2)**:140–149.

66 Quigg M, Broshek DK, Barbaro NM et al. Neuropsychological outcomes after Gamma Knife radiosurgery for mesial temporal lobe epilepsy: a prospective multicenter study. *Epilepsia* 2011; **52(5)**:909–916.

67 Braakman HM, Vaessen MJ, Hofman PA et al.: Cognitive and behavioral complications of frontal lobe epilepsy in children: a review of the literature. *Epilepsia* 2011; **52(5)**:849–856.

68 Exner C, Boucsein K, Lange C et al.: Neuropsychological performance in frontal lobe epilepsy. *Seizure* 2002; **11(1)**:20–32.

69 Patrikelis P, Angelakis E, Gatzonis S: Neurocognitive and behavioral functioning in frontal lobe epilepsy: a review. *Epilepsy Behav* 2009; **14(1)**:19–26.

70 Risse GL: Cognitive outcomes in patients with frontal lobe epilepsy. *Epilepsia* 2006; **47(Suppl. 2)**:87–89.

71 McDonald CR, Delis DC, Norman MA et al.: Discriminating patients with frontal-lobe epilepsy and temporal-lobe epilepsy: utility of a multilevel design fluency test. *Neuropsychology* 2005; **19(6)**:806–813.

72 McDonald CR, Delis DC, Norman MA et al.: Is impairment in set-shifting specific to frontal-lobe dysfunction? Evidence from patients with frontal-lobe or temporal-lobe epilepsy. *J Int Neuropsychol Soc* 2005; **11(4)**:477–481.

73 McDonald CR, Swartz BE, Halgren E et al.: The relationship of regional frontal hypometabolism to executive function: a resting fluoro-deoxyglucose PET study of patients with epilepsy and healthy controls. *Epilepsy Behav* 2006; **9(1)**:58–67.

74 Braakman HM, Vaessen MJ, Jansen JF et al.: Frontal lobe connectivity and cognitive impairment in pediatric frontal lobe epilepsy. *Epilepsia* 2013; **54(3)**:446–454.

75 Centeno M, Thompson PJ, Koepp MJ et al.: Memory in frontal lobe epilepsy. *Epilepsy Res* 2010; **91(2–3)**:123–132.

76 Centeno M, Vollmar C, O'Muircheartaigh J et al.: Memory in frontal lobe epilepsy: an fMRI study. *Epilepsia* 2012; **53(10)**:1756–1764.

77 Dulay MF, Busch RM, Chapin JS et al.: Executive functioning and depressed mood before and after unilateral frontal lobe resection for intractable epilepsy. *Neuropsychologia* 2013; **51(7)**:1370–1376.

78 Bilo L, Santangelo G, Improta I et al.: Neuropsychological profile of adult patients with nonsymptomatic occipital lobe epilepsies. *J Neurol* 2013; **260(2)**:445–453.

79 Gülgönen S, Demirbilek V, Korkmaz B et al.: Neuropsychological functions in idiopathic occipital lobe epilepsy. *Epilepsia* 2000; **41(4)**:405–411.

80 Germanò E, Gagliano A, Magazù A et al.: Benign childhood epilepsy with occipital paroxysms: neuropsychological findings. *Epilepsy Res* 2005; **64(3)**:137–150.

81 Vlooswijk MC, Jansen JF, Jeukens CR et al.: Memory processes and prefrontal network dysfunction in cryptogenic epilepsy. *Epilepsia* 2011; **52(8)**:1467–1475.

82 Widjaja E, Skocic J, Go C et al.: Abnormal white matter correlates with neuropsychological impairment in children with localization-related epilepsy. *Epilepsia* 2013; **54(6)**:1065–1073.

83 Vlooswijk MC, Jansen JF, Majoie HJ et al.: Functional connectivity and language impairment in cryptogenic localization-related epilepsy. *Neurology* 2010; **75(5)**:395–402.

84 Vinţan MA, Palade S, Cristea A et al.: A neuropsychological assessment, using computerized battery tests (CANTAB), in children with benign rolandic epilepsy before AED therapy. *J Med Life* 2012; **5(1)**:114–119.

85 Staden U, Isaacs E, Boyd SG et al.: Language dysfunction in children with Rolandic epilepsy. *Neuropediatrics* 1998; **29(5)**:242–248.

86 Goldberg-Stern H, Gonen OM, Sadeh M et al.: Neuropsychological aspects of benign childhood epilepsy with centrotemporal spikes. *Seizure* 2010; **19(1)**:12–16.

87 Deltour L, Quaglino V, Barathon M et al.: Clinical evaluation of attentional processes in children with benign childhood epilepsy with centrotemporal spikes (BCECTS). *Epileptic Disord* 2007; **9(4)**:424–431.

88 Datta AN, Oser N, Bauder F et al.: Cognitive impairment and cortical reorganization in children with benign epilepsy with centrotemporal spikes. *Epilepsia* 2013; **54(3)**:487–494.

89 Jeong MH, Yum MS, Ko TS et al.: Neuropsychological status of children with newly diagnosed idiopathic childhood epilepsy. *Brain Dev* 2011; **33(8)**:666–671.

90 Northcott E, Connolly AM, Berroya A et al.: The neuropsychological and language profile of children with benign rolandic epilepsy. *Epilepsia* 2005; **46(6)**:924–930.

91 Danielsson J, Petermann F: Cognitive deficits in children with benign rolandic epilepsy of childhood or rolandic discharges: a study of children between 4 and 7 years of age with and without seizures compared with healthy controls. *Epilepsy Behav* 2009; **16(4)**:646–651.

92 Northcott E, Connolly AM, McIntyre J et al.: Longitudinal assessment of neuropsychologic and language function in children with benign rolandic epilepsy. *J Child Neurol* 2006; **21(6)**:518–522.

93 Ay Y, Gokben S, Serdaroglu G et al.: Neuropsychologic impairment in children with rolandic epilepsy. *Pediatr Neurol* 2009; **41(5)**:359–363.

94 Neri ML, Guimarães CA, Oliveira EP et al.: Neuropsychological assessment of children with rolandic epilepsy: executive functions. *Epilepsy Behav* 2012; **24(4)**:403–407.

95 Yung AW, Park YD, Cohen MJ, Garrison TN: Cognitive and behavioral problems in children with centrotemporal spikes. *Pediatr Neurol* 2000; **23(5)**:391–395.

96 Northcott E, Connolly AM, McIntyre J et al.: Longitudinal assessment of neuropsychologic and language function in children with benign rolandic epilepsy. *J Child Neurol* 2006; **21(6)**:518–522.

97 Verrotti A, D'Egidio C, Agostinelli S et al.: Cognitive and linguistic abnormalities in benign childhood epilepsy with centrotemporal spikes. *Acta Paediatr* 2011; **100(5)**:768–772.

98 Tovia E, Goldberg-Stern H, Ben Zeev B et al.: The prevalence of atypical presentations and comorbidities of benign childhood epilepsy with centrotemporal spikes. *Epilepsia* 2011; **52(8)**:1483–1488.

99 Smith AB, Kavros PM, Clarke T et al.: A neurocognitive endophenotype associated with rolandic epilepsy. *Epilepsia* 2012; **53(4)**:705–711.

100 Verrotti A, Matricardi S, Di Giacomo DL et al.: Neuropsychological impairment in children with Rolandic epilepsy and in their siblings. *Epilepsy Behav* 2013; **28(1)**:108–112.

101 Lin JJ, Riley JD, Hsu DA et al.: Striatal hypertrophy and its cognitive effects in new-onset benign epilepsy with centrotemporal spikes. *Epilepsia* 2012; **53(4)**:677–685.

102 Wandschneider B, Thompson PJ, Vollmar C, Koepp MJ: Frontal lobe function and structure in juvenile myoclonic epilepsy: a comprehensive review of neuropsychological and imaging data. *Epilepsia* 2012; **53(12)**:2091–2098.

103 Pascalicchio TF, de Araujo Filho GM, da Silva Noffs MH et al.: Neuropsychological profile of patients with juvenile myoclonic epilepsy: a controlled study of 50 patients. *Epilepsy Behav* 2007; **10(2)**:263–267.

104 Sonmez F, Atakli D, Sari H et al.: Cognitive function in juvenile myoclonic epilepsy. *Epilepsy Behav* 2004; **5(3)**: 329–336.

105 Moschetta SP, Valente KD: Juvenile myoclonic epilepsy: the impact of clinical variables and psychiatric disorders on executive profile assessed with a comprehensive neuropsychological battery. *Epilepsy Behav* 2012; **25(4)**:682–686.

106 Iqbal N, Caswell HL, Hare DJ et al.: Neuropsychological profiles of patients with juvenile myoclonic epilepsy and their siblings: a preliminary controlled experimental video-EEG case series. *Epilepsy Behav* 2009; **14(3)**:516–521.

107 Wandschneider B, Centeno M, Vollmar C et al.: Risk-taking behavior in juvenile myoclonic epilepsy. *Epilepsia* 2013; **54(12)**:2158–2165.

108 Wandschneider B, Kopp UA, Kliegel M et al.: Prospective memory in patients with juvenile myoclonic epilepsy and their healthy siblings. *Neurology* 2010; **75(24)**:2161–2167.

109 Lin K, de Araujo Filho GM, Pascalicchio TF et al.: Hippocampal atrophy and memory dysfunction in patients with juvenile myoclonic epilepsy. *Epilepsy Behav* 2013; **29(1)**:247–251.

110 Vollmar C, O'Muircheartaigh J, Symms MR et al.: Altered microstructural connectivity in juvenile myoclonic epilepsy: the missing link. *Neurology* 2012; **78(20)**: 1555–1559.

111 Vollmar C, O'Muircheartaigh J, Barker GJ et al.: Motor system hyperconnectivity in juvenile myoclonic epilepsy: a cognitive functional magnetic resonance imaging study. *Brain* 2011; **134(Pt 6)**:1710–1719.

112 Fastenau PS, Johnson CS, Perkins SM et al.: Neuropsychological status at seizure onset in children: risk factors for early cognitive deficits. *Neurology* 2009; **73(7)**:526–534.

113 Henkin Y, Sadeh M, Kivity S et al.: Cognitive function in idiopathic generalized epilepsy of childhood. *Dev Med Child Neurol* 2005; **47(2)**:126–132.

114 Pavone P, Bianchini R, Trifiletti RR et al.: Neuropsychological assessment in children with absence epilepsy. *Neurology* 2001; **56(8)**:1047–1051.

115 Masur D, Shinnar S, Cnaan A et al.: Pretreatment cognitive deficits and treatment effects on attention in childhood absence epilepsy. *Neurology* 2013; **81(18)**:1572–1580.

116 Dlugos D, Shinnar S, Cnaan A et al.: Pretreatment EEG in childhood absence epilepsy: associations with attention and treatment outcome. *Neurology* 2013; **81(2)**:150–156.

117 Caplan R, Siddarth P, Stahl L et al.: Childhood absence epilepsy: behavioral, cognitive, and linguistic comorbidities. *Epilepsia* 2008; **49(11)**:1838–1846.

118 Vega C, Vestal M, DeSalvo M et al.: Differentiation of attention-related problems in childhood absence epilepsy. *Epilepsy Behav* 2010; **19(1)**:82–85.

119 Cerminara C, D'Agati E, Casarelli L et al.: Attention impairment in childhood absence epilepsy: an impulsivity problem? *Epilepsy Behav* 2013; **27(2)**:337–341.

120 Hermann BP, Jones JE, Sheth R et al.: Growing up with epilepsy: a two-year investigation of cognitive development in children with new onset epilepsy. *Epilepsia* 2008; **49(11)**:1847–1858.

121 Caplan R, Levitt J, Siddarth P et al.: Frontal and temporal volumes in childhood absence epilepsy. *Epilepsia* 2009; **50(11)**:2466–2472.

122 Aarts JH, Binnie CD, Smit AM, Wilkins AJ: Selective cognitive impairment during focal and generalized epileptiform EEG activity. *Brain* 1984; **107(Pt 1)**:293–308.

123 Binnie CD, Marston D: Cognitive correlates of interictal discharges. *Epilepsia* 1992; **33(Suppl. 6)**:S11–S17.

124 Holmes GL: EEG abnormalities as a biomarker for cognitive comorbidities in pharmacoresistant epilepsy. *Epilepsia* 2013; **54(Suppl. 2)**:60–62.

125 Lv Y, Wang Z, Cui L et al.: Cognitive correlates of interictal epileptiform discharges in adult patients with epilepsy in China. *Epilepsy Behav* 2013; **29(1)**:205–210.

126 Ebus S, Arends J, Hendriksen J et al.: Cognitive effects of interictal epileptiform discharges in children. *Eur J Paediatr Neurol* 2012; **16(6)**:697–706.

127 Kleen JK, Scott RC, Holmes GL, Lenck-Santini PP: Hippocampal interictal spikes disrupt cognition in rats. *Ann Neurol* 2010; **67(2)**:250–257.

128 Kleen JK, Scott RC, Holmes GL et al.: Hippocampal interictal epileptiform activity disrupts cognition in humans. *Neurology* 2013; **81(1)**:18–24.

129 Matsumoto JY, Stead M, Kucewicz MT et al.: Network oscillations modulate interictal epileptiform spike rate during human memory. *Brain* 2013; **136(Pt 8)**: 2444–2456.

130 Zeman AZ, Boniface SJ, Hodges JR: Transient epileptic amnesia: a description of the clinical and neuropsychological features in 10 cases and a review of the literature. *J Neurol Neurosurg Psychiatry* 1998; **64(4)**:435–443.

131 Butler CR, Graham KS, Hodges JR et al.: The syndrome of transient epileptic amnesia. *Ann Neurol* 2007; **61(6)**: 587–598.

132 Butler CR, Zeman AZ: Recent insights into the impairment of memory in epilepsy: transient epileptic amnesia, accelerated long-term forgetting and remote memory impairment. *Brain* 2008; **131(Pt 9)**:2243–2263.

133 Zeman A, Butler C, Muhlert N, Milton F: Novel forms of forgetting in temporal lobe epilepsy. *Epilepsy Behav* 2013; **26(3)**:335–342.

134 Hoefeijzers S, Dewar M, Della Sala S et al.: Accelerated long-term forgetting in transient epileptic amnesia: an acquisition or consolidation deficit? *Neuropsychologia* 2013; **51(8)**:1549–1555.

135 McAuley JW, Elliott JO, Patankar S et al.: Comparing patients' and practitioners' views on epilepsy concerns: a call to address memory concerns. *Epilepsy Behav* 2010; **19(4)**:580–583.

136 Chapieski L, Evankovich K, Hiscock M, Collins R: Everyday verbal memory and pediatric epilepsy. *Epilepsy Behav* 2011; **21(3)**:285–290.

137 Giovagnoli AR: Awareness, overestimation, and underestimation of cognitive functions in epilepsy. *Epilepsy Behav* 2013; **26(1)**:75–80.

138 Vermeulen J, Aldenkamp AP, Alpherts WC: Memory complaints in epilepsy: correlations with cognitive performance and neuroticism. *Epilepsy Res* 1993; **15(2)**:157–170.

139 Elixhauser A, Leidy NK, Meador K et al.: The relationship between memory performance, perceived cognitive function, and mood in patients with epilepsy. *Epilepsy Res* 1999; **37(1)**:13–24.

140 Hall KE, Isaac CL, Harris P: Memory complaints in epilepsy: an accurate reflection of memory impairment or an indicator of poor adjustment? A review of the literature. *Clin Psychol Rev* 2009; **29(4)**:354–367.

141 Baxendale S, Thompson P: Beyond localization: the role of traditional neuropsychological tests in an age of imaging. *Epilepsia* 2010; **51(11)**:2225–2230.

142 Phabphal K, Kanjanasatien J: Montreal Cognitive Assessment in cryptogenic epilepsy patients with normal Mini-Mental State Examination scores. *Epileptic Disord* 2011; **13(4)**:375–381.

143 Witt JA, Alpherts W, Helmstaedter C: Computerized neuropsychological testing in epilepsy: overview of available tools. *Seizure* 2013; **22(6)**:416–423.

144 Walterfang M, Choi Y, O'Brien TJ et al.: Utility and validity of a brief cognitive assessment tool in patients with epileptic and nonepileptic seizures. *Epilepsy Behav* 2011; **21(2)**:177–183.

145 Kurzbuch K, Pauli E, Gaál L et al.: Computerized cognitive testing in epilepsy (CCTE): a new method for cognitive screening. *Seizure* 2013; **22(6)**:424–432.

146 Lutz MT, Helmstaedter C: EpiTrack: tracking cognitive side effects of medication on attention and executive functions in patients with epilepsy. *Epilepsy Behav* 2005; **7(4)**: 708–714.

147 Kadish NE, Baumann M, Pietz J et al.: Validation of a screening tool for attention and executive functions (EpiTrack Junior) in children and adolescents with absence epilepsy. *Epilepsy Behav* 2013; **29(1)**:96–102.

148 MacAllister WS, Bender HA, Whitman L et al.: Assessment of executive functioning in childhood epilepsy: the Tower of London and BRIEF. *Child Neuropsychol* 2012; **18(4)**: 404–415.

149 Rogers SL, Farlow MR, Doody RS et al.: A 24-week, double-blind, placebo-controlled trial of donepezil in patients with Alzheimer's disease. *Neurology* 1998; **50**: 136–145.

150 Noebels J: A perfect storm: converging paths of epilepsy and Alzheimer's dementia intersect in the hippocampal formation. *Epilepsia* 2011; **52(Suppl. 1)**:39–46.

151 Fisher RS, Bortz JJ, Blum DE et al.: A pilot study of donepezil for memory problems in epilepsy. *Epilepsy Behav* 2001; **2**:330–334.

152 Hamberger MJ, Palmese CA, Scarmeas N et al.: A randomized double-blind, placebo-controlled trial of donepezil to improve memory in epilepsy. *Epilepsia* 2007; **48**:1283–1291.

153 Griffith HR, Martin R, Andrews S et al.: The safety and tolerability of galantamine in patients with epilepsy and memory difficulties. *Epilepsy Behav* 2008; **13**:376–380.

154 Cramer JA: Exploration of changes in health-related quality of life after 3 months of vagus nerve stimulation. *Epilepsy Behav* 2001; **2**:460–465.

155 Ghacibeh GA, Shenker JI, Shenal B et al.: The influence of vagus nerve stimulation on memory. *Cogn Behav Neurol* 2006; **19**:119–122.

156 Clark KB, Naritoku DK, Smith DC et al.: Enhanced recognition memory following vagus nerve stimulation in human subjects. *Nat Neurosci* 1999; **2**:94–98.

157 Martin CO, Denburg NL, Tranel D et al.: The effects of vagus nerve stimulation on decision-making. *Cortex* 2004; **40(4–5)**:605–612.

158 Helmstaedter C, Hoppe C, Elger CE: Memory alterations during acute high-intensity vagus nerve stimulation. *Epilepsy Res* 2001; **47**:37–42.

159 Hoppe C, Helmstaedter C, Scherrmann J, Elger CE: No evidence for cognitive side effects after 6 months of vagus nerve stimulation in epilepsy patients. *Epilepsy Behav* 2001; **2**:351–356.

160 McGlone J, Valdivia I, Penner M et al.: Quality of life and memory after vagus nerve stimulator implantation for epilepsy. *Can J Neurol Sci* 2008; **35**:287–296.

161 Sackeim HA, Keilp JG, Rush AJ et al.: The effects of vagus nerve stimulation on cognitive performance in patients with treatment-resistant depression. *Neuropsychiatry Neuropsychol Behav Neurol* 2001; **14(1)**:53–62.

162 Morrell MJ: Responsive cortical stimulation for the treatment of medically intractable partial epilepsy. *Neurology* 2011; **77**:1295–1304.

163 Fisher R, Salanova V, Witt T et al.: Electrical stimulation of the anterior nucleus of thalamus for treatment of refractory epilepsy. *Epilepsia* 2010; **51**:899–908.

164 Oh YS, Kim HJ, Lee KJ et al.: Cognitive improvement after long-term electrical stimulation of bilateral anterior thalamic nucleus in refractory epilepsy patients. *Seizure* 2012; **21**:183–187.

165 McLachlan RS, Pigott S, Tellez-Zenteno JF et al.: Bilateral hippocampal stimulation for intractable temporal lobe epilepsy: impact on seizures and memory. *Epilepsia* 2010; **51(2)**:304–307.

166 Koubeissi MZ, Kahriman E, Syed TU et al.: Low-frequency electrical stimulation of a fiber tract in temporal lobe epilepsy. *Ann Neurol* 2013; **74(2)**:223–231.

167 Suthana N, Haneef Z, Stern J et al.: Memory enhancement and deep-brain stimulation of the entorhinal area. *N Engl J Med* 2012; **366**:502–510.

168 Jacobs J, Lega B, Anderson C: Explaining how brain stimulation can evoke memories. *J Cogn Neurosci* 2012; **24(3)**:553–563.

169 Fregni F, Otachi PTM, Valle A et al.: A randomized clinical trial of repetitive transcranial magnetic stimulation in patients with refractory epilepsy. *Ann Neurol* 2006; **60**: 447–455.

170 Ponds R, Hendriks M: Cognitive rehabilitation of memory problems in patients with epilepsy. *Seizure* 2006; **15**: 267–273.

171 Koorenhof L, Baxendale S, Smith N, Thompson P: Memory rehabilitation and brain training for surgical temporal lobe epilepsy patients: a preliminary report. *Seizure* 2012; **21**:178–182.

172 Bresson C, Lespinet-Najib V, Rougier A et al.: Verbal memory compensation: application to left and right temporal lobe epileptic patients. *Brain Lang* 2007; **102**:13–21.

173 Helmstaedter C, Loer B, Wohlfahrt R et al.: The effects of cognitive rehabilitation on memory outcome after temporal lobe epilepsy surgery. *Epilepsy Behav* 2008; **12(3)**: 402–409.

174 Radford K, Lah S, Thayer Z, Miller LA: Effective group-based memory training for patients with epilepsy. *Epilepsy Behav* 2011; **22**:272–278.

175 Engelberts NHJ, Klein M, Adèr HJ et al.: The effectiveness of cognitive rehabilitation for attention deficits in focal seizures: a randomized controlled study. *Epilepsia* 2002; **43**:587–595.

Attention deficit/hyperactivity disorder, disordered attention, and epilepsy

Introduction

The goal of this section is to review the deficits in attention and the frequency, etiology, and treatment of ADHD in patients with epilepsy. Our discussion will concentrate on ADHD in children and adolescents with epilepsy. It seems reasonable to expect that adults with epilepsy also have an increased risk of ADHD but adequate data are not yet available. We will consider attention as a global, dimensional, neuropsychological construct that can be measured over a population. Scores on measures of attention for the individual can be compared with normative data to allow a determination of relative degree of severity or impairment. ADHD will be considered a categorical diagnosis that is determined by specific criteria such as those found in the Diagnostic and Statistical Manual of Mental Disorders Fifth Edition (DSM-5) [1].

"Attention" is a general term and refers to several different processes involving complex networks in the CNS. The prefrontal cortex is actively involved in shifting focus, divided attention, sustained attention, and inhibition of distracting stimuli. Alerting, vigilance, and sustained attention also require the frontoparietal pathways, thalamus, and cerebellum; orienting in time and space involves the parietal cortex; and both divided and selective attention involve the anterior cingulate gyrus. Dopamine and norepinephrine are the neurotransmitters found most widely in the attention networks (see [2] for a review of attention networks).

The type and degree of attention impairment varies by seizure type. BECTS has been studied extensively, with two reviews finding impairment in sustained, divided, and selective attention [3,4]. Cerminara et al. [5] found impairment in selective and divided attention and in some measures of alertness but no deficits in vigilance. Deficits in sustained attention were found in patients with complex partial epilepsy but selective and divided attention were less consistently affected [3]. In patients with generalized seizures, Tian et al. [6] found deficits in executive control and reaction time but no deficits in alerting or orienting.

Prevalence

Estimates of prevalence of ADHD in samples with epilepsy vary widely depending on the definition used and the sample studied. Some reports use dimensional measures of attention such as the Child Behavior Checklist. Others use a categorical measure of ADHD based on ADHD-specific measures, global structured interviews, or interviews utilizing DSM criteria. The one study that used both dimensional and categorical measures to assess a sample of children with epilepsy found evidence of ADHD in 31% utilizing the Child Behavior Checklist, a dimensional measure, and a probable diagnosis of ADHD in 37% using the Child or Adolescent Symptom Inventories, categorical measures [7].

Studies of prevalence have been population-based or have used convenience samples from clinics. The clinical samples have assessed children with new-onset seizures, all children with epilepsy seen in the clinic, or subsamples of children with specific syndromes or varying degrees of severity.

Four recent population-based studies have found an increased risk of ADHD in children and adolescents with epilepsy. Davies et al. [8] found symptoms of ADHD in 12% of children with complicated epilepsy, compared to 2% of children with diabetes and healthy controls, but did not find symptoms in children with epilepsy only. Turky et al. [9] noted ADHD symptoms in 44% (odds ratio (OR) 9.4) of children with epilepsy and two studies from Norway found significantly more symptoms of ADHD in children and adolescents with epilepsy than in children without seizures [10,11].

Studies that use unstructured or broad-based questionnaires that do not utilize criteria from the DSM-IV [1] find higher prevalence figures than do studies using categorical measures. In the noncategorical studies, prevalence figures range from 8 to 77%, with most in the 20–60% range. The highest prevalence figure is found in children with intractable epilepsy, while the lower figures use very restrictive criteria (see [12] for a review of studies).

Surveys of teachers of children with epilepsy have found substantial numbers of children with symptoms of ADHD. Holdsworth and Whitmore [13] described symptoms of ADHD in 42% of the children with epilepsy they studied and Sturniolo and Galletti [14] in 58%. In a prospective study of teachers' ratings of behavior in children with epilepsy, attention problems were found in 21 and 19% of children with recurring seizures at baseline and at 24 months, respectively, and in 11 and 13% of children with single seizures at baseline and 24 months [15].

Several studies have used DSM criteria to assess the prevalence of ADHD in children with epilepsy, giving a range of prevalence of 10–40% [16–24], with one study of children with severe epilepsy reporting a prevalence of 71% [25]. In contrast to clinical studies of children with ADHD and no epilepsy, which find more ADHD, combined type than ADHD, predominantly inattentive type, studies in children and adolescents with epilepsy more often find more ADHD, inattentive type than ADHD, combined type [18,23,25]. The one recent exception was a study by Gonzalez-Heydrich et al. [26], which reported ADHD, combined type in 58% of participants and ADHD, inattentive type in 42%.

Children with ADHD frequently have other comorbid behavioral difficulties and cognitive problems. A small cross-sectional study of 36 children with ADHD and epilepsy noted a comorbid anxiety disorder in 36% and oppositional defiant disorder (ODD) in 31%, similar to the frequency of comorbidity in children with ADHD without seizures [26]. In contrast, Hermann et al. [23] found more ODD but no increased risk for anxiety, depression, tic disorders, or psychosis in children with epilepsy and ADHD compared to children with epilepsy alone. The most consistent comorbidity has been cognitive problems. In a study of children of 8–15 years of age with a diagnosis of epilepsy, Fastenau et al. [27] showed that ADHD was a risk factor for reading and math learning disorder. Hermann et al. [28], in a 2-year longitudinal study, found that children with epilepsy and no ADHD did not differ from controls in cognitive function, whereas children with epilepsy and ADHD started lower than controls and remained lower at 2 years in all measures of cognitive function.

Etiology

Problems with attention or ADHD might represent true comorbidity of epilepsy and ADHD of genetic origin or, more likely, a secondary or syndromic form of ADHD. We have suggested that there are significant differences between the ADHD seen in patients with epilepsy and

the ADHD apparently resulting from familial or genetic influence [29]. In the familial forms of ADHD there is a gender difference, with more males affected, a difference not found in samples of patients with ADHD and epilepsy. ADHD, combined type, with both inattention and hyperactivity/impulsivity, is more common in familial ADHD, but in patients with epilepsy and ADHD there seems to be more ADHD, predominantly inattentive type. Finally, familial ADHD responds well to stimulant medication, with effect sizes of 0.90–0.95 [30], whereas the response to stimulants is less robust in patients with epilepsy and ADHD [17].

The symptoms of ADHD in patients with epilepsy may result from both CNS damage and epilepsy, the effects of seizures, or epilepsy treatment. CNS damage is a likely risk factor. The prevalence of symptoms of ADHD is higher in children with complicated epilepsy and those with the most severe seizure disorders [8,25]. Symptoms of ADHD are more often found in children with recurrent seizures than in those with single seizures [15] and are more common in those with persistent seizures than in siblings or children whose seizures are in remission [21]. Additional support for considering a possible role of seizure activity comes from Aldenkamp and Arends [31], who found that frequent nonconvulsive seizures were associated with cognitive impairment. With the exception of the epileptic encephalopathies, seizure type and seizure syndrome do not seem to predict symptoms of ADHD [18,23,32]. Symptoms of ADHD are often found in children with absence seizures [33] and in patients with FLE [34]. Symptoms of ADHD are common in the active phase of benign childhood epilepsy with centrotemporal spikes but resolve with the disappearance of the spikes [4]. Treatment is an additional risk factor. Problems with attention and hyperactive behavior are associated with barbiturates and benzodiazepines. Valproic acid has been found to impair attention more than ethosuximide or lamotrigine [33]. Of the newer AEDs, topiramate has been associated with trouble concentrating and other cognitive disturbances [35]. Inattention is more often seen with polypharmacy than monotherapy [20].

Symptoms of ADHD may be present prior to the onset of seizures, suggesting it is a common CNS problem that causes epilepsy and inattention. In a population-based study, ADHD, predominantly inattentive type was significantly more common in children who subsequently developed seizures than in controls [36]. Two additional population-based studies found that children with ADHD had more than twice the risk of epilepsy than controls [37,38]. Austin et al. [39] retrospectively assessed behavior in children with new-onset seizures. They found that 10.7% had symptoms of ADHD in the 6 months prior to first recognized seizure, compared to 3.0% of siblings. They also noted that symptoms of ADHD were more common in children with probable prior unrecognized seizures than in those with apparent true first seizures, suggesting that both CNS dysfunction and seizure activity may contribute to symptoms of ADHD.

Treatment

Evaluation of symptoms of ADHD in patients with epilepsy should start with reassessment of seizure control and AEDs and with an assessment for other possible explanations for inattention and hyperactivity. Improvement in control of seizures may reduce symptoms. Nocturnal seizures can disrupt sleep, leading to inattention during the daytime. Changes in concentration or emergence of hyperactivity after the addition of an AED should prompt consideration of changing the AED. Carbamazepine, oxcarbazepine, lamotrigine, and levetiracetam do not seem to impair attention or other frontal-lobe functions and might be first-choice agents for the child with epilepsy and ADHD [40]. The differential diagnosis includes learning disorders, anxiety, and depression. ADHD and learning disorders are often comorbid but learning disorders may occur in approximately 50% of children with epilepsy and are not always associated with ADHD [27]. Anxiety and depression are associated with epilepsy [7]. The excessive worrying of the child with anxiety may resemble inattention and the restlessness may mimic hyperactivity. Impairment in concentration is a core symptom of depression. Both children and adolescents, and their parents, should be asked about symptoms of anxiety and depression.

If seizures or AEDs do not seem to be causing symptoms of ADHD, medication trials should be considered. The stimulants methylphenidate and amphetamines, atomoxetine, and the extended-release formulations guanfacine and clonidine are approved for the treatment of ADHD. They are also the agents most often used to treat ADHD in patients with epilepsy and ADHD.

Methylphenidate has the most data supporting its efficacy and safety in children with epilepsy and ADHD. Open-label series have shown that children with controlled seizures do not have breakthrough seizures with the addition of methylphenidate [41,42]. Even in samples of children with persistent seizures, there seems to be an equal number of children whose seizures improve and children whose seizures increase in frequency during methylphenidate treatment. Two recent open-label studies have shown that methylphenidate in doses of 0.5–1.0 mg/kg can be used safely without loss of seizure control and with improvement in symptoms of ADHD in 60–70% of children with severe seizures [43,44]. A recent double-blind placebo-controlled crossover trial assessed the efficacy and safety of OROS methylphenidate in children with epilepsy and ADHD [45]. The trial was brief, with each dose (18, 36, or 54 mg) given for 1 week. OROS methylphenidate was more effective than placebo at all doses. Although the trial was too short for an adequate assessment of change in seizure frequency, there seemed to be an increased risk of seizures with increasing dose of OROS methylphenidate.

The data for amphetamines are much more limited. In a retrospective review, Gonzalez-Heydrich et al. [46] found that amphetamines were less effective than methylphenidate. Illicit use of amphetamines has resulted in seizures, often associated with sleep deprivation and additional risk factors for epilepsy [47].

Atomoxetine has been approved for treatment of ADHD in children, adolescents, and adults. Two open-label trials found atomoxetine helpful in some children with epilepsy [48,49]. Torres et al. [49], in a retrospective review of children and adolescents with epilepsy and ADHD that were treated with atomoxetine, found that 37% had an apparent positive response to atomoxetine, 26% discontinued atomoxetine because of inadequate response, and 26% discontinued because of increasing irritability. Wernicke et al. [50] examined two large databases and did not find an increased risk of seizures in patients treated with atomoxetine for ADHD.

Extended-release formulations of clonidine and guanfacine have been approved by the FDA for the treatment of ADHD. A meta-analysis found evidence for the efficacy of both medications as monotherapy and as add-on to stimulants. Sedation and fatigue were common side effects and bradycardia, hypotension, and QTc prolongation were noted [51]. Trials are not available for use in children with epilepsy and ADHD but these agents should be used cautiously in patients on sedative AEDs.

Although other agents have been used to treat ADHD, most have either minimal data in patients with epilepsy or potential side effects limiting their use [52]. Bupropion and the tricyclic antidepressants are effective in treatment of ADHD but can lower seizure threshold. Modafinil, although not approved for use in ADHD, may reduce symptoms of ADHD and improve alertness. There are no trials of modafinil in patients with epilepsy.

Behavioral therapy is an effective treatment of ADHD (although its effect size is typically less than that for medication management) [53] and behavior and environmental modification strategies are commonly used in the clinical and educational settings to manage ADHD symptoms comorbid with epilepsy [54]. Behavior therapy can be combined with medication management in cases where medication has incomplete or limited efficacy. However, there have been no large-scale clinical trials to investigate the efficacy of behavioral therapy specifically in samples of children with comorbid ADHD and epilepsy.

References

1 American Psychiatric Association: *Diagnostic and Statistical Manual of Mental Disorders*, 5 edn. American Psychiatric Association, Arlington, VA, 2013.

2 Bush G: Attention-deficit/hyperactivity disorder and attention networks. *Neuropharmacol Rev* 2010; **35**:278–300.

3 Sánchez-Carpintero R, Neville BGR: Attentional ability in children with epilepsy. *Epilepsia* 2003; **44**:1340–1349.

4 Kavros PM, Clarke T, Strug LJ et al.: Attention impairment in rolandic epilepsy: systematic review. *Epilepsia* 2008; **49**:1570–1580.

5 Cerminara C, D'Agati E, Lange KW et al.: Benign childhood epilepsy with centrotemporal spikes and the multicomponent model of attention: a matched control study. *Epilepsy Behav* 2010; **19**:69–77.

6 Tian Y, Dong B, Ma J et al.: Attention networks in children with idiopathic generalized epilepsy. *Epilepsy Behav* 2010; **19**:513–517.

7 Dunn DW, Austin JK, Perkins SM: Prevalence of psychopathology in children with epilepsy: categorical and dimensional measures. *Dev Med Child Neurol* 2009; **51**: 364–372.

8 Davies S, Heyman I, Goodman R: A population survey of mental health problems in children with epilepsy. *Dev Med Child Neurol* 2003; **45**:918–923.

9 Turky A, Beavis JM, Thapar AK, Kerr MP: Psychopathology in children and adolescents with epilepsy: an investigation of predictive variables. *Epilepsy Behav* 2008; **12**:136–144.

10 Lossius MI, Clench-Aas J, van Roy B et al.: Psychiatric symptoms in adolescents with epilepsy in junior high school in Norway: a population survey. *Epilepsy Behav* 2006; **9**:286–292.

11 Alfstad KÅ, Clench-Aas J, Van Roy B et al.: Psychiatric symptoms in Norwegian children with epilepsy aged 8–13 years: effects of age and gender? *Epilepsia* 2011; **52(7)**:1231–1238.

12 Dunn DW, Kronenberger WG: Attention-deficit hyperactivity disorder, attention problems, and epilepsy. In: Ettinger AB, Kanner AM (eds): *Psychiatric Issues in Epilepsy: A Practical Guide to Diagnosis and Treatment*, 2 edn. Lippincott Williams & Wilkins: Philadelphia, PA, 2007, pp. 272–285.

13 Holdsworth L, Whitmore K: A study of children with epilepsy attending ordinary schools. I: Their seizure patterns, progress and behaviour in school. *Dev Med Child Neurol* 1974; **16**:746–758.

14 Sturniolo MG, Galletti F: Idiopathic epilepsy and school achievement. *Arch Dis Child* 1994; **38**:424–428.

15 Dunn DW, Austin JK, Caffrey HM, Perkins SM: AS prospective study of teachers' ratings of behavior problems in children with new-onset seizures. *Epilepsy Behav* 2003; **4**:26–35.

16 Williams J, Griebel ML, Dykman RA: Neuropsychological patterns in pediatric epilepsy. *Seizure* 1998; **7**:223–228.

17 Semrud-Clikeman M, Wical B: Components of attention in children with complex partial seizures with and without ADHD. *Epilepsia* 1999; **40**:211–215.

18 Dunn DW, Austin JK, Harezlak J, Ambrosius WT: ADHD and epilepsy in childhood. *Dev Med Child Neurol* 2003; **45**:50–54.

19 Thome-Souza S, Kucynski E, Assumpção F et al.: Which factors may play a pivotal role on determining the type of psychiatric disorder in children and adolescents with epilepsy? *Epilepsy Behav* 2004; **5**:988–994.

20 Freilinger M, Reisel B, Reiter E et al.: Behavioral and emotional problems in children with epilepsy. *J Child Neurol* 2006; **21**:939–945.

21 Berg AT, Vickery BG, Testa FM et al.: Behavior and social competency in idiopathic and cryptogenic childhood epilepsy. *Dev Med Child Neurol* 2007; **49**:487–492.

22 Hanssen-Bauer K, Heyerdahl S, Eriksson A-S: Mental health problems in children and adolescents referred to a national epilepsy center. *Epilepsy Behav* 2007; **10**:255–262.

23 Hermann BP, Jones J, Dabbs K et al.: The frequency, complications and aetiology of ADHD in new onset paediatric epilepsy. *Brain* 2007; **130**:3135–3148.

24 Caplan R, Siddarth P, Stahl L et al.: Childhood absence epilepsy: behavioral, cognitive, and linguistic comorbidities. *Epilepsia* 2008; **49**:1838–1846.

25 Sherman EMS, Slick DJ, Connolly MB, Eyrl KL: ADHD, neurological correlates and health-related quality of life in severe pediatric epilepsy. *Epilepsia* 2007; **48**:1083–1091.

26 Gonzalez-Heydrich J, Dodds A, Whitney J et al.: Psychiatric disorders and behavioral characteristics of pediatric patients with both epilepsy and attention-deficit hyperactivity disorder. *Epilepsy Behav* 2007; **10**:384–388.

27 Fastenau PS, Shen J, Dunn DW, Austin JK: Academic underachievement among children with epilepsy: proportion exceeding psychometric criteria for learning disability and associated risk factors. *J Learn Disabil* 2008; **41**:195–207.

28 Hermann BP, Jones JE, Sheth R et al.: Growing up with epilepsy: a two-year investigation of cognitive development in children with new onset epilepsy. *Epilepsia* 2008; **49**:1847–1858.

29 Dunn DW, Kronenberger WG: Is ADHD in epilepsy the expression of a neurological disorder? In: Kanner AM, Schachter SC (eds): *Psychiatric Controversies in Epilepsy*. Academic Press, San Diego, CA, 2008, pp. 141–152.

30 Biederman J, Faraone SV: Attention-deficit hyperactivity disorder. *Lancet* 2005; **366**:237–248.

31 Aldenkamp A, Arends J: The relative influence of epileptic EEG discharges, short nonconvulsive seizures, and type of epilepsy on cognitive function. *Epilepsia* 2004; **45**:54–63.

32 Jones JE, Watson R, Sheth R et al.: Psychiatric comorbidity in children with new onset epilepsy. *Dev Med Child Neurol* 2007; **49**:493–497.

33 Glauser T, Cnaan A, Shinnar S et al.: Ethosuximide, valproic acid, and lamotrigine in childhood absence epilepsy. *N Engl J Med* 2010; **362**:790–799.

34 Braakman HMH, Vaessen MJ, Hofman PAM et al.: Cognitive and behavioral complications in frontal lobe epilepsy in children: a review of the literature. *Epilepsia* 2011; **52**:849–856.

35 Loring DW, Meador KJ: Cognitive side effects of antiepileptic drugs in children. *Neurology* 2004; **62**:872–877.

36 Hesdorffer DC, Ludvigsson P, Olafsson E et al.: ADHD as a risk factor for incident unprovoked seizures and epilepsy in children. *Arch Gen Psychiatry* 2004; **61**:731–736.

37 Davis SM, Katusic SK, Barbaresi WJ et al.: Epilepsy in children with attention-deficit/hyperactivity disorder. *Pediatr Neurol* 2010; **42**:325–330.

38 Cohen R, Senecky Y, Shuper A et al.: Prevalence of epilepsy and attention-deficit hyperactivity (ADHD) disorder: a population-based study. *J Child Neurol* 2013; **28**:120–123.

39 Austin JK, Harezlak J, Dunn DW et al.: Behavior problems in children before first recognized seizures. *Pediatrics* 2001; **107**:115–122.

40 Parisi P, Moavero R, Verrotti A, Curatolo P: Attention deficit hyperactivity disorder in children with epilepsy. *Brain Dev* 2010; **32**:10–16.

41 Gross-Tsur V, Manor O, van der Meere J et al.: Epilepsy and attention deficit hyperactivity disorder: is methylphenidate safe and effective? *J Pediatr* 1997; **130**:670–674.

42 Gucuyener K, Erdemoglu AK, Senol S et al.: Use of methylphenidate for attention-deficit hyperactivity disorder in patients with epilepsy of electroencephalographic abnormalities. *J Child Neurol* 2003; **18**:109–112.

43 Santos K, Palmini A, Radziuk AL et al.: The impact of methylphenidate on seizure frequency and severity in children with attention-deficit-hyperactivity disorder and difficult-to-treat epilepsies. *Dev Med Child Neurol* 2013; **55**:654–660.

44 Fosi T, Lax-Pericall MT, Scott RC et al.: Methylphenidate treatment of attention deficit hyperactivity disorder in young people with learning disability and difficult-to-treat epilepsy: evidence of clinical benefit. *Epilepsia* 2013; **54**:2071–2081.

45 Gonzalez-Heydrich J, Whitney J, Waber D et al.: Adaptive phase I study of OROS methylphenidate treatment of attention deficit hyperactivity disorder with epilepsy. *Epilepsy Behav* 2010; **18**:229–237.

46 Gonzalez-Heydrich J, Hsin O, Hickory M et al.: Comparisons of response to stimulant preparations in pediatric epilepsy. *AACAP Scientific Proceeding* 2004; **31**:107–108.

47 Brown JWL, Dunne JW, Fatovic DM et al.: Amphetamine-associated seizures: clinical features and prognosis. *Epilepsia* 2011; **52**:401–404.

48 Hernández AJC, Barragán PEJ: Efficacy of atomoxetine treatment in children with ADHD and epilepsy [abstract]. *Epilepsia* 2005; **46(Suppl. 6)**:241.

49 Torres A, Whitney J, Rao S et al.: Tolerability of atomoxetine for treatment of pediatric attention-deficit/hyperactivity disorder in the context of epilepsy. *Epilepsy Behav* 2011; **20**:95–102.

50 Wernicke JF, Holdridge KC, Jin L et al.: Seizure risk in patients with attention-deficit-hyperactivity disorder treated with atomoxetine. *Dev Med Child Neurol* 2007; **49**:498–502.

51 Hirota T, Schwartz S, Correll CU: Alpha-2 agonists for attention-deficit/hyperactivity disorder in youth: a systematic review and meta-analysis of monotherapy and add-on trials to stimulant therapy. *J Amer Acad Child Adolesc Psychiatry* 2014; **53**:153–173.

52 Torres A, Whitney J, Gonzalez-Heydrich J: Attention-deficit/hyperactivity disorder in pediatric patients with epilepsy: review of pharmacological treatment. *Epilepsy Behav* 2008; **12**:217–233.

53 MTA Cooperative Group: A 14-month randomized clinical trial of treatment strategies for attention-deficit/hyperactivity disorder. *Arch Gen Psychiatry* 1999; **56**:1073–1086.

54 LaJoie J, Miles DK: Treatment of attention-deficit disorder, cerebral palsy, and mental retardation in epilepsy. *Epilepsy Behav* 2002; **3**:542–548.

Behavioral and developmental disorders in epilepsy

Introduction

Cognitive and behavioral impairments are frequent consequences of epilepsy in the pediatric and adult population. Various contributing factors have been identified, including type of epilepsy and seizures, etiology, age of onset, seizure frequency, duration of epilepsy, and medication(s). However, it is unclear whether seizures themselves cause the deficit or whether the underlying etiology is responsible. More recent information has argued that the impact of etiology is not straightforward, because the underlying pathology may not necessarily coincide with the functional or cognitive impairment. One hypothesis suggests this is the case when activity within a functionally silent ictal zone spreads to a functionally relevant region [1]. Regardless, there are both commonalities and distinctions among the epilepsies and epilepsy syndromes with respect to cognitive and behavioral disturbances.

A study of preschool children with nonspecified epilepsy determined that cognitive impairment was related to intractability, early-onset epilepsy, brain pathology, and age, where age was the significant predictor for cognitive impairment irrespective of duration of epilepsy [2]. However, another study identified that children with new-onset seizures already had neuropsychological deficits at onset [3]. Specific risk factors included multiple seizures, AED use, symptomatic or cryptogenic etiology, and presence of epileptiform activity on initial EEG. The overall risk for neuropsychological deficits, when compared to healthy siblings, was 3.0 times greater for a child with all four risk categories [3]. These children tended to score lower in attention, executive, and construction abilities, verbal memory and learning, and language function compared to unaffected siblings or controls, yet were equivalent in academic achievement [3].

Even untreated children with a second unprovoked seizure demonstrate deficits in attention, construction, and executive functions and those with epileptiform activity on EEG have associated slower psychomotor speed [3]. In children with frequent seizures – even those with short duration or with minimal clinical symptomatology – there may be a cumulative cognitive effect, which can have a substantial impact on daily life and lead to state-dependent learning impairment. Specifically, alertness and short-term memory are the cognitive functions that are most vulnerable to the acute effects of seizures and, in particular, interictal discharges [4]. However, data in the literature are inconsistent and studies have been mostly fraught with small sample sizes, short observation periods, delay in cognitive assessment following seizure onset, retrospective analysis, or exclusion of certain seizure types or etiologies, giving rise to conflicting findings. A newer approach establishes that cognitive impairment in epilepsy is not necessarily a relationship between neuropsychological status and clinical epilepsy characteristics such as seizure frequency, seizure severity, duration of epilepsy, age of onset, etiology, or medications but rather an interrelationship between underlying anatomic, metabolic, and other unidentified neurobiologic correlates of epilepsy with cognitive and behavioral function [5]. It may be that a critical interaction between synaptic development and the pruning process interacting with the epileptic process plays an important role in the permanent cognitive impairment seen in some of the devastating epilepsies of childhood [6,7].

Animal data

In animal models of epilepsy, some of these overlapping factors can be controlled, including etiology, age of onset, and frequency, severity, and duration of seizures. Animal models are designed to tease out the variables that are more likely to be associated with potential cognitive and behavioral impairments. However, the types of assessments used to determine outcomes of cognitive and behavioral impairment are not necessarily validated. Stafstrom [8] summarized various behavioral tests used to assess the effect of seizures on animal models, including tests of sensorimotor function and reflexes, locomotion and exploration, visuospatial learning and memory, anxiety, and social adaptation, and concluded that they are limited in that they measure a specific function and cannot easily be generalized to a broader cognitive/behavioral impairment. The most common model used in the adult animal is that of pharmaco-induced status epilepticus with chemoconvulsants. Use of kainic acid results in pathological neuronal loss within hippocampal structures and in neurological sequelae, including cognitive impairment, as seen in impaired spatial learning and memory, behavioral changes (aggressiveness and hyperactivity), and recurrent seizures [9–12]. Earlier studies did not find similar associations [13–15], but these were notably conducted prior to the development of more sensitive markers that identify neuronal death, synaptic reorganization, and long-term cognitive and behavioral deficits [16–20].

Laboratory evidence from animal data confirms that the immature brain differs from the mature brain in basic mechanisms of epileptogenesis and propagation of seizures. Proposed mechanisms that appear to be protective against structural damage include immature membrane properties, synaptic machinery, ion homeostatic mechanisms, growth factor effects, and possibly neurogenesis [8,21–24]. Nonetheless, the immature brain is prone to imbalances in gamma-aminobutyric acid (GABA), resulting in an imbalance between excitation and inhibition [21]. There are also age-related differences in response to GABAergic agents in the substantia nigra, which is involved in seizure propagation. Immature brain has less damage histologically and less cognitive dysfunction due to prolonged seizures. Early-life seizures are correlated with deficits in long-term spatial memory and behavior, such as anxiety [25]. However, animal models of cortical dysplasia have revealed that early-life seizures do not have a significant impact on cognitive impairment, which result instead from the underlying cortical abnormality. These findings suggest that control of seizures alone is likely not sufficient to minimize cognitive effects [26].

Idiopathic generalized epilepsies and focal epilepsies

Children with IGE or localization-related epilepsy have been found to have higher IQ scores than those with symptomatic or cryptogenic generalized epilepsies or epileptic syndromes [27]. IGE is associated with deficits in frontal-lobe structures, but these are not restricted to this epilepsy type and may also be seen in those with focal epilepsies (temporal, frontal, parietal) [28]. Of the focal epilepsies, TLE is the most common and therefore the most studied. Mesial TLE, the most common cause for TLE, is associated with specific deficits dependent on speech dominance, which translate to moderate impairments of intelligence, academic achievement,

language function, and visuospatial functions [29]. When these are associated with secondarily generalized tonic–clonic seizures they are at risk for deficits of the prefrontal lobe and global intellect [28]. There is also evidence that nonlesional TLE and extratemporal-lobe epilepsy demonstrate reduced functional connectivity in the prefrontal brain [30].

In a study of mesial TLE, patients with unilateral HS were assessed for the influence of duration of seizures, side of pathology, and gender on deficits of memory, intellect, and language domains [31]. All groups had significant deficits in verbal learning and retention scores – greater than in visual learning and retention. Age and duration of epilepsy had no significant effect. With respect to verbal learning tasks, patients with left HS performed worse than those with right HS, but those with right HS performed worse than healthy controls. With respect to gender, female subjects had a more impaired performance in naming tasks and in verbal and performance IQs than males [31]. Based on these findings, the authors suggested that cognitive deficits are established in childhood and show age-related gradients of decline throughout adulthood. Helmstaedter [32] also demonstrated that epilepsy patients start with an already impaired level of cognitive proficiency. This is paradoxical to previously accepted assumptions that patients experience a progressive decline in cognitive domains.

Neuropsychological studies in children with childhood absence are complicated by small sample size, poor separation between juvenile and childhood absence, and medication effects. In a small but well-controlled study, Pavone [33] showed that 81% of absence patients had IQs that were in the normal range but lower than those of their matched controls. The study concluded that absence patients showed slight but statistically significant impairments in global cognition, nonverbal memory, and visual spatial skills but that verbal memory and skills were less affected [33]. A later study replicated these general conclusions [34].

Despite remission of their epilepsy, patients with CAE suffer a poorer psychosocial outcome than controls with other chronic illness (juvenile rheumatoid arthritis). Those with absence are more likely to be high-school dropouts, have unplanned pregnancies, and abuse drugs.

Patients with JME have demonstrated impairments of prospective memory when compared with their unaffected siblings or controls. This specific type of memory is needed to fulfill previously planned intentions and is dependent on executive functions, which have been shown to be impaired in this group [35]. Overall, patients with JME demonstrate abnormal cognition, intellectual level, short-term memory, and executive dysfunction compared to controls [35]. Another study identified neuropsychological dysfunctions in verbal fluency, comprehension, and expression, as well as nonverbal memory and mental flexibility. Neuroimaging studies (structural and tractography) have identified various anatomical pathways for these functions, including mesial frontal cortex – specifically the supplementary motor area – and PCC [36].

Age-acquired syndromes

ESES is frequently encountered in age-acquired pediatric epilepsy syndromes associated with cognitive and language dysfunction. This electrographic pattern can present at any point along various stages of a spectrum of diseases, including continuous spikes and waves during slow-wave sleep syndrome (CSWS), LKS, and the initial presenting period of BECTS. These epilepsy syndromes present during critical development of tertiary association cortices and are primarily centered in the tertiary association cortex. In CSWS, the EEG abnormality is maximal in the prefrontal association cortex, presenting with a behavioral disorder, frontal dementia, and an expressive language disorder. The parietal–temporal–occipital (PTO) association cortex is maximally involved in LKS, presenting as loss of comprehension and auditory agnosia followed by loss of expressive speech [37,38]. The overlap in these syndromes can cause difficulty in proper diagnosis early in the disease, as some benign conditions can transition into a more complicated and progressive course. Therefore, it is important to distinguish more devastating syndromes such as LKS and CSWS from BECTS by identifying atypical neuropsychiatric and cognitive dysfunctions.

LKS is a functional disorder characterized by self-limiting seizures that are relatively easy to treat, an acquired aphasia, EEG abnormalities consisting of unilateral or bilateral epileptiform discharges over the temporal regions, and absence of any brain pathology [6,37,39]. Children affected by this disorder have typically developed normal language until onset and

later improve in language when the EEG abnormalities resolve. However, permanent language deficits and other neuropsychological sequelae persist, particularly if the paroxysmal EEG begins early in childhood [40] and continues during the critical period of language development [6,37]. One hypothesis for the persistent language deficit after resolution of the epileptiform activity is that the epileptiform activity interferes with the normal synaptic pruning during the critical period of language development. It is thought that those synapses that are actively involved in both synaptic activity and epileptic activity are spared the normal pruning process, allowing nonfunctional synapses to persist through the developmental process [6].

CSWS is also a functional childhood disorder, characterized by severe paroxysmal EEG abnormalities dominating >85% of sleep recordings, self-limited clinical seizures, behavioral and cognitive dysfunction with or without premorbid developmental disturbances, and no brain pathology [41]. Spontaneous resolution of epileptiform activity occurs by the midteen years and often the behavioral and neuropsychological deficits stabilize or improve. However, the severity of these deficits is dependent on the age of onset and the duration of the active phase of EEG abnormalities [42]. Again, the permanent deficits result from the persistence of nonfunctional synapses after the critical developmental period.

BECTS is characterized by infrequent nocturnal seizures and centrotemporal spikes on EEG and often spontaneously remits in the midteen years. Small studies have revealed transient disturbances related to interictal EEG abnormalities [43,44]. In one group, patients demonstrated full-scale IQ scores within the normal range but significantly below those of matched controls. When these patients were tested during periods of marked interictal epileptiform activity, neuropsychological deficits were identified in areas including visuospatial short-term memory, attention, cognitive flexibility, picture naming, word fluency, visuoperceptual skills, and visuomotor coordination. Once patients achieved remission from the interictal activity, they demonstrated notable improvement in IQ scores and significant improvement in neuropsychological deficits [43,44]. However, other studies have identified a subset of these patients who do not have a benign course (as the name would suggest) and develop mild intellectual disability, behavioral dysfunction, specific learning disabilities, and language delay or regression [45]. Concurrent with this, one study identified deficits in measures of impulsivity and inhibition, reflecting poor frontal-lobe functioning [44].

Catastrophic epilepsies

Catastrophic epilepsies such as West syndrome, LGS, and myoclonic epilepsies are characterized by intractable seizures, cognitive arrest or decline in a child with previously normal early development, neurological abnormalities, normal neuroimaging studies, and a progressive course. West syndrome is associated with early signs of cognitive impairment, including deterioration of responsiveness and sensory abilities and poor social contact [46]. Studies assessing infants have reported impaired hand–eye coordination [47] and impaired visual functioning involving acuity, ocular motility, visual field, visual attention, and visual scanning skills [48–50]. Patients with the idiopathic form of West syndrome in which spasms resolved within the first year underwent immediate and delayed evaluations that revealed deficits in attention, learning, and memory [51]. Learning disability has been reported in 71–80%, of which it is severe in more than half [52]. Disturbances in behavior followed autistic features in about 15% of patients [46], especially in those whose disease was secondary to tuberous sclerosis [53].

Multiple seizure types are characteristic of LGS, including brief tonic, atonic, myoclonic, and atypical absence seizures. The typical abnormal EEG demonstrates diffuse slow spike–wave discharges in the waking portion, with fast rhythms in sleep. Approximately 20–60% of children with LGS have a history of infantile spasms. Poor outcome is predicted when onset occurs before 3 years of age and there is a prior history of West syndrome [54]. Over the long term, these patients also show perseverative behavior, psychomotor slowing, and apathy [55]. Still, controlled studies have not been pursued and information regarding cognitive and behavioral disturbances is sparse and lacking.

Dravet syndrome (severe myoclonic epilepsy, SME) and myoclonic–astatic epilepsy (MAE) are epileptic encephalopathies characterized by myoclonic seizures and other seizure types that typically predominate with onset in infancy and early childhood and are associated with cognitive and behavioral disturbances

with no known etiology. SME is typically characterized by prolonged febrile and nonfebrile convulsive seizures in infancy and subsequent cognitive decline. In 30% of cases, it is associated with a mutation of the *SCN1A* gene [56]. Children with SME have poor outcomes and epilepsy that is difficult to control, with apparent behavioral issues including attention deficit and hyperactivity. The majority of these children achieve unsteady ambulation and severely impaired language, where they are categorized as moderately to severely retarded [57]. MAE presents in childhood with episodes of nonconvulsive status and generalized tonic–clonic seizures, which have an unpredictable course and outcome. Children with MAE can either achieve remission within a few years (with normal cognition) or have chronic intractable epilepsy (with cognitive impairments). The classification of this specific group of epilepsies is variable in the literature as the term "MAE" has been used to designate all primary generalized epilepsies of childhood whose main clinical manifestations include myoclonic and/or astatic seizures and it is best to identify these syndromes as representative of a spectrum of myoclonic disorders rather than as a single entity. In general, mild behavioral problems such as hyperactivity can be observed but, because of the unpredictable course and the lack of consistent classification, cognitive and behavioral disturbances are variable and can range from mild to severe impairments [56]. Interpersonal relationships rarely exceed the developmental level of 2 years of age and behavior is marked by hyperactivity, psychotic-type relationships, and sometimes autistic traits [58].

Conclusion

Cognitive and behavioral impairments are the rule rather than the exception in childhood epilepsy syndromes. With increasingly sensitive neuropsychological testing, mild impairments are found even in the "benign" childhood syndromes. Cognitive and behavioral impairments can at times be predicted by the source of the epileptic process (e.g., short-term memory deficits in hippocampal epilepsy). It appears that early onset, increased severity, longer duration, and intractability are associated with more severe cognitive and behavioral impairments. The etiologies of these impairments are multifocal and interactive. They include but are not limited to: underlying neuronal/synaptic pathology present before the epilepsy begins; the excitotoxic effects of seizures, causing neuronal death and neuronal reorganization; the effects of the epileptiform activity on the developing cortex and during critical periods of synaptogenesis and synaptic pruning; the effects of AEDs on cognition, learning, and behavior; and the psychosocial stigma that labels these children as outsiders and "losers" in modern society. It is only by rapid and complete control of the epileptic seizures and normalization of the EEG that these children can achieve disease remission and the cognitive and behavioral impairments of childhood epilepsy can be ameliorated.

References

1 Jokeit H, Schacher M: Neuropsychological aspects of type of epilepsy and etiological factors in adults. *Epilepsy Behav* 2004; **5(Suppl. 1)**:S14–S20.

2 Rantanen K, Eriksson K, Nieminen P: Cognitive impairment in preschool children with epilepsy. *Epilepsia* 2011; **52(8)**: 1499–1505.

3 Fastenau PS, Johnson CS, Perkins SM et al.: Neuropsychological status at seizure onset in children: risk factors for early cognitive deficits. *Neurology* 2009; **73(7)**:526–534.

4 Aldenkamp AP, Arends J, de la Parra NM, Migchelbrink EJ: The cognitive impact of epileptiform EEG discharges and short epileptic seizures: relationship to characteristics of the cognitive tasks. *Epilepsy Behav* 2010; **17(2)**:205–209.

5 Hermann BP, Lin JJ, Jones JE, Seidenberg M: The emerging architecture of neuropsychological impairment in epilepsy. *Neurol Clin* 2009; **27(4)**:881–907.

6 Morrell F, Whisler WW, Smith MC et al.: Landau-Kleffner syndrome: treatment with subpial intracortical transection. *Brain* 1995; **118**:1529–1546.

7 Huttenlocher PR, de Courten C: The development of synapses in striate cortex of man. *Hum Neurobiol* 1987; **6(1)**: 1–9.

8 Stafstrom CE: Assessing the behavioral and cognitive effects of seizures on the developing brain. *Prog Brain Res* 2002; **135**:377–390.

9 Ben-Ari Y: Limbic seizure and brain damage produced by kainic acid: mechanisms and relevance to human temporal lobe epilepsy. *Neuroscience* 1985; **14**:375–403.

10 Cronin J, Dudek FE: Chronic seizures and collateral sprouting of dentate mossy fibers after kainic acid treatment in rats. *Brain Res* 1988; **474**:181–184.

11 Milgram NW, Isen DA, Mandel D et al.: Deficits in spontaneous behavior and cognitive function following systemic administration of kainic acid. *Neurotoxicology* 1988; **9**: 611–624.

12 Stafstrom CE, Chronopoulos A, Thurber S et al.: Age-dependent cognitive and behavioral deficits after kainic acid seizures. *Epilepsia* 1993; **34**:420–435.

13 Cavalheiro E, Silva D, Turski W et al.: The susceptibility of rats to pilocarpine-induced seizures is age-dependent. *Brain Res* 1987; **465**:43–58.

14 Albala B, Moshe S, Okada R: Kainic acid induced seizures: a developmental study. *Dev Brain Res* 1984; **13**:139–148.

15 Stafstrom CE, Thompson JL, Holmes GL: Kainic acid seizures in the developing brain: status epilepticus and spontaneous recurrent seizures. *Dev Brain Res* 1992; **65**:227–236.

16 Holmes GL, Gaiarsa J-L, Chevassus-Au-Louis N, Ben-Ari Y: Consequences of neonatal seizures in the rat: morphological and behavioral effects. *Ann Neurol* 1998; **44**:845–857.

17 Holmes GL, Sarkisian M, Ben-Ari Y, Chevassus-Au-Louis N: Mossy fiber sprouting after recurrent seizures during early development in rats. *J Comp Neurol* 1999; **404**:537–553.

18 Sankar R, Shin D, Liu H et al.: Patterns of status epilepticus-induced neuronal injury during development and long-term consequences. *J Neurosci* 1998; **18**:8382–8393.

19 Thompson K, Holm A, Schousboe A et al.: Hippocampal stimulation produces neuronal death in the immature brain. *Neuroscience* 1998; **82**:337–348.

20 Chen K, Baram T, Soltesz I: Febrile seizures in the developing brain result in persistent modification of neuronal excitability in limbic circuits. *Nat Med* 1999; **5**:888–894.

21 Holmes GL: Epilepsy in the developing brain: lessons from the laboratory and clinic. *Epilepsia* 1997; **38**:12–30.

22 Stafstrom CE, Lynch M, Sutula TP: Consequences of epilepsy in the developing brain: implications for surgical management. *Semin Pediatr Neurol* 2000; **7**:147–157.

23 Ben-Ari Y: Developing networks play a similar melody. *Trends Neurosci* 2001; **24**:353–360.

24 Sanchez RM, Jensen FE: Maturational aspects of epilepsy mechanisms and consequences for the immature brain. *Epilepsia* 2001; **42**:577–585.

25 Sayin U, Sutula TP, Stafstrom CE: Seizures in the developing brain cause adverse long-term effects on spatial learning and anxiety. *Epilepsia* 2004; **45(12)**:1539–1548.

26 Lucas MM, Lenck-Santini PP, Holmes GL, Scott RC: Impaired cognition in rats with cortical dysplasia: additional impact of early-life seizures. *Brain* 2011; **134(Pt 6)**: 1684–1693

27 Bulteau C, Jambaque I, Viguier D et al.: Epileptic syndromes, cognitive assessment and school placement: a study of 251 children. *Dev Med Child Neurol* 2000; **42(5)**:319–327.

28 Jokeit H, Seitz RJ, Markowitsch HJ et al.: Prefrontal asymmetric interictal glucose hypometabolism and cognitive impairment in patients with temporal lobe epilepsy. *Brain* 1997; **120**:2283–2294.

29 Hermann BP, Seidenberg M, Schoenfeld J, Davies K: Neuropsychological characteristics of the syndrome of mesial temporal lobe epilepsy. *Arch Neurol* 1997; **54**:369–376.

30 Vlooswijk MC, Jansen JF, Jeukens CR et al.: Memory processes and prefrontal network dysfunction in cryptogenic epilepsy. *Epilepsia* 2011; **52(8)**:1467–1475.

31 Baxendale S, Heaney D, Thompson PJ, Duncan JS: Cognitive consequences of childhood-onset temporal

lobe epilepsy across the adult lifespan. *Neurology* 2010; **75(8)**:705–711.

32 Helmstaedter C, Kemper B, Elger CE: Neuropsychological aspects of frontal lobe epilepsy. *Neuropsychologia* 1996; **34**: 399–406.

33 Pavone P, Bianchini R, Trifiletti RR et al.: Neuropsychological assessment in children with absence epilepsy. *Neurology* 2001; **56(8)**:1047–1051.

34 Nolan MA, Redoblado MA, Lah S et al.: Intelligence in childhood epilepsy syndromes. *Epilepsy Res* 2003; **53(1–2)**: 139–150.

35 Wandschneider B, Kopp UA, Kliegel M et al.: Prospective memory in patients with juvenile myoclonic epilepsy and their healthy siblings. *Neurology* 2010; **75(24)**:2161–2167.

36 O'Muircheartaigh J, Vollmar C, Barker GJ et al.: Focal structural changes and cognitive dysfunction in juvenile myoclonic epilepsy. *Neurology* 2011; **76(1)**:34–40.

37 Morrell F: Electrophysiology of CSWS in Landau-Kleffner syndrome. In: Beaumanoir A, Bureau M, Deonna T et al (eds): *Continuous Spikes and Waves During Slow Sleep: Electrical Status Epilepticus During Slow Sleep*. John Libbey, London, 1995, pp. 77–90.

38 Huttenlocher PR, de Courten C, Garey LJ, Van der Loos H: Synaptogenesis in human visual cortex: evidence for synapse elimination during normal development. *Neurosci Lett* 1982; **33(3)**:247–252.

39 Deonna T, Roulet E: Acquired epileptic aphasia (AEA): definition of the syndrome and current problems. In: Beaumanoir A, Bureau M, Deonna T et al (eds): *Continuous Spikes and Waves During Slow Sleep: Electrical Status Epilepticus During Slow Sleep*. John Libbey, London, 1995, pp. 37–45.

40 Bishop DVM: Age of onset and outcome in "acquired aphasia with convulsive disorder" (Landau-Kleffner syndrome). *Dev Med Child Neurol* 1985; **27**:705–712.

41 Bureau M: Continuous spikes and waves during slow sleep (CSWS): definition of the syndrome. In: Beaumanoir A, Bureau M, Deonna T et al (eds): *Continuous Spikes and Waves During Slow Sleep: Electrical Status Epilepticus During Slow Sleep*. John Libbey, London, 1995, pp. 17–26.

42 Smith MC, Hoeppner TJ: Epileptic encephalopathy of late childhood: Landau-Kleffner syndrome and the syndrome of continuous spikes and waves during slow-wave sleep. *J Clin Neurophysiol* 2003; **20(6)**:462–472.

43 Baglietto MG, Battaglia FM, Nobili L et al.: Neuropsychological disorders related to interictal epileptic discharges during sleep in benign epilepsy of childhood with centrotemporal or Rolandic spikes. *Dev Med Child Neurol* 2001; **43(6)**: 407–412.

44 Deonna T, Zesiger P, Davidoff V et al.: Benign partial epilepsy of childhood: a longitudinal neuropsychological and EEG study of cognitive function. *Dev Med Child Neurol* 2000; **42(9)**:595–603.

45 Yung AW, Park YD, Cohen MJ, Garrison TN: Cognitive and behavioral problems in children with centrotemporal spikes. *Pediatric Neurology* 2000; **23(5)**:391–395.

46 Guzzetta F: Cognitive and behavioral outcome in west syndrome. *Epilepsia* 2006; **47(Suppl. 2)**:49–52.

47 Randò T, Baranello G, Ricci D et al.: Cognitive competence at the onset of west syndrome: correlation with EEG patterns and visual function. *Dev Med Child Neurol* 2005; **47(11)**: 760–765.

48 Guzzetta F, Frisone MF, Ricci D et al.: Development of visual attention in West syndrome. *Epilepsia* 2002; **43(7)**:757–763.

49 Jambaque I, Dellatolas G, Dulac O et al.: Verbal and visual memory impairment in children with epilepsy. *Neuropsychologia* 1993; **31(12)**:1321–1337.

50 Randò T, Bancale A, Baranello G et al.: Visual function in infants with west syndrome: correlation with EEG patterns. *Epilepsia* 2004; **45(7)**:781–786.

51 Gaily E, Appelqvist K, Kantola-Sorsa E et al.: Cognitive deficits after cryptogenic infantile spasms with benign seizure evolution. *Dev Med Child Neurol* 1999; **41(10)**: 660–664.

52 Jambaque I: Neuropsychological aspects. In: Dulac O, Chugani HT, Dalla Bernadina B (eds): *Infantile Spasms and West Syndrome*. Saunders, London, 1994, pp. 82–87.

53 Hunt A, Dennis J: Psychiatric disorder among children with tuberous sclerosis. *Dev Med Child Neurol* 1987; **29**:190–198.

54 Wirrell E, Farrell K, Whiting S: The epileptic encephalopathies of infancy and childhood. *Can J Neurol Sci* 2005; **32(4)**:409–418.

55 Kieffer-Renaux V, Kaminska A, Dulac O: Cognitive deterioration in Lennox–Gastaut and Doose epilepsy. In: Jambaque I, Lassonde M, Dulac O (eds): *Neuropsychology of Childhood Epilepsy*. Kluwer, New York, NY, 2001, pp. 185–190.

56 Guerrini R, Aicardi J: Epileptic encephalopathies with myoclonic seizures in infants and children (severe myoclonic epilepsy and myoclonic-astatic epilepsy). *J Clin Neurophysiol* 2003; **20(6)**:449–461.

57 Aicardi J: Myoclonic epilepsies in childhood. *Int Pediatr* 1991; **6**:195–200.

58 Casse-Perrot C, Wolf M, Dravet C: Neuropsychological aspects of severe myoclonic epilepsy in infancy. In: Jambaque I, Lassonde M, Dulac O (eds): *Neuropsychology of Childhood Epilepsy*. Kluwer Academic/Plenum Publishers, New York, NY, 2001, pp. 131–140.

CHAPTER 5

Cognitive effects of epilepsy therapies

Beth A. Leeman and Kimford J. Meador

Department of Neurology, Emory University, USA

Introduction

Patients with epilepsy often demonstrate cognitive dysfunction in areas such as attention, language, and memory, in the setting of otherwise normal intelligence. Cognitive deficits have been documented in both newly diagnosed patients and those with long-standing seizures [1–3]. Although controversial, some data suggest that cognitive difficulties may progress over time [4], particularly in the setting of generalized convulsions.

Cognitive deficits are likely multifactorial in etiology, due to factors including underlying brain injuries, frequent seizures, ongoing interictal epileptiform discharges [1], comorbid depression, and disrupted sleep. Function may be further compromised by epilepsy therapy, such as the use of anticonvulsant medications [5], anterior temporal lobectomy (ATL) for the treatment of medically refractory temporal-lobe epilepsy [6,7], and other surgical interventions (Box 5.1). While the magnitude of deficits due to epilepsy treatments may be small in comparison to that of the underlying disease state, recognition of treatment effects is important, as they may be predicted and in some cases prevented. In this chapter, we will review the cognitive effects of specific epilepsy therapies, methods for evaluating cognitive deficits and predicting their occurrence, and options for the management of cognitive dysfunction.

Cognitive effects of anticonvulsant medications

While the contribution of antiepileptic drugs (AEDs) to cognitive impairment may be small compared to other

Box 5.1 Factors affecting cognition in patients with epilepsy.

- Etiology/preexisting brain injury
- Type of seizure
- Effects of seizures: ictal, interictal, postictal
- Interictal epileptiform discharges
- Medications
- Surgical resection
- Vagal nerve stimulation/device implantation
- Psychosocial/psychiatric factors

factors, identification of drug effects is important, as medication regimen is a modifiable factor. These agents are used chronically, both in otherwise healthy adults and in the elderly, children, and those with underlying cognitive or behavioral issues, who may be particularly sensitive to adverse effects. The balance between seizure control and the risk of cognitive adverse effects must be weighed in each patient. In general, the deficits are more pronounced with rapid titration, higher dosage, and polypharmacy and are reversible upon discontinuation of the drug (Box 5.2). Unfortunately, studies detailing the cognitive profiles of each medication are limited, in that they often are of small sample size, lack controls, randomization, or blinding, and fail to account for drug levels or medication interactions. Studies are also frequently conducted in healthy volunteers rather than epilepsy patients, such that results may not be generalizable to the population of interest. Trials often compare the effects of one drug to those of another, which provides no information regarding effects compared to a non-drug baseline. Finally, investigations may rely upon subjective measures and the concordance between objective and subjective cognitive

Epilepsy and the Interictal State: Co-Morbidities and Quality of Life, First Edition.
Edited by Erik K. St. Louis, David M. Ficker, and Terence J. O'Brien.
© 2015 John Wiley & Sons, Ltd. Published 2015 by John Wiley & Sons, Ltd.

Box 5.2 Factors associated with cognitive effects of anticonvulsants.

- Titration rate
- Time for habituation
- Dose
- Blood level
- Polytherapy
- Type of anticonvulsant
- Individual susceptibility

abilities is only 63–70% [8]. Bearing these limitations in mind, this section discusses the cognitive effects of the commonly used AEDs.

First-generation AEDs
The older AEDs, including carbamazepine, phenytoin, and valproate, have similar cognitive profiles [9–11], generally causing greater negative effects compared to the newer medications (Box 5.3). The older drugs may impair response inhibition, verbal fluency, attention, psychomotor speed, P3 potentials, and verbal recall. They may also lead to subjective reports of confusion and memory, speech, and attentional deficits [10–12], although the magnitude of effects is small. Phenobarbital can cause more impairment than other older agents, with greater declines in psychomotor speed, response inhibition, and attention [9,11] compared to carbamazepine, valproate, and phenytoin. Benzodiazepines in particular also produce significant impairment across many domains, including reaction time, sensory discrimination, vigilance, short-term memory, and divided attention, when compared to placebo [12].

Eslicarbazepine acetate
A new drug recently approved in Europe, eslicarbazepine acetate is a novel voltage-gated sodium channel blocker closely related to oxcarbazepine and carbamazepine. In healthy volunteers, oxcarbazepine and eslicarbazepine acetate had similar cognitive profiles [13]. Neither caused clinically meaningful impairments on multiple objective measures, including reaction time, attention, memory, and psychomotor speed, when administered as a single 900 mg dose or over 3 weeks of daily dosing (eslicarbazepine acetate 800 and 1200 mg/day, oxcarbazepine 300 and 600 mg twice/day). With both drugs, there were minimal

Box 5.3 Differential anticonvulsant effects: likelihood of cognitive deficits.

Least
- Gabapentin
- Lamotrigine
- Levetiracetam
- Tiagabine
- Vigabatrin

Moderate
- Carbamazepine
- Phenytoin
- Pregabalin
- Oxcarpazepine
- Valproate

Most
- Benzodiazepines
- Phenobarbital
- Topiramate
- Zonisamide

Uncertain due to inadequate data:
- Eslicarbazepine acetate
- Felbamate
- Lacosamide
- Rufinamide

declines in choice reaction time, vigilance, and verbal memory and increases in verbal fluency. Patients taking oxcarbazepine also had improved performance on the Trail Making Test. Isolated complaints of attentional or memory deficits with these agents resolved with continued treatment.

Felbamate
Anecdotal reports suggest felbamate has an alerting effect. Potential side effects of aplastic anemia and hepatotoxicity have restricted the investigation of cognitive adverse events, however. Hence, no human neuropsychological studies of felbamate have been performed.

Gabapentin
While higher doses of gabapentin (i.e., 2400 mg/day) may cause sedation [14], results from objective cognitive measures are variable. Some data suggest

improvement on isolated measures of verbal learning and frontal-executive function. Adjunctive gabapentin at 1200–2400 mg/day in patients with refractory partial seizures caused no measurable changes in psychomotor speed, response inhibition, or working memory, with some improvement of paired associate learning compared to placebo [14]. Patients with epilepsy tested pre- and 1–2 months post-treatment with adjunctive gabapentin compared to those with stable medication regimens had no significant changes in central integrative ability, verbal memory, or attention at a mean dosage of 1428.6 mg, although patients receiving gabapentin performed better on a selected measure of the Stroop Neuropsychological Screening Test [15]. Similarly, there were no effects of acute dosing or 4 weeks of daily treatment, with 17 and 35 mg/kg, respectively, in healthy adults completing tests of psychomotor and visuomotor processing speed, learning and memory, and verbal fluency. With 2–4 weeks of treatment, however, there was improvement on an attentional task [16].

Conversely, Meador et al. [17] documented deficits in attention and processing speed in healthy volunteers taking 2400 mg/day of gabapentin compared to a non-drug baseline, although fewer cognitive effects were evident when compared to carbamazpine. Salinsky et al. [18] also demonstrated EEG slowing with gabapentin doses titrated to 3600 mg/day, as well as more subjective cognitive deficits and poorer performance on objective tests of psychomotor speed and response inhibition when compared to untreated controls. These data suggest that gabapentin may not be as benign with respect to cognitive clouding as previously believed.

Lacosamide

The manufacturer reported memory impairment in 2% of patients taking lacosamide 200–600 mg/day, similar to that seen with placebo. Higher rates of memory complaints (6%) were noted in those taking 600 mg/day in their double-blind placebo-controlled trials. No systematic investigations of cognition with use of lacosamide have been conducted to date.

Lamotrigine

At 300 mg/day (mean blood level 4.41 μg/mL) in healthy volunteers, lamotrigine led to improvements in tests of attention and phonemic fluency but to relative impairments in semantic fluency, psychomotor speed, and response inhibition compared to a non-drug baseline [19]. No negative effects on psychomotor and visuomotor processing speed, attention, learning and memory, or verbal fluency were noted with higher levels in healthy adults taking 7.1 mg/kg for up to 4 weeks (mean blood level 8.1 μg/mL) [16]. Overall, lamotrigine is considered to cause fewer adverse reactions than the older generation of AEDs and may have slightly beneficial effects [20].

Levetiracetam

Levetiracetam rapidly gained popularity due to its ease of administration and relatively benign side-effect profile. It is generally considered to be a "nootropic" or cognition-enhancing medication. In patients tested before and up to 6 months after treatment with levetiracetam, subjective improvement was reported in 58%, objective improvement in 23–29%, and documented decline in 5–6%, across a broad neuropsychological battery, including measures of executive function, memory, fluency, comprehension, and visuospatial skills. Positive outcomes were predicted by greater baseline function, later-onset seizures, fewer concurrent AEDs, and better seizure control [8]. In a nonrandomized, blinded study in which subjects completed assessments of attention, memory, language, visuospatial skills, and executive function after 1 year of treatment with either add-on levetiracetam or topiramate, no change was detected after use of levetiracetam [21]. Levetiractam add-on therapy also demonstrated a trend for improved visual short-term memory and subjective increases in alertness, with no change in other measures of episodic memory, executive function, or attention, suggesting a favorable neuropsychological profile after 2 weeks of treatment [22]. In a double-blind, placebo-controlled study, levetiracetam led to improvements in attention span, with no changes in motor speed, EEG frequencies, or visual evoked potentials, at daily doses of 1500 mg [23]. Overall, levetiracetam has compared favorably to other regimens, such as oxcarbazepine and carbamazepine [23,24].

Oxcarbazepine

Although an estimated 23% of patients taking oxcarbazepine will have mild cognitive complaints, and some patients will have EEG slowing, subjective confusion, and/or objective drowsiness [25], most data suggest that oxcarbazepine does not impair objective cognitive function [20,26,27]. The drug may have some beneficial neuropsychological effects, including improved list learning and executive function in adolescents and adults [20] and improved processing speed, attention, and IQ testing in children and adolescents [27]. Changes do not appear to relate to patient characteristics, features of the epilepsy syndrome, EEG findings, structural abnormalities, or dosage/blood level [20,26].

Oxcarbazepine is a new agent that is closely related to carbamazepine but is believed to have fewer serious adverse reactions. Subjective complaints, including somnolence, ideomotor slowing, poor concentration, memory loss, and language difficulties were more commonly reported with carbamazepine. With oxcarbazepine and carbamazepine at daily doses of 1200 and 800 mg, respectively, carbamazepine also led to greater objective impairments of motor speed, slowing of the EEG, and more consistently increased visual evoked potential P1 latencies. Both agents were associated with improvements in attention span. Overall, however, oxcarbazepine appeared to be better tolerated [23].

Pregabalin

Data regarding the cognitive effects of pregabalin are limited to short-term outcome studies, primarily in healthy volunteers. Results suggest a benign cognitive profile. Adverse effects may be more frequent than with the closely related agent gabapentin, perhaps due to pregabalin's greater alpha-2-delta protein affinity.

In healthy volunteers, pregabalin at 150 mg three times/day led to mild, transient negative effects on measures of sensory discrimination and divided attention, with improvement on a reaction-time task. No significant differences from placebo were evident with choice reaction time, short-term memory, or attentional tasks. Hindmarch et al. [12] suggested that pregabalin might be useful for patients in whom sedation or cognitive clouding is a concern. In a longer-term study, its cognitive effects (up to 300 mg twice/day) were assessed in healthy volunteers after 12 weeks of treatment in a randomized, double-blind, placebo-controlled trial. Subjects receiving pregabalin had mild declines on measures of psychomotor speed, response inhibition, and verbal fluency, as well as subjective cognitive toxicity. Impairments were associated with higher blood levels. Immediate story recall, however, favored pregabalin

over placebo, and other tests of learning, memory, IQ, and divided attention were not significantly changed with treatment [28]. In the one published study of pregabalin and cognition in patients with medically refractory partial epilepsy, pregabalin was compared with levetiracteam add-on therapy in a nonrandomized, open-label trial. Cognitive testing was performed at baseline and after 1 week of treatment at the target doses, but dosing and titration schedules were unclear [22]. With pregablin, there were impairments of episodic memory for verbal and visual information and some patients reported difficulty concentrating for prolonged periods. No effects were noted on measures of IQ, vocabulary, nonverbal skills, executive function, phonemic fluency, attention, concentration, or nonverbal and verbal short-term and working memory. These results may reflect temporary impairment during titration, however, and long-term studies in patients are needed.

Rufinamide

The one published human investigation of the cognitive effects of rufinamide employed a double-blind, randomized, placebo-controlled add-on parallel study design with rufinamide dosages of 200–1600 mg/day in patients with partial seizures [29]. Cognitive testing was performed at baseline and after 3 months of treatment. Assessments included measures of information processing speed and reaction time, psychomotor speed and motor fluency, and verbal and nonverbal working memory. No measure demonstrated a decline with treatment. The authors concluded that there were no serious cognitive adverse events of these dose ranges, but longer-term studies are needed.

Tiagabine

Although there are isolated reports of nonconvulsive status with a confusional state induced by tiagabine, the drug typically does not have negative cognitive effects. In an open-label trial followed by a double-blind, placebo-controlled, cross-over study at median doses of 24–32 mg/day, tiagabine had no significant effects on cognitive (verbal learning and memory, response inhibition, semantic processing, processing speed, psychomotor speed) or EEG measures but there were occasional subjective reports of cognitive improvement [30]. In a 12-week double-blind, add-on, placebo-controlled, dose-ranging study at

16, 32, or 56 mg/day, results showed no clinically significant effects on tests of psychomotor speed, response inhibition, verbal fluency, verbal learning and memory, IQ, or attention [31]. Long-term studies in patients with epilepsy, with follow-up over 1–2 years, also failed to demonstrate any significant negative effects on learning and memory, attention, response inhibition, verbal fluency, psychomotor speed, or overall intellectual abilities, or any consistent EEG changes, at doses ranging from 5 to 80 mg/day [32–34], and variable improvements were noted in list learning and memory, auditory reaction times, fluency, and attention [32–34].

Topiramate

Language deficits are a prominent cognitive complaint with use of topiramate, with anomia or other expressive difficulties reported by up to 50% of patients. Patients may also complain of cognitive or psychomotor slowing (7–9%), memory loss (5–18%), confusion (5–6%), and decreased concentration (4–9%) [35,36]. Objective deficits may be significant even in patients who do not experience subjective changes [37], and while deficits have been rated as mild to moderate in most patients [35], they may be of sufficient severity to impact daily life [38]. Data suggest that at 50 mg/day, with 50 mg/day weekly increases to 400 mg/day, 10–15% of patients will have clinically relevant cognitive side effects [36]. In a dose-ranging study using a slower titration schedule, Loring et al. [39] found that cognitive risks increased as healthy subjects approached 200 mg/day, and 35% of participants had deficits at 400 mg/day, even in monotherapy.

Effects may be seen shortly after initiation and are reversible upon drug discontinuation [37,38,40]. The duration of effects after discontinuation is unclear, however, and deficits may require 1 day to many weeks for resolution. While there is some suggestion that the adverse effects may resolve with continued treatment [35], a longer-term study with 6 months of treatment indicated that deficits persist [39]. While some studies have shown no significant dysfunction due to topiramate [21], this is rare, and adverse effects have usually been documented by direct testing of IQ, verbal comprehension, verbal and nonverbal memory, verbal and nonverbal fluency, response inhibition, working memory, attention, processing and psychomotor speed, visuospatial skills, naming, and problem-solving at average doses typically ranging from approximately 200 to 400 mg/day in patients with epilepsy and healthy volunteers [16,19,36,37,40,41]. In Thompson et al. [38], the most significant difficulties were noted with verbal IQ, verbal fluency, and verbal learning. It has also been suggested that the Symbol Digit Modalities Test is particularly sensitive to the adverse effects of topiramate and may be used as a screening tool [36]. Although there are some inconsistencies across studies, difficulties tend to be associated with primary generalized seizure disorders, higher initial or target doses and blood levels, faster titrations, and polypharmacy (particularly coadministration of lamotrigine) [35,39–41]. Individual susceptibility may also play a prominent role. In general, however, topiramate is considered to have similar, or perhaps more negative, effects than the older-generation AEDs [19,36].

Vigabatrin

While there are subjective reports of memory and concentration deficits with vigabatrin, direct testing has generally failed to substantiate these findings. Studies typically show no cognitive impairment or a suggestion of minimal improvement with use of the drug. Results may be affected by small sample sizes, low doses, and short periods of follow-up, however. Cognitive performance in epilepsy patients receiving 2 g/day of adjunctive vigabatrin, for example, was compared to that in matched controls whose regimens remained unchanged [42]. Subjects were tested at baseline and 4 weeks after treatment with measures of attention, mental speed, motor speed, central cognitive processing, and perceptuomotor performance and no adverse effects were noted. Although there was improvement in speed on a test of arithmetic, it was unclear given the multiple comparisons whether this result was due to chance.

Addressing these limitations of sample size, dosage, and duration of follow-up, a larger double-blind, add-on, placebo-controlled study of patients with intractable focal-onset seizures was conducted, in which subjects were treated with either placebo or 1, 3, or 6 g of vigabatrin for 12 weeks [43]. Decline in performance of a digit cancellation test with increasing doses was evident but 95% of the measures, including tests of psychomotor speed, visual scanning, response inhibition, spatial memory, verbal fluency, verbal memory, IQ, and attention, were not impaired. Overall, the drug has little impact on cognitive performance.

Zonisamide

Up to nearly 50% of patients taking zonisamide report mild cognitive complaints [44], including speech difficulty, memory loss, poor attention, and dyscalculia, even at therapeutic blood levels. Conversely, patients may also be unaware of relatively large objective deficits.

As with topiramate, language dysfunction is commonly reported with zonisamide use [40]. It is unclear whether this relates to their common sulfa moiety, increases in GABA, effects on glutamate, sodium, or calcium channel activity, carbonic anhydrase-inhibiting effects, or other mechanisms. Effects appear to be dose-related and may resolve with dosage reduction [40,44,45]. A pilot study demonstrated deficits in verbal intelligence on zonisamide monotherapy compared to carbamazepine monotherapy, but this was at supratherapeutic doses with levels greater than 30 µg/mL [40]. An uncontrolled pilot study with cognitive testing pretreatment and 12 and 24 weeks post-treatment demonstrated impairment of verbal learning and delayed verbal and nonverbal memory at levels greater than 30 µg/mL but no effect on retention of previously learned material, attention, perceptual orientation, psychomotor speed, or nonverbal encoding [45]. Declines evident at 12 weeks were resolving upon retest at 24 weeks, although the finding of tolerance was not replicated in a longer-term study. A randomized trial of zonisamide monotherapy demonstrated dose-related impairment on measures of verbal and nonverbal memory, attention, executive function, and verbal fluency after 1 year of treatment at 300–400 mg/day [44]. Park et al. [44] have suggested an initial target dose of ≤100 mg/day, particularly in patients with newly diagnosed seizures, in order to minimize cognitive adverse effects.

Cognitive effects of surgical epilepsy treatments

Evaluation of cognitive performance in patients undergoing epilepsy surgery

Neuropsychological testing

Neuropsychological testing may be performed when there is concern for cognitive deficits. It is administered routinely pre- and post-epilepsy surgery. Batteries typically include measures of verbal memory (e.g., word list memorization tasks such as the Rey Auditory Verbal Learning Test or Paired Associates), naming (i.e., the Boston Naming Test), spatial memory (e.g., Visual Reproduction, Rey Osterrieth Complex Figure Test), verbal and performance IQ, frontal/executive function (e.g., Wisconsin Card Sorting, Trails A and B), and behavior (e.g., Minnesota Multiphasic Personality Inventory (MMPI), Personality Assessment Inventory).

The expected pattern of deficits reflects the impairment of functions normally served by the site of seizure onset. In temporal-lobe epilepsy of the language-dominant hemisphere, for example, patients will likely demonstrate deficits in verbal-based tasks such as word list learning, naming, and verbal IQ, while nonverbal task performance remains intact. Conversely, patients with nondominant temporal-lobe epilepsy will likely have deficits in nonverbal memory and performance IQ. Patients with frontal-lobe epilepsy may have difficulties with tasks requiring attention and planning. When the expected patterns are obtained, there is less risk for postoperative impairment, as the tissue to be removed was not functioning normally at baseline (Table 5.1). It is also reassuring with respect to hypotheses regarding seizure localization.

Concern is raised, however, when test results are normal or unexpected patterns are observed. When all testing is normal or above average, there is greater risk for postoperative deficits, as functional tissue will

Table 5.1 Neuropsychological testing: typical patterns of deficits after temporal lobectomy.

		Left TL	Right TL[a]
Verbal	Rey Auditory Verbal Learning Test	↓	Normal
	Paired Associates	↓	Normal
	Boston Naming Test	↓	Normal
	Verbal IQ	↓	Normal
Nonverbal	Rey Osterrieth	Normal	↓
	Visual Reproduction	Normal	↓
	Performance IQ	Normal	↓

TL, temporal lobectomy. Arrows indicate impairment.
[a]Nonverbal changes for right TL are more variable. Changes after left TL are more predictable, with less risk of decline if there is poor performance at baseline (see text for details).

be removed. Moreover, such results do not provide any information regarding seizure localization. Even more worrisome are cases in which the opposite testing patterns are observed; that is, nonverbal memory is impaired but verbal memory is intact in dominant temporal-lobe epilepsy. This suggests that functional tissue will be removed and nonfunctional tissue will remain. Alternatively, such results may suggest reorganization of function or erroneous seizure localization. A limitation, however, is the lack of testing available to specifically tap nondominant temporal-lobe function. Tests for nonverbal memory are less lateralizing than those for verbal memory, and further research and test development in this area are needed.

Wada testing

Wada testing has been the "gold standard" for assessing risk to cognitive function after surgical resection. When further information regarding language lateralization and memory is desired, Wada testing may be performed. This involves administration of cognitive testing during selective anesthetization of the anterior circulation of each hemisphere, which produces deafferentation of the hippocampus and renders cortical language areas nonfunctional for a limited period of time. Injecting the surgical side indicates what tasks can be performed in the absence of that tissue (functional reserve). Injecting the nonsurgical side demonstrates what functions the to-be-resected tissue performs (functional adequacy). If the surgical side is inactivated by amobarbital or a similar anesthetic and concurrent neuropsychological testing suggests that the contralateral hemisphere is unable to adequately support memory functions, resection would pose a great risk of postoperative amnesia [46].

Testing begins with angiography, to ensure patency and flow of contrast in the carotid, middle cerebral, and anterior cerebral arteries. It is also performed to ensure there is no significant cross-filling; if anesthetic injected into one hemisphere crossed into the opposite one and the patient performed poorly on testing, it would be unclear which hemisphere produced the deficit. The surgical side is typically injected first, commonly using amobarbital. While protocols may vary across centers, doses commonly range from 100 to 125 mg. Alternative agents include methohexital, propofol, and etomidate. EEG is recorded during Wada testing primarily to monitor for seizures during the procedure, which could intefere with patient performance and thus alter the results. EEG after the injection, in the absence of cross-filling, will demonstrate slowing restricted to the injected hemisphere. The patient will also exhibit a flaccid paralysis of the contralateral arm. If these signs are not achieved, injection of additional amobarbital may be indicated. Once adequate anesthesia is obtained, cognitive testing is performed. While protocols are variable, testing at our center includes measures of counting, naming, repetition of phrases, and reading, with notations made of any hesitations, aphasia, dysarthria, or paraphasias. Objects are shown and recall and recognition are tested after a 10-minute delay. After 30 minutes, testing is repeated with injection of the opposite hemisphere.

While Wada testing has the advantage of reversibly inactivating tissue to simulate outcomes of resection, several disadvantages should be noted. First, there is no single Wada protocol shared by all centers. Examiners may use different memory assessments (recall versus recognition), scoring procedures, stimuli (e.g., objects, pictures, designs, words, or sentences), criteria for anesthesia (EEG slowing versus strength), medications, or dosages and have differing interpretations of results (pass versus fail). Hence, findings may be difficult to interpret and compare across examiners or institutions. Second, the procedure is invasive, with complication rates of 0–20% [47], and carries the risk of bleeding, infection, and stroke. Third, testing may be limited by patient- and medication-related factors, such as agitation, sedation, and cross-filling of vessels. Carbonic anhydrase inhibitors, including topiramate and zonisamide, may induce metabolism of the anesthetics, leading to rapidly decreased drug effect and a limited testing window. Finally, this procedure is informative with respect to hemispheric function but lacks more detailed spatial resolution.

Functional MRI

Attempts to develop less invasive protocols for assessment of language and memory using functional magnetic resonance imaging (fMRI) hold promise. This technique uses blood oxygenation level-dependent (BOLD) fMRI imaging to detect the changes in local magnetic fields induced by an increased ratio of oxygenated to deoxygenated blood, an indirect marker of increased local neuronal activity. The changes in magnetic field during cognitive activity can be compared to a baseline and statistical maps can be generated to represent the foci in the brain that have been activated by the task. These maps have predicted postoperative Boston Naming Test performance [48]. Limited group data also suggest that left-hippocampal fMRI activation during encoding tasks predicts poor cognitive outcomes from left ATL, as functional tissue would be removed. At present, however, it is unclear how well fMRI will predict individual outcomes [49]. Results were based on small numbers of subjects and varied by the neuropsychological batteries employed. It is also possible that identification of individual active regions is less important than identification of coherent networks underlying a given task. At this stage, the clinical utility of fMRI is limited.

Cortical mapping

Patients implanted with intracranial electrodes present an opportunity to map cortical function through direct stimulation of the electrodes. Mapping may be performed intra- or extraoperatively, with an applied electrical current gradually increased until there is disruption of the function of the underlying tissue. With concurrent cognitive testing, the regions subserving various tasks can be determined. This allows a more tailored surgery, avoiding resection of eloquent cortex [50]. Sparing language cortex in dominant-hemisphere surgeries is often of concern, and precisely defining the boundaries of language cortex in each individual is important, as the classical maps of language areas are an artifact of averaging. An individual's language cortex may lie outside of these regions, as a normal variant or consequence of reorganization of function. A patient's language cortex may also encompass a much smaller area than that evident on published atlases – as small as $1\,cm^2$ [51] – and have indistinct boundaries. Individuals may also have multiple cortical regions subserving a given task, with great variability evident across patients [52]. Intraoperative mapping also demonstrates functional separation of languages in bilingual patients [53].

Testing may be limited by epileptiform discharges ("afterdischarges") or seizures elicited by electrical stimulation of epileptogenic tissue. The EEG is monitored continuously for these events throughout the procedure. Such discharges may prevent further increase of stimulation parameters, such that the threshold for disruption of function cannot be reached. It is also possible for function to be impaired

by these discharges or their spread to neighboring regions, clouding interpretation of the testing. The risk of afterdischarges or seizures may be mitigated by administration of anticonvulsant medications prior to testing. Stimulation parameters may also be adjusted, using lower current for a shorter duration of time, with increments of smaller intervals in epileptogenic regions.

Other factors can also limit testing. Testing is constrained by time when performing intraoperative mapping and is restricted to those areas implanted or exposed by surgery. The spread of stimulation to neighboring regions may confound results. Finally, patients must be alert and cooperative, which may be difficult after anesthesia, following sleep deprivation, or during a postictal state.

The cognitive assessments performed during mapping are not standardized, which limits comparison across centers. At our institution, memory is tested by presentation of word pairs during stimulation, with immediate recall of the items when each stimulation ends. Language is evaluated by naming of simple line drawings presented one-by-one on a computer screen during stimulation, with notes made of nonresponses, hesitations, and paraphasias. The type of error may be characteristic of certain brain regions; for example, phonological errors are associated with stimulation of the superior temporal area [54]. Baseline testing prior to stimulation mapping is essential in order to distinguish a true deficit due to stimulation from underlying naming difficulty. Objects that cannot be named at baseline are removed from the test battery for that individual.

Effects of surgery on cognition

ATL is the most common surgical procedure performed for the treatment of medically refractory epilepsy. Assessing the risk to cognitive function is an important aspect of the presurgical evaluation, allowing the clinician to predict postoperative dysfunction, prevent deficits (when possible), and counsel patients appropriately. Available data regarding cognitive outcomes are limited, controlled long-term follow-up studies are rare, there is considerable individual variation in pre- and postoperative performance, and test performance may be masked by the strategies used [55]. Nevertheless, some general patterns have emerged.

Overall IQ tends to remain stable following ATL [56], with one study noting slight improvement [57]. Patients may suffer from word-finding difficulties after language-dominant temporal lobectomy [58]. This persists in approximately 25% of patients when tested 1 year after surgery. Perhaps of greatest concern, however, are the effects of ATL on memory. Standard anterior temporal-lobe resections place the patient at risk for postoperative memory dysfunction, which may significantly impact quality of life (QOL) [7]. This is particularly true in the setting of dominant-hemisphere resections [56,59]. While approximately 22% of patients may experience some variable – often minor – decline in nonverbal memory after nondominant ATL [60], all patients are at significant risk for postoperative verbal memory dysfunction following dominant-hemisphere ATL. Verbal memory decline is evident in up to approximately 20% of patients undergoing nondominant temporal lobectomy, while deficits occur in as much as 48–60% of dominant-hemisphere ATL patients [59]. In 21%, the decline is severe, with performance decrements of >60% from baseline [6]. Memory deficits are considered disabling in 1–4% of patients [61]. Furthermore, deficits in those undergoing dominant ATL tend to persist, with data suggesting continued verbal memory decline at testing >9 years postoperatively [7].

Although data are variable, within 1–2 years after right ATL, verbal and nonverbal memory tends to improve from the preoperative baseline [62]. Stroup et al. [59] noted that 3% of dominant and 7% of nondominant ATL patients had improvement of verbal memory. Other data suggest improvement in up to 25% of patients [63–65]. This may be due to the removal of nociferous tissue, allowing the remaining tissue to function more effectively.

Various factors may confer a greater risk of postoperative memory decline. Better preoperative memory, intact memory performance following Wada injections contralateral to the seizure focus, normal preoperative structural MRI, and normal cellular appearance of the resected region increase risk, as they suggest that functional tissue is removed [59,66–69]. Abnormal MRI findings other than unilateral mesial temporal sclerosis [59] and poor memory following Wada injections ipsilateral to the seizure focus also pose some risk, suggesting that the remaining tissue may have less functional reserve. Bilateral abnormalities on EEG may also indicate greater risk, in that removal of the epileptogenic region leaves behind abnormally functioning contralateral tissue [70]. Older age at the time of ATL or later age at seizure onset may also confer

increased risks to postoperative function, in that there is less time for reorganization of neural networks that subserve memory prior to resection, although this is controversial [68,71]. Sex may be a relevant factor, as men have demonstrated poorer verbal recall than women, both pre- and postoperatively, regardless of the extent of hippocampal injury [72]. While data are conflicting, continued seizures may also be associated with postsurgical memory decline [56,73]. The most predictive factors appear to be side of resection and MRI findings [59].

Additional variables may confound postoperative test performance. Cognitive changes following the initial surgical trauma may be evident, resolving in the first few months after surgery. Postoperative depression can affect attention, concentration, and memory encoding. The patient should be reassured that with time and treatment of depression, test performance may improve. In addition, if the dosage of AEDs is decreased after surgery, patients may experience fewer cognitive side effects, with improved memory, processing speed, and language skills [55].

It should be noted that the correlation between objective and subjective performance is not perfect. In Stroup et al. [59], only 39% of those with verbal memory decline reported a change and 12% with no decline reported worsening. Hence, in most patients, decline was not detectable in everyday life. Objective findings, however, should be documented in any patient with memory complaints.

A more limited resection may help to preserve cognitive function. A logical hypothesis is that the less tissue is removed, the less function should be affected. Data, however, suggest that this may not always be the case. An extreme example is that of functional hemispherectomy in children, in which the temporal and parietal lobes of the affected hemisphere are resected and connections of the frontal and occipital lobes to the opposite hemisphere are severed. While the procedure is extensive, an estimated 70% have no change in postoperative intelligence and 7% may improve in IQ. Across studies using a variety of cognitive batteries, deficits are seen in visual spatial skills, attention, verbal fluency, and visual memory. About half of patients will have no change in performance, however, and approximately 25% will improve [74–82]. As in ATL, outcomes tend to be better in those who become seizure-free. In addition, patients who had a shorter duration of epilepsy prior to surgery and greater preoperative development have better cognitive outcomes [76,77,79]. Etiology may also play a role, with vascular causes of epilepsy having more favorable outcomes. The mechanisms for improvement are unknown but may involve use and refinement of ipsilateral networks.

In many patients with temporal-lobe epilepsy, more restricted resections are performed in hopes of attaining seizure freedom while minimizing adverse cognitive effects. While some studies have documented better neuropsychological outcomes with selective amygdalo-hippocampectomy in which lateral cortex remains intact [83], data are conflicting [84]. Although less tissue is resected, the surgical approach may still disrupt connecting fibers or neighboring tissue, leading to cognitive deficits. Thus, various surgical approaches for selective amygdalohippocampectomy, which affect different connecting fibers, may have different cognitive effects [85].

Surgical lesions may be further restricted by using gamma knife radiosurgery, which focuses gamma radiation using stereotaxic guidance to create lesions confined to the amygdala, anterior hippocampus, and parahippocampal gyrus. Verbal memory was evaluated 1 and 2 years post-treatment and 25% of patients with dominant surgeries and 7% of patients with nondominant surgeries showed impairment. Significant improvements were evident in 16% of patients with dominant surgeries and 7% of patients with nondominant surgeries. Notably, performance was not associated with seizure freedom or dose of radioactivity [86]. Regis et al. [87] followed patients 2 years after treatment and found no decline in visual or verbal memory, with 20% experiencing improvements. Nor were subjective deficits reported. Overall, data suggest relative preservation of verbal memory with radiosurgery compared to standard ATL, but larger randomized comparative trials are needed.

Device implantation provides another option for the treatment of refractory epilepsy. As no tissue is removed in such procedures, better cognitive outcomes may be expected. In a double-blind randomized trial of bilateral stimulation of the anterior nuclei of the thalamus for epilepsy (SANTE), no cognitive effects of stimulation were demonstrated at 2-year follow-up [88]. Although subjects receiving active stimulation reported subjective memory impairments more frequently, all complaints ultimately resolved. With vagus nerve stimulation (VNS), animal studies showed cognitive improvement but human trials demonstrated mixed results. Investigations in epilepsy patients have generally documented no overall adverse effects on cognition but positive effects have not been confirmed [89]. When counseling patients, the lower likelihood of cognitive deficits must be balanced against the likelihood of seizure freedom on a case-by-case basis.

Treatment of cognitive deficits

Unfortunately, treatment options for cognitive dysfunction in epilepsy patients are limited. The first step is to remove any agents that may cause deficits, if possible. The type of AED may be changed to one with fewer cognitive side effects, for example, or the dose or number of AEDs may be reduced. Cognitive therapy is also a common approach. Patients can learn techniques for aiding memory, such as writing down items to be remembered and keeping notes in a single notebook, calendar, or computerized device. Therapy may help patients to cope but it does not treat the memory loss or address the underlying pathologic process.

No pharmacologic agents have been approved for the treatment of cognitive deficits in epilepsy. Two studies examined the pharmacologic management of memory dysfunction in epilepsy patients using donepezil (Aricept), but results were inconsistent and the drug of questionable benefit. A pilot study by Fisher et al. [90] showed some promise for use of the drug, although the mechanism of its possible effect was unclear. The study found improved immediate recall and consistent long-term retrieval scores on the Buschke Selective Reminding Test after 3 months of open-label treatment when compared to a pretreatment baseline. A more recent randomized, double-blind, placebo-controlled cross-over trial of donepezil showed no effect on memory as measured by delayed recall on the Hopkins Verbal Learning Test, however [91]; nor did a trial of galantamine demonstrate an effect on verbal or nonverbal memory in patients with epilepsy [92].

Use of acetylcholinesterase inhibitors may also pose a risk of seizure exacerbation in this population. Fisher et al. [90] reported a significant increase in the frequency of generalized tonic–clonic seizures during donepezil treatment. Cholinergic agents have been shown to cause seizures in animal models as well [93]. Given isolated case reports of seizures associated with donepezil use, the manufacturer issued an advisory note warning of a possible relationship, although data have been insufficient to establish causality. While an increase in seizures was not noted in the Hamberger et al. [91] study, seizure exacerbation remains a concern regarding the use of this drug in patients with epilepsy.

Current trials are examining other agents for treatment of memory deficits in epilepsy. These compounds include memantine (an NMDA antagonist prescribed for treatment of moderate to severe Alzheimer's disease [94–96]) and the dietary supplement vinpocetine (a synthetic ethyl ester of a vinca alkaloid obtained from the leaves of the lesser periwinkle, *Vinca minor*). Both compounds have neuroprotective properties against glutamate and NMDA-mediated excitotoxicity, as well as possible anticonvulsant effects. Theoretically, protection against NMDA receptor activity would block the pathway of excitotoxicity that leads to hippocampal injury and memory loss [97]. In addition, vinpocetine may enhance long-term potentiation [98] and improve memory in animal models [99] and young healthy human volunteers [100]. Data collection in these trials is ongoing.

Conclusion

Many patients with epilepsy experience cognitive deficits. Although largely due to the underlying etiology of the seizures, medical and surgical therapies for epilepsy may also play a role. Dysfunction may be characterized by neuropsychological assessments and deficits sustained with surgical resection may be predicted by neuropsychological, Wada, fMRI, and cortical-stimulation testing. While cognitive difficulties can be managed by cognitive or behavioral therapy, better strategies are needed. Future research may focus on identifying the underlying mechanisms of cognitive dysfunction in epilepsy and developing rational mechanisms for treatment of these deficits, which will improve the QOL of our patients.

References

1 Aarts JH, Binnie CD, Smit AM et al.: Selective cognitive impairment during focal and generalized epileptiform EEG activity. *Brain* 1984; **107(Pt 1)**:293–308.

2 Aikia M, Salmenpera T, Partanen K et al.: Verbal memory in newly diagnosed patients and patients with chronic left temporal lobe epilepsy. *Epilepsy Behav* 2001; **2(1)**: 20–27.

3 Pulliainen V, Kuikka P, Jokelainen M: Motor and cognitive functions in newly diagnosed adult seizure patients before antiepileptic medication. *Acta Neurol Scand* 2000; **101(2)**:73–78.

4 Helmstaedter C, Elger CE: Chronic temporal lobe epilepsy: a neurodevelopmental or progressively dementing disease? *Brain* 2009; **132(Pt 10)**:2822–2830.

5 Ortinski P, Meador KJ: Cognitive side effects of antiepileptic drugs. *Epilepsy Behav* 2004; **5(Suppl. 1)**: S60–S65.

6 Ivnik RJ, Sharbrough FW, Laws ER Jr.: Anterior temporal lobectomy for the control of partial complex seizures: information for counseling patients. *Mayo Clin Proc* 1988; **63(8)**:783–793.

7 Rausch R, Kraemer S, Pietras CJ et al.: Early and late cognitive changes following temporal lobe surgery for epilepsy. *Neurology* 2003; **60(6)**:951–959.

8 Helmstaedter C, Witt JA: The effects of levetiracetam on cognition: a non-interventional surveillance study. *Epilepsy Behav* 2008; **13(4)**:642–649.

9 Meador KJ, Loring DW, Huh K et al.: Comparative cognitive effects of anticonvulsants. *Neurology* 1990; **40(3 Pt 1)**: 391–394.

10 Meador KJ, Loring DW, Allen ME et al.: Comparative cognitive effects of carbamazepine and phenytoin in healthy adults. *Neurology* 1991; **41(10)**:1537–1540.

11 Meador KJ, Loring DW, Moore EE et al.: Comparative cognitive effects of phenobarbital, phenytoin, and valproate in healthy adults. *Neurology* 1995; **45(8)**:1494–1499.

12 Hindmarch I, Trick L, Ridout F: A double-blind, placebo- and positive-internal-controlled (alprazolam) investigation of the cognitive and psychomotor profile of pregabalin in healthy volunteers. *Psychopharmacology (Berl)* 2005; **183(2)**: 133–143.

13 Milovan D, Almeida L, Romach MK et al.: Effect of eslicarbazepine acetate and oxcarbazepine on cognition and psychomotor function in healthy volunteers. *Epilepsy Behav* 2010; **18(4)**:366–373.

14 Leach JP, Girvan J, Paul A et al.: Gabapentin and cognition: a double blind, dose ranging, placebo controlled study in refractory epilepsy. *J Neurol Neurosurg Psychiatry* 1997; **62(4)**:372–376.

15 Mortimore C, Trimble M, Emmers E. Effects of gabapentin on cognition and quality of life in patients with epilepsy. *Seizure* 1998; **7(5)**:359–364.

16 Martin R, Kuzniecky R, Ho S et al.: Cognitive effects of topiramate, gabapentin, and lamotrigine in healthy young adults. *Neurology* 1999; **52(2)**:321–327.

17 Meador KJ, Loring DW, Ray PG et al.: Differential cognitive effects of carbamazepine and gabapentin. *Epilepsia* 1999; **40(9)**:1279–1285.

18 Salinsky MC, Binder LM, Oken BS et al.: Effects of gabapentin and carbamazepine on the EEG and cognition in healthy volunteers. *Epilepsia* 2002; **43(5)**:482–490.

19 Meador KJ, Loring DW, Vahle VJ et al.: Cognitive and behavioral effects of lamotrigine and topiramate in healthy volunteers. *Neurology* 2005; **64(12)**:2108–2114.

20 Seo JG, Lee DI, Hwang YH et al.: Comparison of cognitive effects of lamotrigine and oxcarbazepine in epilepsy patients. *J Clin Neurol* 2007; **3(1)**:31–37.

21 Huang CW, Pai MC, Tsai JJ: Comparative cognitive effects of levetiracetam and topiramate in intractable epilepsy. *Psychiatry Clin Neurosci* 2008; **62(5)**:548–553.

22 Ciesielski AS, Samson S, Steinhoff BJ: Neuropsychological and psychiatric impact of add-on titration of pregabalin versus levetiracetam: a comparative short-term study. *Epilepsy Behav* 2006; **9(3)**:424–431.

23 Mecarelli O, Vicenzini E, Pulitano P et al.: Clinical, cognitive, and neurophysiologic correlates of short-term treatment with carbamazepine, oxcarbazepine, and levetiracetam in healthy volunteers. *Ann Pharmacother* 2004; **38(11)**:1816–1822.

24 Meador KJ, Gevins A, Loring DW et al.: Neuropsychological and neurophysiologic effects of carbamazepine and levetiracetam. *Neurology* 2007; **69(22)**:2076–2084.

25 Salinsky MC, Spencer DC, Oken BS et al.: Effects of oxcarbazepine and phenytoin on the EEG and cognition in healthy volunteers. *Epilepsy Behav* 2004; **5(6)**:894–902.

26 Aikia M, Kalviainen R, Sivenius J et al.: Cognitive effects of oxcarbazepine and phenytoin monotherapy in newly diagnosed epilepsy: one year follow-up. *Epilepsy Res* 1992; **11(3)**:199–203.

27 Donati F, Gobbi G, Campistol J et al.: The cognitive effects of oxcarbazepine versus carbamazepine or valproate in newly diagnosed children with partial seizures. *Seizure* 2007; **16(8)**:670–679.

28 Salinsky M, Storzbach D, Munoz S: Cognitive effects of pregabalin in healthy volunteers: a double-blind, placebo-controlled trial. *Neurology* 2010; **74(9)**:755–761.

29 Aldenkamp AP, Alpherts WC: The effect of the new antiepileptic drug rufinamide on cognitive functions. *Epilepsia* 2006; **47(7)**:1153–1159.

30 Sveinbjornsdottir S, Sander JW, Patsalos PN et al.: Neuropsychological effects of tiagabine, a potential new antiepileptic drug. *Seizure* 1994; **3(1)**:29–35.

31 Dodrill CB, Arnett JL, Sommerville KW et al.: Cognitive and quality of life effects of differing dosages of tiagabine in epilepsy. *Neurology* 1997; **48(4)**:1025–1031.

32 Aikia M, Jutila L, Salmenpera T et al.: Comparison of the cognitive effects of tiagabine and carbamazepine as monotherapy in newly diagnosed adult patients with partial epilepsy: pooled analysis of two long-term, randomized, follow-up studies. *Epilepsia* 2006; **47(7)**:1121–1127.

33 Aikia M, Jutila L, Salmenpera T et al.: Long-term effects of tiagabine monotherapy on cognition and mood in adult patients with chronic partial epilepsy. *Epilepsy Behav* 2006; **8(4)**:750–755.

34 Kalviainen R, Aikia M, Mervaala E et al.: Long-term cognitive and EEG effects of tiagabine in drug-resistant partial epilepsy. *Epilepsy Res* 1996; **25(3)**:291–297.

35 Reife R, Pledger G, Wu SC: Topiramate as add-on therapy: pooled analysis of randomized controlled trials in adults. *Epilepsia* 2000; **41(Suppl. 1)**: S66–S71.

36 Meador KJ, Loring DW, Hulihan JF et al.: Differential cognitive and behavioral effects of topiramate and valproate. *Neurology* 2003; **60(9)**:1483–1488.

37 Lee S, Sziklas V, Andermann F et al.: The effects of adjunctive topiramate on cognitive function in patients with epilepsy. *Epilepsia* 2003; **44(3)**:339–347.

38 Thompson PJ, Baxendale SA, Duncan JS et al.: Effects of topiramate on cognitive function. *J Neurol Neurosurg Psychiatry* 2000; **69(5)**:636–641.

39 Loring DW, Williamson DJ, Meador KJ et al.: Topiramate dose effects on cognition: a randomized double-blind study. *Neurology* 2011; **76(2)**:131–137.

40 Ojemann LM, Ojemann GA, Dodrill CB et al.: Language disturbances as side effects of topiramate and zonisamide therapy. *Epilepsy Behav* 2001; **2(6)**:579–584.

41 Burton LA, Harden C: Effect of topiramate on attention. *Epilepsy Res* 1997; **27(1)**:29–32.

42 McGuire AM, Duncan JS, Trimble MR: Effects of vigabatrin on cognitive function and mood when used as add-on therapy in patients with intractable epilepsy. *Epilepsia* 1992; **33(1)**:128–134.

43 Dodrill CB, Arnett JL, Sommerville KW et al.: Effects of differing dosages of vigabatrin (Sabril) on cognitive abilities and quality of life in epilepsy. *Epilepsia* 1995; **36(2)**: 164–173.

44 Park SP, Hwang YH, Lee HW et al.: Long-term cognitive and mood effects of zonisamide monotherapy in epilepsy patients. *Epilepsy Behav* 2008; **12(1)**:102–108.

45 Berent S, Sackellares JC, Giordani B et al.: Zonisamide (CI-912) and cognition: results from preliminary study. *Epilepsia* 1987; **28(1)**:61–67.

46 Jokeit H, Ebner A, Holthausen H et al.: Individual prediction of change in delayed recall of prose passages after left-sided anterior temporal lobectomy. *Neurology* 1997; **49(2)**:481–487.

47 Haag A, Knake S, Hamer HM et al.: The Wada test in Austrian, Dutch, German, and Swiss epilepsy centers from 2000 to 2005: a review of 1421 procedures. *Epilepsy Behav* 2008; **13(1)**:83–89.

48 Sabsevitz DS, Swanson SJ, Hammeke TA et al.: Use of preoperative functional neuroimaging to predict language deficits from epilepsy surgery. *Neurology* 2003; **60(11)**: 1788–1792.

49 Grote CL, Meador K: Has amobarbital expired? Considering the future of the Wada. *Neurology* 2005; **65(11)**: 1692–1693.

50 Shimizu H, Suzuki I, Ishijima B et al.: Modifications of temporal lobectomy according to the extent of epileptic foci and speech-related areas. *Surg Neurol* 1990; **34(4)**: 229–234.

51 Sanai N, Mirzadeh Z, Berger MS. Functional outcome after language mapping for glioma resection. *N Engl J Med* 2008; **358(1)**:18–27.

52 Ojemann G, Ojemann J, Lettich E et al.: Cortical language localization in left, dominant hemisphere: an electrical stimulation mapping investigation in 117 patients. 1989. *J Neurosurg* 2008; **108(2)**:411–421.

53 Lucas TH 2nd, McKhann GM 2nd, Ojemann GA: Functional separation of languages in the bilingual brain: a comparison of electrical stimulation language mapping in 25 bilingual patients and 117 monolingual control patients. *J Neurosurg* 2004; **101(3)**:449–457.

54 Corina DP, Loudermilk BC, Detwiler L et al.: Analysis of naming errors during cortical stimulation mapping: implications for models of language representation. *Brain Lang* 2010; **115(2)**:101–112.

55 Baxendale S: The impact of epilepsy surgery on cognition and behavior. *Epilepsy Behav* 2008; **12(4)**:592–599.

56 Tellez-Zenteno JF, Dhar R, Hernandez-Ronquillo L et al.: Long-term outcomes in epilepsy surgery: antiepileptic drugs, mortality, cognitive and psychosocial aspects. *Brain* 2007; **130(Pt 2)**:334–345.

57 Keogan M, McMackin D, Peng S et al.: Temporal neocorticectomy in management of intractable epilepsy: long-term outcome and predictive factors. *Epilepsia* 1992; **33(5)**:852–861.

58 Langfitt JT, Rausch R: Word-finding deficits persist after left anterotemporal lobectomy. *Arch Neurol* 1996; **53(1)**:72–76.

59 Stroup E, Langfitt J, Berg M et al.: Predicting verbal memory decline following anterior temporal lobectomy (ATL). *Neurology* 2003; **60(8)**:1266–1273.

60 Paglioli E, Palmini A, da Costa JC et al.: Survival analysis of the surgical outcome of temporal lobe epilepsy due to hippocampal sclerosis. *Epilepsia* 2004; **45(11)**:1383–1391.

61 Spencer SS. Long-term outcome after epilepsy surgery. *Epilepsia* 1996; **37(9)**:807–813.

62 Grammaldo LG, Di Gennaro G, Giampa T et al.: Memory outcome 2 years after anterior temporal lobectomy in patients with drug-resistant epilepsy. *Seizure* 2009; **18(2)**: 139–144.

63 Leijten FS, Alpherts WC, Van Huffelen AC et al.: The effects on cognitive performance of tailored resection in surgery for nonlesional mesiotemporal lobe epilepsy. *Epilepsia* 2005; **46(3)**:431–439.

64 Cukiert A, Buratini JA, Machado E et al.: Seizure-related outcome after corticoamygdalohippocampectomy in patients with refractory temporal lobe epilepsy and mesial temporal sclerosis evaluated by magnetic resonance imaging alone. *Neurosurg Focus* 2002; **13(4)**:ecp2.

65 Sanyal SK, Chandra PS, Gupta S et al.: Memory and intelligence outcome following surgery for intractable

temporal lobe epilepsy: relationship to seizure outcome and evaluation using a customized neuropsychological battery. *Epilepsy Behav* 2005; **6(2)**:147–155.

66 Trenerry MR, Jack CR Jr, Ivnik RJ et al.: MRI hippocampal volumes and memory function before and after temporal lobectomy. *Neurology* 1993; **43(9)**:1800–1805.

67 Sass KJ, Spencer DD, Kim JH et al.: Verbal memory impairment correlates with hippocampal pyramidal cell density. *Neurology* 1990; **40(11)**:1694–1697.

68 Hermann BP, Seidenberg M, Haltiner A et al.: Relationship of age at onset, chronologic age, and adequacy of preoperative performance to verbal memory change after anterior temporal lobectomy. *Epilepsia* 1995; **36(2)**:137–145.

69 Seidenberg M, Hermann B, Wyler AR et al.: Neuropsychological outcome following anterior temporal lobectomy in patients with and without the syndrome of mesial temporal lobe epilepsy. *Neuropsychology* 1998; **12(2)**:303–316.

70 Tuunainen A, Nousiainen U, Hurskainen H et al.: Preoperative EEG predicts memory and selective cognitive functions after temporal lobe surgery. *J Neurol Neurosurg Psychiatry* 1995; **58(6)**:674–680.

71 Davies KG, Bell BD, Bush AJ et al.: Prediction of verbal memory loss in individuals after anterior temporal lobectomy. *Epilepsia* 1998; **39(8)**:820–828.

72 Berenbaum SA, Baxter L, Seidenberg M et al.: Role of the hippocampus in sex differences in verbal memory: memory outcome following left anterior temporal lobectomy. *Neuropsychology* 1997; **11(4)**:585–591.

73 Helmstaedter C, Kurthen M, Lux S et al.: Chronic epilepsy and cognition: a longitudinal study in temporal lobe epilepsy. *Ann Neurol* 2003; **54(4)**:425–432.

74 Samargia SA, Kimberley TJ: Motor and cognitive outcomes in children after functional hemispherectomy. *Pediatr Phys Ther* 2009; **21(4)**:356–361.

75 Devlin AM, Cross JH, Harkness W et al.: Clinical outcomes of hemispherectomy for epilepsy in childhood and adolescence. *Brain* 2003; **126(Pt 3)**:556–566.

76 Basheer SN, Connolly MB, Lautzenhiser A et al.: Hemispheric surgery in children with refractory epilepsy: seizure outcome, complications, and adaptive function. *Epilepsia* 2007; **48(1)**:133–140.

77 Jonas R, Nguyen S, Hu B et al.: Cerebral hemispherectomy: hospital course, seizure, developmental, language, and motor outcomes. *Neurology* 2004; **62(10)**:1712–1721.

78 Lettori D, Battaglia D, Sacco A et al.: Early hemispherectomy in catastrophic epilepsy: a neuro-cognitive and epileptic long-term follow-up. *Seizure* 2008; **17(1)**:49–63.

79 Maehara T, Shimizu H, Kawai K et al.: Postoperative development of children after hemispherotomy. *Brain Dev* 2002; **24(3)**:155–160.

80 Vining EP, Freeman JM, Pillas DJ et al.: Why would you remove half a brain? The outcome of 58 children after hemispherectomy – the Johns Hopkins experience: 1968 to 1996. *Pediatrics* 1997; **100(2 Pt 1)**:163–171.

81 Battaglia D, Chieffo D, Lettori D et al.: Cognitive assessment in epilepsy surgery of children. *Childs Nerv Syst* 2006; **22(8)**:744–759.

82 Pulsifer MB, Brandt J, Salorio CF et al.: The cognitive outcome of hemispherectomy in 71 children. *Epilepsia* 2004; **45(3)**:243-254.

83 Morino M, Uda T, Naito K et al.: Comparison of neuropsychological outcomes after selective amygdalo-hippocampectomy versus anterior temporal lobectomy. *Epilepsy Behav* 2006; **9(1)**:95–100.

84 Wolf RL, Ivnik RJ, Hirschorn KA et al.: Neurocognitive efficiency following left temporal lobectomy: standard versus limited resection. *J Neurosurg* 1993; **79(1)**:76–83.

85 Lutz MT, Clusmann H, Elger CE et al.: Neuropsychological outcome after selective amygdalohippocampectomy with transsylvian versus transcortical approach: a randomized prospective clinical trial of surgery for temporal lobe epilepsy. *Epilepsia* 2004; **45(7)**:809–816.

86 Barbaro NM, Quigg M, Broshek DK et al.: A multicenter, prospective pilot study of gamma knife radiosurgery for mesial temporal lobe epilepsy: seizure response, adverse events, and verbal memory. *Ann Neurol* 2009; **65(2)**: 167–175.

87 Regis J, Rey M, Bartolomei F et al.: Gamma knife surgery in mesial temporal lobe epilepsy: a prospective multicenter study. *Epilepsia* 2004; **45(5)**:504–515.

88 Fisher R, Salanova V, Witt T et al.: Electrical stimulation of the anterior nucleus of thalamus for treatment of refractory epilepsy. *Epilepsia* 2010; **51(5)**:899–908.

89 Boon P, Moors I, De Herdt V et al.: Vagus nerve stimulation and cognition. *Seizure* 2006; **15(4)**:259–263.

90 Fisher RS, Bortz JJ, Blum DE et al.: A pilot study of donepezil for memory problems in epilepsy. *Epilepsy Behav* 2001; **2(4)**:330–334.

91 Hamberger MJ, Palmese CA, Scarmeas N et al.: A randomized, double-blind, placebo-controlled trial of donepezil to improve memory in epilepsy. *Epilepsia* 2007; **48(7)**:1283–1291.

92 Griffith HR, Martin R, Andrews S et al.: The safety and tolerability of galantamine in patients with epilepsy and memory difficulties. *Epilepsy Behav* 2008; **13(2)**:376–380.

93 Turski L, Ikonomidou C, Turski WA et al.: Review: cholinergic mechanisms and epileptogenesis. The seizures induced by pilocarpine: a novel experimental model of intractable epilepsy. *Synapse* 1989; **3(2)**:154–171.

94 Tariot PN, Farlow MR, Grossberg GT et al.: Memantine treatment in patients with moderate to severe Alzheimer disease already receiving donepezil: a randomized controlled trial. *JAMA* 2004; **291(3)**:317–324.

95 Reisberg B, Doody R, Stoffler A et al.: Memantine in moderate-to-severe Alzheimer's disease. *N Engl J Med* 2003; **348(14)**:1333–1341.

96 Reisberg B, Doody R, Stoffler A et al.: A 24-week open-label extension study of memantine in moderate to severe Alzheimer disease. *Arch Neurol* 2006; **63(1)**:49–54.

97 Kelsey JE, Sanderson KL, Frye CA: Perforant path stimulation in rats produces seizures, loss of hippocampal neurons, and a deficit in spatial mapping which are reduced by prior MK-801. *Behav Brain Res* 2000; **107(1–2)**:59–69.

98 Molnar P, Gaal L: Effect of different subtypes of cognition enhancers on long-term potentiation in the rat dentate gyrus in vivo. *Eur J Pharmacol* 1992; **215(1)**:17–22.

99 DeNoble VJ: Vinpocetine enhances retrieval of a step-through passive avoidance response in rats. *Pharmacol Biochem Behav* 1987; **26(1)**:183–186.

100 Coleston DM, Hindmarch I: Possible memory-enhancing properties of vinpocetine. *Drug Develop Res* 1988; **14(3–4)**: 191–193.

CHAPTER 6

Autism and epilepsy

Vladimír Komárek

Department of Pediatric Neurology, 2nd Faculty of Medicine, Charles University, Motol University Hospital, Czech Republic

Introduction

The quality of life (QOL) of people with epilepsy depends on many objective and subjective factors, including ictal factors (frequency and severity of epileptic seizures) and interictal cognitive or socioemotional difficulties. These factors may in turn be influenced by the nature of any present comorbidity, by the quality of medical and social care, and, in some patients, by covert interictal subclinical epileptiform EEG abnormalities. Simultaneous occurrence of two medically and socially burdening disorders (e.g., epilepsy plus autism) significantly affects a patient's QOL. Among individuals with an autism spectrum disorder (ASD), 15–30% suffer from epileptic seizures and up to 50% have specific epileptiform changes in EEG [1–6]. Whether this is by chance or a consequence of a comorbidity with causal relationship to epilepsy is unclear. Recent research confirms that the common denominator is probably a genetically determined neurodevelopmental disorder affecting early synaptogenesis and connectivity of the developing brain, resulting in a multileveled pathophysiologic disturbance spanning from clinical symptoms through electrophysiological and neuroimaging studies to molecular genetics focusing on cell adhesion molecule (CAM)-related and other genes [7,8]. Interictal cognitive and emotional dysfunction in patients with epilepsy and autism is determined not only by the severity of the ASD but also by the types and severities of epileptic seizures.

The ASD includes low-functioning forms with severe mental retardation and an inability to verbally communicate, high-functioning forms without mental delay, and Asperger syndrome, with relatively normal language development. The epileptic spectrum in ASD includes various types of epileptic encephalopathies (West syndrome, Landau–Kleffner syndrome (LKS), temporal and frontal epilepsies with complex seizures), as well as benign idiopathic epilepsy syndromes that are relatively rare in autistic persons. Appropriate treatment of epilepsy undoubtedly contributes to improving the QOL of autistic patients but cannot "cure" autism, and whether antiepileptic drugs (AEDs) should be used in autistic patients with epileptiform EEG without clinical manifestations of epilepsy is debatable [2,3]. Current research in epilepsy and autism focuses on the hypothesis that improved understanding of the molecular basis of autism and developmental epilepsy might enable us to prevent the condition from developing, rather than just to treat the symptoms.

Autism: definition, subtypes, and etiology

Autism is a complex pervasive developmental disorder (PDD). Its prevalence rate is 0.5–1.0% and it is three to four times more common in males than in females. According to the DSM-IV and the ICD-10, the definition of autism includes impairment and disability in three broad areas: 1) social reciprocal interaction abilities; 2) reciprocal communicative abilities; and 3) behavior, including a narrow range of stereotypic behaviors, activities, and interests [9]. ASD is synonymous with PDD and includes the diagnoses autistic disorder (AD), Rett syndrome, disintegrative disorder, Asperger syndrome, and PDD not otherwise specified (equivalent to the terms "atypical autism" and "autism-like conditions")

Epilepsy and the Interictal State: Co-Morbidities and Quality of Life, First Edition.
Edited by Erik K. St. Louis, David M. Ficker, and Terence J. O'Brien.

[4,6]. Developmental abnormalities are present from the first years of life in the majority of cases, but about one-third of parents of children diagnosed with AD report that their child first seemed to develop normally but then had a loss of already acquired language and social skills in the second or third year of life (i.e., an **autistic regression**). The regression is rarely documented except by parents' reports, so may be disputed [10]. Recent data suggest that most children with ASD also demonstrate previous, subtle developmental delays of social and communicative behaviors [11]. There is a high prevalence of comorbid **intellectual impairment (mental retardation)** and psychiatric disorders (specific phobia, obsessive–compulsive disorder (OCD), and attention deficit/hyperactivity disorder (ADHD)) in children with autism. In a population-based study on autism in preschool children, the prevalence of mental delay was 29.8%; in children with AD, 66.7%; in children with PDD not otherwise specified, 12%; and in children with Asperger syndrome, 0% [4]. The presence of mental delay and the level of language impairment are key in the development of cognitive dysfunction and impaired QOL in patients with epilepsy as well as autism. The various combinations of the four main comorbidities – epilepsy, ASD, mental delay, and language impairment – are presented in Figure 6.1.

Inadequate language is a defining feature of autism. Persistent lack of speech in some individuals is attributed to the severity of their autism and may result in lower QOL. Prevalence rates of language regression and associated findings in 255 children aged 9–14 years participating in a population-based study of ASD were 20.7% with narrowly defined autism, 41.2% with broader ASD, and 38% with non-ASD neurodevelopmental problems, drawn from those with special-education needs within a population of 56 946 children [12]. Language regression was reported in 30% with narrowly defined autism, 8% with broader ASD, and less than 3% with developmental problems without ASD.

Autism has a multitude of different **etiologies**. In 12–35% of subjects with autism, an underlying medical disorder can be identified [13]. Associated medical conditions in autism are chromosomal abnormalities, neurocutaneous disorders (e.g., tuberous sclerosis), Rett syndrome, fetal valproate syndrome, Möbius syndrome, central nervous system (CNS) infections, and some metabolic disorders. Studies of congenital anomalies

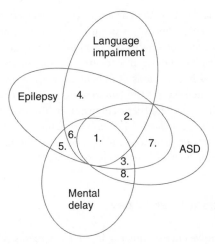

Figure 6.1 Spectrum of comorbidities in epilepsy and autism: 1) combination of epilepsy, ASD, MD, and LI; 2) epilepsy with ASD and LI; 3) epilepsy with ASD and MD; 4) epilepsy with LI (e.g. LKS); 5) epilepsy with MD (e.g. LGS); 6) epilepsy with MD, and LI (e.g., CSWS/ESES) ; 7) epilepsy with ASD; 8) ASD with MD. ASD, autism spectrum disorder; CSWS, continuous spike wave in slow wave sleep; ESES, electrical status epilepticus in sleep; LGS, Lennox–Gastaut syndrome; LI, language impairment; LKS, Landau–Kleffner syndrome; MD, mental delay.

associated with autism have shown that there seem to be critical periods during embryogenesis [14,15]. Some experts have suggested that studies on autism etiology and brain morphology should be limited to children with "essential" autism, excluding those with "complex" autism (i.e., children with microcephaly and/or abnormal physical features). This would allow analysis of a more uniform population, and the group with "essential" autism is probably the more heritable [16]. Ongoing research into the relationship between neurophysiology, neuroanatomy, neurochemistry, and genetic factors is likely to increase our understanding of the **complex etiology of autism**. There is strong evidence supporting a neurobiological basis [17]. Twin and family studies suggest that most cases of autism arise because of a combination of genetic factors [18,19]. Underconnectivity in the brain appears to be an important substrate for autism, since both MRI and fMRI studies have shown thinning of the corpus callosum and reduced connectivity in the frontal and temporal fusiform areas, among other regions [20]. Our study [21] used nonlinear analysis of sleep EEG in 27 patients with autism and 20 mentally non-retarded controls and showed a significant decrease of distant synchronization through all three NREM stages in the autistic group in comparison to control subjects. Mini-columnar pathology in the prefrontal cortex and the middle temporal gyrus has been found, which may be the result of a different circuitry or spatial morphologic features in the brains of individuals with autism [22]. Mirror neurons are thought to be essential for empathy, which is considered deficient in autism; this explains the difficulty in understanding and predicting the behavior or emotions of others and possibly also the impaired imitation ability often seen in autism [23].

Autism in epilepsy

The prevalence of epilepsy in autistic patients is better described than the prevalence of autism in patients with epilepsy, since relevant data and studies remain generally lacking. The frequency of epilepsy appears to be lower in children with autism because epilepsy is often diagnosed at an older age than is autism [4]. Comorbid autism is perhaps best described in patients with West syndrome, especially in association with tuberous sclerosis complex (TSC), although other studies have focused on refractory epilepsies, complex partial seizures (CPS), and, most recently, Dravet syndrome. Some patients with LKS exhibit autism-like behavior, including avoidance of eye contact or contact with family and friends, extreme pickiness over food, prominently disturbed sleep, attacks of rage and aggression, insensitivity to pain, or bizarre, inappropriate, and repetitive play. Many parents report highly unpredictable behavior in their autistic children, similar to "getting a different child" every day or even every hour. LKS may also be overlooked where a diagnosis of an ASD is present [24–26]. Whether frequent or even continuous epileptiform EEG discharges cause intellectual and behavioral disorders directly (via prolonged, transient cognitive impairment) or indirectly remains unclear, with possible mechanisms for cognitive impairment occurring through impairment of memory consolidation during sleep and developmental pruning and sprouting. There are few studies on the prevalence of autism in individuals with epilepsy, but autism and ADHD are probably the two most common neuropsychiatric disorders in children with epilepsy [4,27], especially if the epilepsy is drug-resistant. Autism was seen in 16% of children with epilepsy and neurologic deficits, but in none with uncomplicated epilepsy [28].

In a recent community-based study of newly diagnosed childhood epilepsy, 28 (5%) of 460 children had autism [29]. In a population-based study of children with mental retardation and epilepsy, autism was found in 38% [30]. Conversely, a retrospective descriptive study from a rehabilitation and epilepsy unit found that only 48 of 573 (8%) children with epilepsy had autism, but another 86 (15%) were excluded from assessment for autism given mental decline [31]. In a tertiary pediatric epilepsy clinic, the prevalence of autism was 32% when using an autism screening questionnaire [32]. Among children with therapy-resistant epilepsy being assessed before resective epilepsy surgery, autism was diagnosed in 19–38% of subjects [33].

West syndrome and intellectual impairment are frequently associated with ASD. In 90 children with West syndrome assessed using the Autism Behavior Checklist (ABC), 17 (18.9%) with a total score above 66 were considered to have a "high probability" for autism; when 14 with borderline scores of 54–67 were added, the frequency of autism was 34.5% [32]. Autism in **Dravet syndrome** has rarely been investigated. In one study, 9 (24.3%) of 37 patients met the criteria for autism [35]. All patients with autism showed speech delay, no emotional reciprocity, and narrow interests, whereas in patients without autism, 89.3% had speech delay, 46.4% short temper, and 39.9% narrow interests. Mental retardation was observed in 94.6% of patients with Dravet syndrome, with more frequent severe or profound mental retardation in those with autism [35].

In a retrospective study of 86 patients with childhood-onset CPS, 36 (42%) also had autism [36]. CPS without secondary generalization was more common in patients with autism (69%), who also manifested more frequent frontal paroxysms on EEG (54.5 versus 30.0%, respectively). In the non-ASD group, 82% of cases had been seizure-free for 2 or more years, in comparison to 50% in the ASD group. In 16 children and adolescents treated surgically for temporal-lobe epilepsy, 12 had psychopathology, most often developmental behavioral disorder (DBD) and/or autism [14]. All children with autism had mental retardation and three had problems with hyperactivity. Behavioral change postoperatively was assessed in 13 of these children, and in 11 of the 13 there was either a positive change or no behavioral change. One out of five children with autism became seizure-free. Parents reported a positive behavioral change in three children (calmer, less aggressive), no change in one, and increased symptoms of autism in one. Postsurgical significant cognitive improvement was seen in two seizure-free individuals, one of whom had autism.

In a recent study of 127 patients with idiopathic autism (96 male, 31 female), the mean age was 16.5 ± 9.4 years (range 3–49 years) and the age of seizure onset was 8.2 ± 6.8 years (range 3 weeks to 39 years) [37]; 33.9% were treatment-resistant, 27.5% were seizure-free, and 38.6% had an undetermined seizure outcome due to insufficient data or limited AED trials.

Epilepsy and epileptiform EEG abnormalities in autism

The **prevalence of epilepsy in autism** ranges from 7 to 46% and is increased with greater intellectual disability, symptomatic versus idiopathic autism, age, and history of cognitive or developmental regression [3,4,6,37–42]. In our study [38], we investigated 77 autistic children (61 boys, 16 girls) using clinical interview, evaluation of epilepsy types, IQ testing, and 24-hour video-EEG monitoring. Epilepsy was found in 22.1%. Autistic regression and mental retardation were significantly more frequent in patients with epilepsy. In a series of 72 patients (57 male, 15 female; 4–21 years of age), the overall prevalence of epilepsy was 7.4% in primary autism and 55% in secondary [39]. A population-based cohort found at least a 38% occurrence of epilepsy in subjects up to age 38 years [4]. A retrospective follow-up study on a clinical series of 130 individuals aged 18–35 years diagnosed with autism in childhood found epilepsy in 25% [42]. A recent review considered 13 studies published since 2000 that examined the prevalence of epilepsy in ASD populations (total samples and special populations within samples, such as those with and without intellectual disability or male versus female), taking into account sample characteristics (samples size, age, ascertainment methods, diagnoses, whether the samples included nonidiopathic autism) [6]. Nine population-based studies reported epilepsy prevalence with a median of 17% and a range of 5–26%. Another long-term follow-up study of a population-based sample reported a substantially higher lifetime epilepsy prevalence of 38%.

Studies of children with autism found an overall prevalence of interictal **epileptiform EEG abnormalities** ranging from 6 to 64% (a prevalence significantly greater than the 2.4–3.5% reported in normal children): the lowest rates when only routine EEG was used and the highest with 24-hour ambulatory EEG [4,38,43,44]. Studies have shown that a history of autistic regression versus nonregression does not predict the presence of EEG epileptiform activity. Our data [38] also do not support the hypothesis that epileptiform abnormalities occurring during wakefulness or sleep EEG play a significant role in autistic regression or in the severity of impairment in cognitive or emotional functioning. The type and localization of sleep epileptiform EEG abnormalities were different than those found in LKS or electrical status epilepticus in sleep (ESES); discharges were focal with maximum (26 from 42) without tendency to continuous generalized spike and wave. There are studies showing normalization of EEGs with valproic acid treatment in children with autism, but none showing whether future epilepsy can be prevented by treatment or if there is a positive influence on the core symptoms and prognosis of autism, so whether treating subclinical epileptic spikes in this population improves behavior remains dubious [37,41,44].

Epileptiform abnormality rates are approximately 30% in ASD patients without clinical seizures, although one video-EEG monitoring study found interictal epileptiform abnormalities in 59% [6]. A retrospective review of almost 900 children with ASD who had no known history of epilepsy found 61% with epileptiform EEG activity in sleep [6]. In another study of 57 children (86% male) with ASD (mean age 82 ± 36.2 months), the frequency of interictal epileptiform EEG abnormalities was 24.6% and the frequency of epilepsy 14.2% [5].

Interictal cognitive disabilities (ICD), epilepsy, and autism can result from the same pathophysiological mechanisms (e.g., genetic impairment of synaptic plasticity resulting in a developmental imbalance of excitation and inhibition) [8,45]. This occurs in the developing brain in disorders with common dual features of ASD, ICD, and epilepsy, such as fragile X syndrome (FXS), Rett syndrome, cyclin-dependent kinase-like 5 (CDKL5) mutations, neuroligin mutations, and "interneuronopathies" resulting from aristaless-related homeobox, X-linked (ARX) and neuropilin 2 (NRP2) gene mutations. **Four main clusters of autism subtypes** were differentiated by cluster analysis based on structural MRI data in 64 autistic patients, and the lowest frequency of epilepsy was found to correlate with the least abnormal psychomotor development during the first year of life and with the largest size of amygdalo-hippocampal complex and the least abnormal visual response on the Childhood Autism Rating Scale (CARS), cluster 2 [46]. In contrast, cluster 4 showed hypogenesis of the corpus callosum, small amygdala, and caput of the nucleus caudatus, the most abnormal visual response in CARS, abnormal psychomotor development during the first year of life, and the highest frequency of epilepsy. **TSC has been described as a model of common mechanisms** of cognitive impairment, autism, and epilepsy [46], including genetic, electrophysiological, and neuroanatomical risk factors. ASDs were diagnosed in 40% of 103 patients in this TSC cohort; individuals with ASD had earlier age at seizure onset and a lower IQ (p < 0.001). There was a trend for patients with ASD to have the largest tuber burden in the left temporal lobe and mutations inactivating the hamartia domain of the *TSC2* gene, suggesting that autism in TSC may be associated with early and persistent seizure activity in specific brain regions, particularly in the left temporal lobe, where the areas responsible for social communication are localized. Inherited **mitochondrial dysfunction** is another possible common pathophysiological mechanism for comorbid autism, epilepsy, and cognitive impairment [59,60].

Conclusion

Poor QOL in patients suffering from autism and epilepsy mostly results from the high incidence of intellectual and language impairment. A genetically determined disorder of synaptogenesis, plasticity, and brain connectivity appears to be the common underlying pathology in the majority of these patients. In a relatively smaller group of patients, an epileptic process within the limbic structures contributes to the development of autistic symptomatology. In these patients, early antiepileptic therapy may reduce both epileptic and autistic symptoms and thus improve QOL. Abnormal epileptiform EEG activity is not assumed to be the cause of autism and, therefore, antiepileptic treatment is unlikely to improve the QOL of patients with ASD having abnormal EEGs without a clinical history of epilepsy.

References

1 Volkmar FR, Nelson DS: Seizure disorders in autism. *J Am Acad Child Adolesc Psychiatry* 1990; **29**:127–129.

2 Tuchman RF, Rapin I: Regression in pervasive developmental disorders: seizures and epileptiform electroencephalogram correlates. *Pediatrics* 1997; **99**:560–566.

3 Deonna T, Roulet E: Autistic spectrum disorder: evaluating a possible contributing or causal role of epilepsy. *Epilepsia* 2006; **47(Suppl. 2)**:79–82.

4 Danielsson S, Gillberg IC, Billstedt E et al.: Epilepsy in young adults with autism: a prospective population-based follow-up study of 120 individuals diagnosed in childhood. *Epilepsia* 2005; **46**:918–923.

5 Ekincia O, Ayşe RA, Işık U et al.: EEG abnormalities and epilepsy in autistic spectrum disorders: clinical and familial correlates. *Epilepsy & Behavior* 2010; **17(2)**: 178–182.

6 Spence SJ, Schneider MI: The role of epilepsy and epileptiform EEGs in autism spectrum disorders. *Pediatr Res* 2009; **65(6)**:599–606.

7 Brooks-Kaya A: Molecular mechanisms of cognitive and behavioral comorbidities of epilepsy in children. *Epilepsia* 2011; **52(Suppl. 1)**:13–20.

8 Ye H, Liu J, Wu JY: Cell adhesion molecules and their involvement in autism spectrum disorder. *Neurosignals* 2010; **18**:62–71.

9 American Psychiatric Association: *Diagnostic and Statistical Manual of Mental Disorders*, 4 edn (DSM-IV). American Psychiatric Association: Washington, DC, 1994.

10 Rapin I: Autistic regression and disintegrative disorder: how important the role of epilepsy? *Sem Ped Neurol*, 1995; **2**: 278–285.

11 Rogers SJ, DiLalla DL: Age of symptom onset in young children with pervasive developmental disorders. *J Am Acad Child Adolesc Psychiatry* 1990; **29**:863–872.

12 Baird G, Charman T, Pickles A et al.: Regression, developmental trajectory and associated problems in disorders in the autism spectrum: the SNAP study. *Journal of Autism and Developmental Disorders*, (2008). **38**, 1827–1836.

13 Gillberg C, Coleman M. Autism and medical disorders: a review of the literature. *Dev Med Child Neurol* 1996; **38(3)**: 191–202.

14 Arndt TL, Stodgell CJ, Rodier PM: The teratology of autism. *Int J Dev Neurosci* 2005; **23(2–3)**:189–199.

15 Johansson M, Gillberg C, Rastam M: Autism spectrum conditions in individuals with Mobius sequence, CHARGE syndrome and oculo-auriculo-vertebral spectrum: diagnostic aspects. *Res Dev Disabil* 2010; **31**:9–24.

16 Miles HL, Hofman PL, Cutfield WS: Fetal origins of adult disease: a paediatric perspective. *Rev Endocr Metab Disord* 2005; **6(4)**:261.

17 Volkmar FR, Pauls D: *Autism Lancet* 2003; **362(9390)**: 1133–1141.

18 Bailey A, Le Couter A, Gottesman I et al.: Autism as a strongly genetic disorder, evidence from a British twin study. *Psychol Med* 1995; **25**:63–78.

19 Acosta MT, Pearl PL: The neurobiology of autism: new pieces of the puzzle. *Curr Neurol Neurosci Rep* 2003; **3(2)**:149–156.

20 Hughes JR: Autism: the first firm finding = underconnectivity? *Epilepsy & Behavior* 2007; **11(1)**:20–22.

21 Kulisek R, Hrncir Z, Hrdlicka M: Nonlinear analysis of the sleep EEG in children with pervasive developmental disorder. *Neuro Endocrinol Lett* 2008; **29(4)**:512–517.

22 Casanova M, van Kooten IA, Switala AE et al.: Minicolumnar abnormalities in autism. *Acta Neuropathologica* 2002; **112(3)**:287–303.

23 Oberman LM, Pineda JA, Ramachandran VS. The human mirror neuron system: a link between action observation and social skills. *Soc Cogn Affect Neurosci* 2007; **2(1)**:62–66.

24 St. Aubin G: Landau-Kleffner Syndrome is a form of epilepsy that can mimic Autism. http://www.examiner.com/article/landau-kleffner-syndrome-is-a-form-of-epilepsy-that-can-mimic-autism (last accessed July 15, 2014).

25 Mantovani JF: Autistic regression and Landau-Kleffner syndrome: progress or confusion? *Dev Med Child Neurol* 2000; **42(5)**:349–353.

26 Gordon N: Acquired aphasia in childhood: the Landau–Kleffner syndrome. *Dev Med Child Neurol* 1990; **32**: 267–274.

27 Besag FM: Childhood epilepsy in relation to mental handicap and behavioural disorders. *J Child Psychol Psychiatry* 2002; **43(1)**:103–131.

28 Davies S, Heyman I: A population survey of mental health problems in children with epilepsy. *Dev Med Child Neurol* 2003; **45(5)**:292–295.

29 Berg AT, Plioplys S, Tuchman R: Risk and correlates of autism spectrum disorder in children with epilepsy: a community-based study. *J Child Neurol* 2011; **26(5)**: 540–547.

30 Steffenburg U, Hagberg G, Kyllerman M: Characteristics of seizures in a population-based series of mentally retarded children with active epilepsy. *Epilepsia* 1996; **37(9)**: 850–856.

31 Boel MJ: Behavioural and neuropsychological problems in refractory paediatric epilepsies. *Eur J Paediatr Neurol* 2004; **8(6)**:291–297.

32 Clarke DF, Roberts W, Daraksan M et al.: The prevalence of autistic spectrum disorder in children surveyed in a tertiary care epilepsy clinic. *Epilepsia* 2005; **46(12)**:1970–1977.

33 McLellan A, Davies S, Heyman I et al.: Psychopathology in children with epilepsy before and after temporal lobe resection. *Dev Med Child Neurol* 2005; **47(10)**:666–672.

34 Hançerli S, Çalışkan M, Mukaddes NM et al.: Autistic spectrum in West syndrome. *Turk Arch Ped* 2011; **46**:68–74.

35 Li BM, Liu XR, Yi YH et al.: Autism in Dravet syndrome: prevalence, features, and relationship to the clinical characteristics of epilepsy and mental retardation. *Epilepsy Behav* 2011; **21(3)**:291–295.

36 Matsuo M, Maeda T, Ishii K et al.: Characterization of childhood-onset complex partial seizures associated with autism spectrum disorder. *Epilepsy Behav* 2011; **20(3)**: 524–527.

37 Sansa G, Carlson C, Doyle W et al.: Medically refractory epilepsy in autism. *Epilepsia* 2011; **52**:1071–1075.

38 Hrdlicka M, Komarek V, Propper L et al.: Not EEG abnormalities but epilepsy is associated with autistic regression and mental functioning in childhood autism. *Eur Child Adolesc Psychiatry* 2004; **13**:209–213.

39 Pavone P, Incorpora G, Fiumara A et al.: Epilepsy is not a prominent feature of primary autism. *Neuropediatrics* 2004; **35(4)**:207–210.

40 Gabis L, Pomeroy J, Andriola MR: Autism and epilepsy: cause, consequence, comorbidity, or coincidence? *Epilepsy Behav* 2005; **7**:652–656.

41 Hughes JR, Melyn M: EEG and seizures in autistic children and adolescents: further findings with therapeutic implications. *Clin EEG Neurosci* 2005; **36**:15–20.

42 Hara H: Autism and epilepsy: a retrospective follow-up study. *Brain Dev* 2007; **29**:486–490.

43 Chez MG, Chang M, Krasne V et al.: Frequency of epileptiform EEG abnormalities in a sequential screening of autistic patients with no known clinical epilepsy from 1996 to 2005. *Epilepsy Behav* 2006; **8**:267–271.

44 Kim HL, Donnelly JH, Tournay AE et al.: Absence of seizures despite high prevalence of epileptiform EEG abnormalities in children with autism monitored in a tertiary care center. *Epilepsia* 2006; **47**:394–398.

45 Brooks-Kayal J Molecular mechanisms of cognitive and behavioural comorbidities of epilepsy in children. *Epilepsia* 2011; **52(Suppl. 1)**:13–20.

46 Hrdlicka M, Dudova I, Beranova I et al.: Subtypes of autism by cluster analysis based on structural MRI data. *Eur Child Adolesc Psychiatry* 2005; **14**:138–144.

47 Curatolo P, Moavero R: Autism in tuberous sclerosis: are risk factors identifiable and preventable? *Future Neurology* 2011; **6(4)**:451–454.

48 Filiano JJ, Gpldental MJ: Mitochondrial dysfunction in patients with hypotonia, epilepsy, autism, and developmental delay: HEADD syndrome. *Child Neurol* 2002; **17**: 435–439.

49 Holtzman D: Autistic spectrum disorders and mitochondrial encephalopathies. *Acta Pædiatrica* 2008; **97**:859–860.

50 Frye RE, Rossigno DL: Mitochondrial dysfunction can connect the diverse medical symptoms associated with autism spectrum disorders. *Pediatr Res* 2011; **69**:41–47.

CHAPTER 7

Cognitive rehabilitation strategies in epilepsy

Cher Stephenson[1] and Robert D. Jones[2]

[1] *Stephenson Counseling LLC, USA*
[2] *Department of Neurology, University of Iowa, USA*

Introduction

Pharmacologic treatments for the management of epilepsy have increased in number over time but progress in neuropsychological/cognitive rehabilitation has received somewhat less attention as an ameliorative intervention in complications of epilepsy, including cognitive, affective, and social deficits. This chapter will provide insight into the primary deficit areas seen in the epilepsies and an introduction to compensatory strategies utilized to minimize the impact of these deficits on daily life, maximize functioning, and improve quality of life (QOL) for persons living with epilepsy. Factors related to "the burden of normalcy" will also be explored.

Background

Epilepsy is one of the most common neurological conditions, impacting approximately 1.4% of the US population, or 2.3 million people [1,2]. It is a chronic and often disabling disorder in several domains of life, including cognitive, affective, and social areas. People living with epilepsy have more cognitive and behavioral problems than those without the condition. Cognitive deficits in epilepsy are varied, but those generally captured in neuropsychological evaluation include the domains of memory, attention, processing speed, language, and executive functions [3]. When considering the implications of these deficits for real-world functioning, multiple factors affect the extent to which any given set of difficulties may be present (e.g., age of onset,

type and severity of seizure, well-controlled versus refractory, pharmacotherapy side effects, comorbid psychiatric diagnoses, and coping/skills development) [4]. Deficits associated with epilepsy are evident not only during seizures but especially during interictal periods [5]. Despite awareness of the impact these deficits have on individuals with epilepsy, cognitive rehabilitation interventions are not as commonly applied as they could and should be in epilepsy patients, since alleviating the impact of deficits on a patient's daily functioning and psychosocial opportunities may improve their QOL. The efficacy of cognitive rehabilitation has been well demonstrated in other neurologic conditions (traumatic brain injury, multiple sclerosis, Parkinson's disease, demyelinating diseases, and encephalopathies), but use in epilepsy has been more limited [6–8].

Cognitive rehabilitation

Given the multiple cognitive domains that can be affected by epilepsy and the cognitive side effects of antiepileptic medications, rehabilitation planning must necessarily be customized to the needs of the individual. This makes implementing cognitive rehabilitation interventions a challenging task.

Historically, cognitive rehabilitation was exclusively focused on remediation of brain dysfunction (i.e., return of function). More recently, cognitive rehabilitation has focused on behavioral compensation to reduce everyday difficulties encountered as a result of brain dysfunction. Cognitive rehabilitation may be defined as "the therapeutic process of increasing or improving

Epilepsy and the Interictal State: Co-Morbidities and Quality of Life, First Edition.
Edited by Erik K. St. Louis, David M. Ficker, and Terence J. O'Brien.
© 2015 John Wiley & Sons, Ltd. Published 2015 by John Wiley & Sons, Ltd.

an individual's capacity to process and use incoming information so as to allow increased functioning in everyday life" [9]. A holistic approach to patient care is encouraged.

When initiating cognitive rehabilitation with people living with epilepsy, the influence of epilepsy-related and non-epilepsy-related variables such as neuropsychological factors, psychosocial factors, environmental factors, and societal issues on functioning and QOL must be considered [10]. Individualized treatment planning and execution of strategies offers a better fit to the real-world conditions, needs, and wants of the patient. When exploring deficit areas, both the patient's subjective complaints (i.e., their perception of their deficits) and their objective deficits (based on thorough evaluation) have importance and value, as both may contribute to a worsening in functioning and emotional well-being. Perceptions also influence focus, motivation, effort, and selection of tasks or activities [3].

Assessment

Background
Rehabilitation is preceded by assessment, which serves to outline the strengths, weaknesses, and needs of any given patient with epilepsy. Neuropsychological assessment of patients with epilepsy must necessarily assume a broad-based approach, given the myriad of problems that such patients may experience [11,12]. For example, particularly in cases of focal brain dysfunction, patients may experience specific difficulties with an area of cognition such as memory, language, executive functions, or vision. The prevalence of psychological and psychiatric disturbance necessitates use of examination materials aimed at depression, anxiety, and other aspects of psychological disturbances. There are often medication side effects that must be accounted for, especially in medication-resistant epilepsy patients on drug polytherapy. Finally, given the practical daily difficulties associated with epilepsy, such as restricted driving privileges, the possible need for supervision, and restricted opportunities, the examination of a patient's QOL is an important part of an assessment.

Connection to rehabilitation
In neuropsychological assessment of epilepsy, the referral question is a primary consideration guiding the nature of the examination and the tailoring of specific testing for each individual patient. For presurgical assessment, the primary interests of the examination might be localization of a "focal" cognitive deficit, while examination for medication adverse effects would instead emphasize tests of attention and processing speed. Since rehabilitation may focus on accommodation of daily problems associated with epilepsy, assessment of psychological and psychiatric problems and QOL is typically the primary interest of the examination.

Approach
Although there are several schools of assessment, a broad-based approach is needed, with flexibility to attend to the particular needs and concerns of the patient [13,14]. In our examinations of patients with epilepsy, we have utilized the Iowa Benton Model, which stresses the use of a small core battery of measures followed by flexible assessment, which varies based on numerous other factors, including the referral question, the patient's complaints, and the results of the core battery. Examinations may take anywhere between 1 and 6 hours, depending on the nature of the referral question, the patient, and other factors. In the context of patients with epilepsy who will be receiving neuropsychological rehabilitation, examinations are typically oriented toward emotional aspects of the conditions, identification of cognitive deficits and cognitive strengths, and the extent to which the underlying medical condition affects the patient's daily activities and QOL.

Monitoring
Patients with epilepsy may be seen on multiple occasions and at different points in time, depending on the clinical situation. For example, a patient who is to undergo surgery will be seen both pre- and post-surgical intervention, for assessment of possible changes, and for adjustments in the rehabilitation approach. Patients are regularly seen at annual or biannual periods to monitor changes in cognition and emotional functioning. The frequency of evaluations is guided by the patient's clinical needs as they are perceived by the rehabilitation counselor, in addition to the underlying medical condition and previous psychological assessments.

Common measures

A large armamentarium of assessment tools is available in the assessment of patients with epilepsy. Common measures are shown in Box 7.1, but these are constantly evolving based on new scientific findings, updated instruments, and new domains of inquiry.

Nonepileptic events and psychological factors

Diagnostic assessment of patients with epilepsy must take into account multiple aspects of the patient's examination. A significant minority of patients may have nonepileptic events or "pseudoseizures" [17], which may be caused by psychological factors. Differential diagnosis of which specific factors is helpful for rehabilitation. Nonepileptic events may be caused by stress, including symptoms of anxiety or depression, or by a conversion or somatization disorder. If pseudoseizures are volitional, malingering should be included in the differential diagnosis. Depending on the results of neuropsychological and psychological testing, the approach to rehabilitation will be significantly different in each of these cases.

Comorbidities and dual diagnoses

Dual diagnoses of both epilepsy and related but distinct other conditions is common, including both nonepileptic events and psychiatric comorbidities [18]. The nature of the neuropsychological assessment is guided in part by the results of previous testing, including medical assessments. In patients diagnosed with nonepileptic events or "pseudoseizures," the nature of the neuropsychological assessment will be appropriately aimed at possible underlying etiologies for these events, which will help to guide rehabilitation. The results of long-term video-EEG monitoring may be helpful in determining the nature of the assessment. In addition, patients with nonepileptic events frequently have comorbid epileptic seizures, complicating the diagnostic picture and leading to more complicated interventions from a rehabilitation perspective. Finally, comorbid psychiatric conditions may well need attention; these can be identified through interview and psychological assessment, with appropriate referral to psychiatric specialists.

Box 7.1 Common measures of assessment used in the Benton neuropsychology laboratory. Note: References for tests can be found in [15,16].

- Temporal Orientation Questionnaire
- Orientation to Personal Information
- Orientation to Place
- Presidential Face Naming
- Wechsler Adult Intelligence Scale IV:
  ○ Similarities
  ○ Digit span
  ○ Vocabulary
  ○ Arithmetic
  ○ Information
  ○ Letter number sequencing
  ○ Comprehension
  ○ Block design
  ○ Matrix reasoning
  ○ Symbol search
  ○ Visual puzzles
  ○ Coding
- Wide Range Achievement Test IV:
  ○ Reading
- Rey Auditory Verbal Learning Test
- Wechsler Memory Scale III:
  ○ Faces
  ○ Logical memory
- Complex Figure Test
- Benton Visual Retention Test
- Ratings of Speech and Language:
  ○ Word finding
  ○ Fluency
  ○ Paraphasias
  ○ Articulation
  ○ Prosody
  ○ Comprehension
- Controlled Oral Word Association Test
- Boston Naming Test
- MAE Sentence Repetition
- Token Test
- Visual Acuity Screen
- Facial Discrimination Test
- Judgment of Line Orientation Test
- Grooved Pegboard Test
- Trail Making Test
- Wisconsin Card Sorting Test
- Beck Depression Inventory
- Beck Anxiety Inventory
- Minnesota Multiphasic Personality Inventory II
- Iowa Scales of Personality Change
- Quality of Life in Epilepsy

Primary cognitive complaints

The most common patient-reported cognitive complaints in epilepsy are in the realms of memory, attention, and slowed processing speed. Localized and generalized epilepsy patients perform worse than controls in varied cognitive domains [19]. Between 20 and 50% of refractory epilepsy patients have memory problems, and over half of epilepsy patients referred for neuropsychological evaluation report difficulties in daily living as a result of memory problems [3]. However, subjective memory complaints may reflect differing degrees of depression rather than actual memory impairments, especially in those with temporal-lobe epilepsy and depression, and memory performance may improve after treatment of depression [4,19]. The most common memory complaints in patients are similar to those in the general population, but typically more severe (i.e., forgetting names, word-finding problems, forgetting new verbal information, and forgetting plans) [3].

In general, repetition and rehearsal in new learning are beneficial; this is a fundamental principle of cognitive rehabilitation planning and the application of various compensatory strategies. One specific benefit of cognitive rehabilitation participation is a positive interactive impact of one intervention on other areas of deficit [20]. For example, the use of external aids for the management of memory difficulties often also has an ameliorative impact on problems with attention and executive functioning. Opinions vary on the benefit of utilizing internal versus external memory strategies. Determining what works best for each individual is important, taking into account their deficit areas and strengths, as well as their own natural inclination for particular compensatory strategies and skills.

Memory

Cognitive rehabilitation for memory deficits utilizes external aids, environmental modifications, and cuing. Strategies for addressing memory deficits vary based on the type of memory impairment, but efforts are made to use a combination of strategies when possible for maximum benefit [21]. Environmental modifications include organizational strategies, strategic placement of items in the environment, and logical categorization or association of new with previously learned information. External aids include a variety of calendar and agenda systems (paper/pencil or electronic format), checklists, to-do lists, verbal and visual cues, sequenced instructions, and chunking of information. Self-monitoring (internalized) memory strategies include repetition of routines, acronyms, associations, and visual imagery. Two strategies used in remembering reading material that can be generalized to other life situations are PQRST (preview, question, read, state, test) and SQR3 (survey, question, read, recall, review). All strategies will require adequate training and repetition to become an integrated and automatic part of daily life routines [3,5,7,20,21].

Attention

Attention is a foundation of cognitive functioning and attentional deficits are often present in people with epilepsy [5]. Attention is quite susceptible to disruption related to brain dysfunction but tends to benefit quite well from treatment strategies. Strategies for reducing the negative impact of attention defects on functioning include attention process training (APT), use of external aids, environmental modifications, and self-management strategies. APT is a specific process-oriented therapy that aims to improve sustained, alternating, and divided attention [7]. External aids include the use of written or electronic systems to logically order tasks, stay on-task, track task completion, and enable cueing. External aids can include calendar/agenda systems, list-making, note-taking, and verbal or visual reminders. Environmental modifications include environment organization, reduction of distractions, allowing time to refocus between shifts in tasks, and chunking like items or tasks together. Self-management involves pacing (making best use of time, increasing time spent on-task, gradually increasing task complexity as tolerated), associations (pairing tasks that fit well together with already established routines), and self-talk (walking oneself through tasks from beginning to completion) [7,20,22]. In the rehabilitation setting, attentional difficulties also create problems with information processing speed.

Processing speed

Generally, slowed thinking/processing speed impacts all other cognitive and communication capacities, increasing the risk of emotional and behavioral reactions in coping with problematic educational, occupational, and social environments [8]. If slowed processing speed is the primary deficit, simply extending the time allowed to respond or to complete tasks, offering step-by-step structure to tasks, making use of repetition, and slowing the rate at which information is presented or expected in response can be beneficial across many settings [20].

Other deficit areas

Other possible deficit areas must be explored in order to maximize functioning and QOL. In the epilepsies, deficits in general intellect, executive functions, and language are common. These deficits tend to vary based on type of epilepsy, location of epileptogenic lesion, side effects of medications, and severity of mood symptoms. A pattern of relatively generalized cognitive dysfunction has been described in patients with temporal-lobe epilepsy. General intellect deficits that are resistant to rehabilitation and are critical for daily activities or roles may require specific accommodations for academic and occupational functioning. Environmental modifications and external aids utilized for deficits in attention or memory are often able to minimize the negative impact of executive dysfunction on daily living.

One intervention specific to executive dysfunction is Goal Management Training (GMT). This strategy is utilized to assist individuals with task completion. It follows a five-stage process to help patients engaged in a specific multistep task intentionally consider each step. It offers patients training in the use of an internal dialogue (i.e., self-talk) to facilitate goal selection, task breakdown and sequence, follow-through, problem-solving (mid-process, if difficulties arise), and monitoring of outcome (to allow revisions to be made as needed). The stages involved in GMT are: 1) **stop** (having the patient ask themselves what they are doing: "the main goal") and **define** (defining the specific task at hand); 2) **list** (writing out each individual step needed to complete the main goal); 3) **learn** (asking themselves if they know each of the steps in the task); 4) **do it** (performing the entire task); and 5) **check** (asking themselves if they are doing what they planned to do and in the order they listed). This particular strategy has been noted to be most effective in persons who have some level of awareness and insight into their deficits and those who are motivated to improve their functioning [7]. The purpose

of all strategies for executive dysfunction is to address challenges with planning, sequencing, organizing, initiation, follow-through, and awareness [20].

Language is an essential part of human interaction and addressing language complaints helps minimize disruptions in social interaction and emotional reactions. Strategies for language include allowing ample time to respond, use of circumlocution (talking around the word), visualization, gestures, written format, hints/cues from others, asking questions, and use of synonyms or antonyms [20]. Referral to speech therapists can be critical. When establishing expectations for communication, longitudinal changes over time must be considered, especially following surgery (i.e., patients may initially be worse in some cognitive and emotional domains, with variability in the clinical course and extent of recovery, since some patients identify almost immediate improvement while others may have long-term residual deficits). Some cognitive domains may improve and others decline following surgical intervention and repeated neuropsychological assessments and ongoing rehabilitation efforts are necessary in many patients.

Other important factors

Cognitive deficits are not the only factors contributing to patient reports of poor functioning or poor adjustment. Psychosocial factors are a significant aspect of disability for people living with epilepsy, including mood state (depression and anxiety), sleep, stress, self-esteem, stigma, and occupational status. Assisting patients in learning to compensate for cognitive deficits, seeking support and treatment (pharmacotherapy and psychotherapy) for mood symptoms, appreciating the value of basic health maintenance (adequate and regular sleep schedules, stress-management skills, healthy eating habits), and fostering an attitude of self-efficacy and empowerment has been shown to have a positive accumulative effect on functioning, treatment compliance, and QOL in the long term [23].

The value of exploring the interaction between the person, brain dysfunction, skill set, and life context has recently been encouraged in treatment interventions. In order for people to adjust well to a life with epilepsy (or a life of becoming epilepsy-free), addressing these various psychosocial, psychological, sociological, and cognitive factors will be vital to maximizing functioning and developing a more positive sense of self [6,9,21].

Health care providers should recognize that people with epilepsy may be quite complicated from a psychosocial perspective. Patients are often impacted by their upbringing: how supportive their family has been, what opportunities were provided for inclusion in typical rites of passage (sleepovers, participation in competitive sports, driving, intimate relationships), and what limitations were imposed (reasonable versus overprotective and restrictive). All health care providers need to recognize that the academic and occupational functioning of an individual patient is affected by their cognitive abilities and interpersonal skills, the extent of social stigma they have experienced, and the accommodations they have been offered and utilized. These factors may help a patient to overcome possible obstacles to "normal" functioning and life experiences and may be further developed by the process of cognitive rehabilitation.

Burden of normalcy

Although one might assume that becoming seizure-free is reason to celebrate, this is not always the case. A patient may be relieved of seizures (e.g., through outgrowing a juvenile form of epilepsy or through surgical intervention) but continue to struggle in day-to-day functioning, in part due to difficulty adjusting to life without a chronic medical condition and all of the changes this brings. "The burden of normalcy" is a psychosocial syndrome in which a patient struggles with the transition from being chronically ill to well. Consideration must be given to the perceptions and expectations involved in this process and the ability of the individual and their family to cope with the role changes brought about a result of their becoming well, in order to minimize maladjustment. Exploring the psychosocial dynamics involved in chronic illness and in overcoming chronic illness is vital to decreasing the risk of developing the burden of normalcy. Psychosocial dynamics include interpersonal relationships, affective functioning, social interactions, and educational/occupational activities involved in living with (and overcoming) seizures.

When a patient decides to pursue surgical intervention for epilepsy, setting practical and realistic

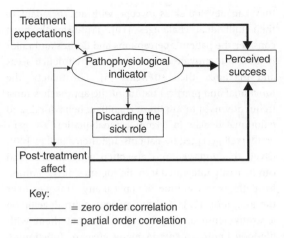

Key:
——— = zero order correlation
—— = partial order correlation

Figure 7.1 Model of perceived treatment success. Thick lines denote partial-order correlation, thin lines zero-order correlation.

expectations about the likely outcome will yield a more positive response postoperatively. For example, a person who opts for surgery might desire complete seizure freedom, decreased restrictions on activities, increased independence, increased social interactions, better educational and occupational opportunities, or decreased medication use [24]. Figure 7.1 shows a model of perceived treatment success.

Adjustment
Healthy and adaptive adjustment involves the individual's ability (and that of their family) to transition from "the sick role" to a capable and more independently functioning person. Previous restrictions may impact subsequent skill development and life experiences and new demands may affect their ability to adjust to their new status. Seizure freedom may not eliminate, and may worsen, anxiety and depression, even when reducing cognitive complaints [24]. These changes warrant close monitoring over time in order to maximize functioning and QOL.

Conclusion

For cognitive rehabilitation to be beneficial, patients need to recognize and understand their deficit areas and accept that it can be helpful for them. They also need to be provided with accurate explanations about how these deficits can impact their lives and how they can develop skills to cope with and/or adapt to their individual challenges [10]. Professionals must consider the patient's perceptions and desires and tailor treatment to provide improvement in their deficit areas and maximize their strengths [5]. Fortunately, the functional and practical nature of the approaches most frequently used to minimize cognitive, behavioral, and emotional deficits in cognitive rehabilitation are generally well accepted by patients and their families [20]. Given that interventions are often generalizable and can be easily integrated into life routines, it is common for patients to continue to apply many strategies over the long term [22]. Assisting patients with developing a strong sense of empowerment can aid them with life-long improvements in many areas of functioning and help them sustain the courage to tackle additional challenges as they occur throughout life, whether with or without epilepsy.

References

1 Strine T, Kobau R, Chapman DP et al.: Psychological distress, comorbidities, and health behaviors among US citizens with seizures: results from the 2002 National Health Interview Survey. *Epilepsia* 2005; **46(7)**:1133–1139.

2 National Institute of Neurological Diseases and Stroke (2011) Curing the epilepsies: the promise of research. Available from: http://www.ninds.nih.gov/disorders/epilepsy/epilepsy_research.htm (last accessed July 15, 2014).

3 Ponds RWHM, Hendriks M: Cognitive rehabilitation of memory problems in patients with epilepsy. *Seizure* 2006; **15**:267–273.

4 Shulman M, Barr W: Treatment of memory disorders in epilepsy. *Epilepsy Behav* 2002; **3**:S30–S34.

5 Devinsky O: Therapy for neurobehavioral disorders in epilepsy. *Epilepsia* 2004; **45(Suppl. 2)**: 34–40.

6 Helmstaedter C, Loer B, Wohlfahrt R et al.: The effects of cognitive rehabilitation on memory outcome after temporal lobe epilepsy surgery. *Epilepsy Behav* 2008; **12(3)**:402–409.

7 Sohlberg MM, Mateer CA: *Cognitive Rehabilitation: An Integrative Neuropsychological Approach*. The Guilford Press: New York, NY, 2001.

8 Engelberts NHJ, Klein M, Kasteleijn-Nolst Trenité DG et al.: The effectiveness of psychological interventions for patients with relatively well-controlled epilepsy. *Epilepsy & Behavior* 2002; **3**:420–426.

9 Prigatano GP: *Principles of Neuropsychological Rehabilitation*. Oxford University Press: New York, NY, 1999.

10 Baker GA, Goldstein LH: The dos and don'ts of neuropsychological assessment in epilepsy. *Epilepsy Behav* 2004; **5**: S77–S80.

11 Benton AL: Neuropsychological assessment. *Ann Rev Psychol* 1994; **45**:1–23.

12 Reitan RM, Wolfson D: Theoretical, methodological, and validational bases of the Halstead Reitan Neuropsychological Test Battery. In: Grant I, Adams K (eds): *Neuropsychological Assessment of Neuropsychiatric Disorders*. Oxford University Press: New York, NY, 1996.

13 Tranel D: The Iowa Benton school of neuropsychological assessment. In: Grant I, Adams K (eds): *Neuropsychological Assessment of Neuropsychiatric Disorders*. Oxford University Press: New York, NY, 1996.

14 Jones RD: Neuropsychological assessment of patients with traumatic brain injury: the Iowa Benton approach. In: Rizzo M, Tranel D: *Head Injury and Postconcussive Syndrome*. Churchill Livingstone: New York, NY, 1996.

15 Lezak M, Howieson DB, Loring DW: *Neuropsychological Assessment*. Oxford University Press: New York, NY, 2004.

16 Benton Neuropsychology Laboratory: *Manual of Operations*. Benton Neuropsychology Laboratory, Iowa City, IA, 2010.

17 Reuben M, Elger CE: Psychogenic nonepileptic seizures: review and update. *Epilepsy Behav* 2003; **4**:205–216.

18 Swinkels W, Kyuk J, van Dyck R, Spinhover P: Psychiatric comorbidity in epilepsy. *Epilepsy Behav* 2005; **7**:37–50.

19 Hermann B, Seidenberg M: Epilepsy and cognition. *Epilepsy Curr* 2007; **7(1)**:1–6.

20 Johnstone B, Stonnington HH: *Rehabilitation of Neuropsychological Disorders: A Practical Guide for Rehabilitation Professionals*. Psychology Press: Philadelphia, PA, 2001.

21 Kreutzer JS, Wehman PH: *Cognitive Rehabilitation for Persons with Traumatic Brain Injury*. Imaginart Press: Bisbee, AZ, 1991.

22 Engelberts NHJ, Klein M, Adèr HJ et al.: The effectiveness of cognitive rehabilitation for attention deficits in focal seizures: a randomized controlled study. *Epilepsia* 2002; **43(6)**:587–595.

23 Pramuka M, Hendrickson R, Zinski A, Van Cott AC: A psychosocial self-management program for epilepsy: a randomized pilot study in adults. *Epilepsy Behav* 2007; **11**:533–545.

24 Wilson SJ, Bladin PF, Saling MM: Paradoxical results in the care of chronic illness: the "burden of normalcy" as exemplified following seizure surgery. *Epilepsy Behav* 2004; **5**:13–21.

SECTION III
Adverse effects of epilepsy therapies

CHAPTER 8

Adverse effects in epilepsy: recognition, measurement, and taxonomy

Frank G. Gilliam,[1] Laura S. Snavely,[1] and Piero Perucca[2]

[1] *Department of Neurology, Penn State University, Hershey, USA*
[2] *The Montreal Neurological Institute, Canada*

Introduction

The goal of balancing adverse the side effects of a medication with its efficacy for seizures has been a primary topic in the epilepsy community since the discussion of bromide therapy by Sieveking and Locock at a meeting of the Royal Medical Society in London in 1857 [1]. Although reducing seizure rate has been the major focus of epilepsy treatment for decades, recent efforts by international health organizations have emphasized a more comprehensive approach to determining outcomes [2]. The International League Against Epilepsy (ILAE) Commission on Outcome Measurement in Epilepsy has emphasized the importance of including adverse medication effects in every study of epilepsy treatment and effects of health status [3]. This chapter will review the available evidence supporting this approach and the methods used to accurately assess, classify, and quantify clinically relevant seizure medication effects.

Assessing antiepileptic medication adverse effects: a historical perspective

The conventional means of identifying adverse medication effects has been direct questioning of the patient in the clinic setting. Although the clinician–patient encounter is necessary for delivery of optimal care,

investigators acknowledged more than 2 decades ago that more objective quantification was required to more fully understand the adverse effects of medication for epilepsy [4–6]. The VA Cooperative studies were among the first research teams to utilize a standardized inquiry into medication effects in a clinical trial, employing a questionnaire and neurological exam to estimate the adverse effects of a drug and combining this adverse-effects score with the degree of seizure control to determine a composite score for overall clinical outcome [7]. Interestingly, the composite outcome scores for carbamazepine, phenytoin, phenobarbital, and primidone were each closer to the previously determined "poor outcome" category than the good category. The authors concluded that "The outcome of this project underscores the unsatisfactory status of antiepileptic therapy with the medications currently available. Most patients whose epilepsy is reasonably controlled must tolerate some side effects. These observations emphasize the need for new AEDs and other approaches to treatment" [7].

A large European study of quality of life (QOL) in epilepsy [8] used a reliable and valid instrument, the Adverse Events Profile (AEP), to comprehensively assess patient-oriented outcomes. The sample consisted of over 5000 patients from 15 countries identified through regional epilepsy organizations. Between 38 and 55% of those taking phenytoin, carbamazepine, or valproate reported significant tiredness, difficulty concentrating, or sleepiness. These studies suggest that

Epilepsy and the Interictal State: Co-Morbidities and Quality of Life, First Edition.
Edited by Erik K. St. Louis, David M. Ficker, and Terence J. O'Brien.

many antiepileptic medications cause problematic side effects in a substantial proportion of patients. Although some clinical studies indicate better tolerability of some newer drugs compared to more established medications, this is not consistent across all agents and no drugs are without any adverse effects [9].

The impact of adverse medication effects on QOL has been evaluated in several studies in the past decade. An early investigation of a large sample of outpatients in a tertiary epilepsy center found a very strong correlation of the AEP with the Quality of Life in Epilepsy-89 (QOLIE-89), which was later replicated as illustrated in Figure 8.1 [10]. Interestingly, there was no significant association of self-reported seizure rate with QOL, as shown in Figure 8.2. Another study demonstrated that the QOLIE-89 was more strongly correlated with adverse effects of seizure medications than comorbid symptoms of depression, as indicated in Figure 8.3 [11]. The combination of adverse medication effects and depression together explained 72% of the variance in QOLIE-89 scores in a large sample of epilepsy patients from five academic medical centers in the United States.

Available instruments for assessment of seizure medication adverse effects

Several instruments have been developed to assess seizure medication adverse effects in a reliable and valid manner. In the VA Cooperative randomized trials, adverse effects were determined by a standardized neurological exam and interview [7,12]. This method was comprehensive and thorough but required more time to complete than was practical for most clinicians to utilize regularly in clinic settings. The Neurotoxicity Scale, a self-report instrument used to assess the central nervous system (CNS) effects of common seizure medications, has been validated [13]. Small group interviews were utilized to develop a relatively brief but comprehensive assessment of all types of common adverse effects of seizure medications [14], the AEP, which had excellent psychometric properties of reliability and validity and was demonstrated to be easy to use in systematic evaluations of large samples of epilepsy patients [8,14].

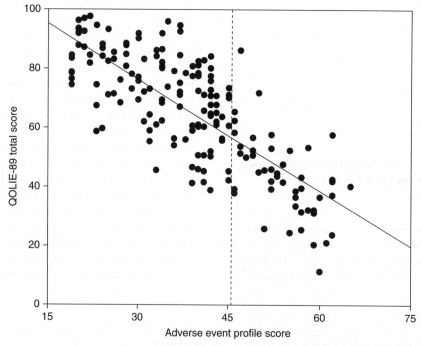

Figure 8.1 Scatterplot of baseline Quality of Life in Epilepsy-89 (QOLIE-89) scores with baseline Adverse Event Profile (AEP) scores. Source: Gilliam et al., 2004 [10]. Reproduced with permission of Lippincott Williams & Wilkins.

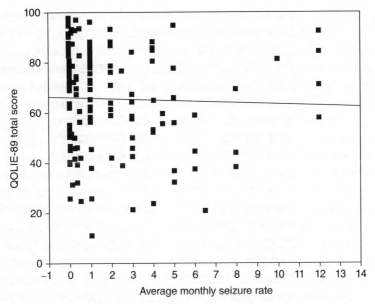

Figure 8.2 Comparison of baseline Quality of Life in Epilepsy-89 (QOLIE-89) score with baseline average monthly seizure rates. Source: Gilliam et al., 2004 [10]. Reproduced with permission of Lippincott Williams & Wilkins.

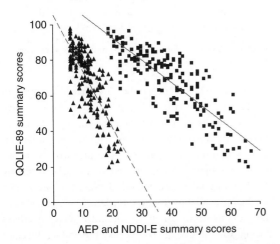

Figure 8.3 Comparison of Quality of Life in Epilepsy-89 (QOLIE-89) scores with Adverse Event Profile (AEP) score and Neurological Disorders Depression Inventory for Epilepsy (NDDI-E) score. Source: Gilliam et al., 2006 [11]. Reproduced with permission of Elsevier.

Classification and taxonomy of adverse seizure medication effects

Medication side effects have typically been presented in clinical studies as lists of symptoms or medical problems [9,15]. This approach can cause difficulty in interpreting the rates of certain categories of symptoms and in communicating the risks of adverse effects to patients. For example, most clinical trials of newer drugs list dizziness and vertigo as separate entities, when they are both very likely to describe the same patient experience. Similarly, unsteadiness and ataxia are often included as separate problems. This approach may also limit the understanding of the pharmacological basis of adverse effects, which is necessary to design improved compounds with reduced potential for specific common effects such as sedation, dizziness, fatigue, and poor concentration.

A recent study utilized a statistical approach to categorize adverse effects of seizure medications in a more understandable manner that is clinically relevant [15]. A more rational approach to classification may also facilitate advances in the pharmacology of adverse effects and lead to development of medications with less toxicity to specific neuronal aggregates subserving functions related to adverse effects. The study analyzed the items in the AEP from 200 patients in a tertiary epilepsy clinic [15]. After evaluating rates of specific adverse effects as listed in Figure 8.4, the investigators determined correlations of each item with the other, as illustrated in Figure 8.5. Factor analysis then demonstrated which items correlated with each other, identifying categories

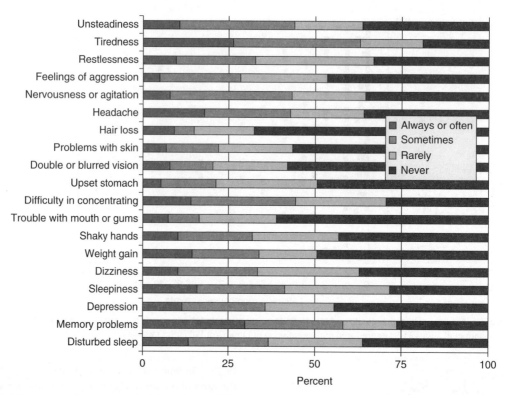

Figure 8.4 Percentage of occurrence of adverse effects included in the Adverse Event Profile (AEP) questionnaire. Source: Perucca et al., 2009 [15]. Reproduced with permission of Lippincott Williams & Wilkins.

of adverse effects that aggregate and may have potential to aid the study of the neurobiology of symptoms arising from dysfunction in specific neuronal systems. Figure 8.6 shows the radial plot of the segregation of individual adverse effects into more general classes. The classes of adverse effects were neurobiologically plausible and clinically relevant; these classes were cognition/coordination, sleep, tegument/mucosa, mood/emotion, and weight/cephalgia.

Clinical utility of systematic screening for adverse effects

Another study evaluated the clinical utility of the AEP in the outpatient epilepsy clinic setting [5]. As illustrated in Figure 8.7, the investigators attempted to screen a consecutive sample of epilepsy patients to identify 60 subjects who scored in the predetermined "toxic" range of >45. Only 200 patients were screened in order

to identify 62 subjects, indicating that over 30% of the screened outpatients were experiencing excessive adverse effects. The scatterplot of the correlation of increased adverse effect burden with worsened QOL is again presented in Figure 8.1. The protocol then randomized subjects to either their neurologist receiving the AEP to guide management decisions or the profile not being available to the clinician. The participating neurologists were asked to minimize adverse effects during the following 16 weeks if possible, without risking worsened seizure control, using their professional judgment. No other instructions were given. The results indicate that the AEP allows significant reductions in the toxic burden of seizure medications, as shown in Figure 8.8. Significantly more subjects in the AEP-available group had a >15 point improvement in AEP score during the course of the trial. Furthermore, Figure 8.9 shows this degree of improvement was associated with an average increase in QOLIE-89 composite score of 21 points at the conclusion of the trial. Use of

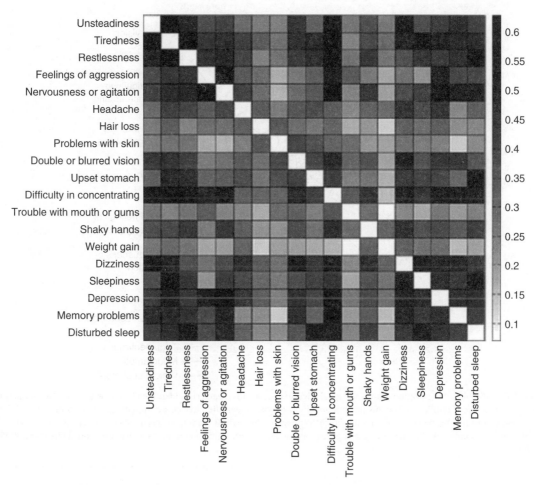

Figure 8.5 Correlations among the adverse effects listed in the Adverse Event Profile (AEP) questionnaire for the entire cohort. Correlation strength is indicated by a gray scale (right bar of the y axis), ranging from white (r = 0.05, lowest correlation) to black (r = 0.63, highest correlation). As shown, many of the correlations are significant. Source: Perucca et al., 2009 [15]. Reproduced with permission of Lippincott Williams & Wilkins.

the AEP resulted in a 2.8-fold increase in alteration of a seizure medication. Eighteen different combinations of seizure medications were used, indicating that tailoring of the medication regimen to the patients' unique situation was needed to improve outcomes. Seizure rates did not significantly change in either group and no patient had an unexpected generalized tonic–clonic seizure during the period of drug alteration to minimize adverse effects.

In summary, adverse medication effects appear to be the single most important factor in determining QOL in pharmacoresistant epilepsy, much more so than seizure rates [16]. The combination of medication side effects and comorbid mood disorders explains the large majority of variance in QOL and thus it is pertinent for the treating clinician to accurately assess and effectively address the patient's medication burden in order to maximize QOL. Use of reliable and valid instruments to systematically assess adverse effects in clinical care and research should allow improvement in individual outcomes and provide a platform for future advances in epilepsy care.

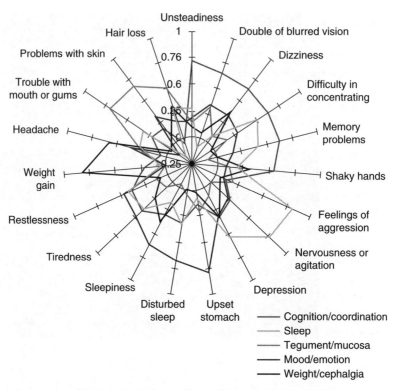

Figure 8.6 Radial plot of segregation of the individual adverse effects within each class identified by factor analysis. Factor analysis of the 19 Adverse Event Profile (AEP) items (represented by the spokes) identified five classes of segregation: cognition/coordination, sleep, tegument/mucosa, mood/emotion, and weight/cephalgia. The highest loading on each spoke depicts the specific class into which the corresponding AEP item is segregated. Source: Perucca et al., 2009 [15]. Reproduced with permission of Lippincott Williams & Wilkins.

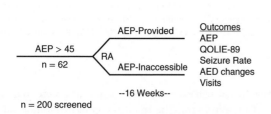

Figure 8.7 Schematic showing study design with randomization of patients and the outcome measures used to evaluate the clinical utility of the Adverse Events Profile (AEP). For the study, 62 patients with an AEP >45 were enrolled. Patients were randomized into two groups: one had physicians who had access to the AEP results, the other had physicians who did not. Outcome measures at 16 weeks post the initial visit included the AEP, QOLIE-89, seizure rate, AED changes, and visits. Source: Novelly et al., 1986 [5]. Reproduced with permission of Wiley.

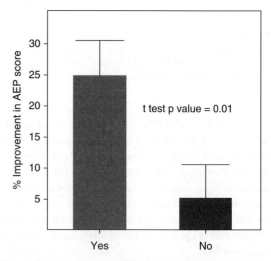

Figure 8.8 Bar graph depicting the change in the mean Adverse Event Profile (AEP) scores for the AEP-accessible and AEP-inaccessible groups. Source: Gilliam et al., 2004 [10]. Reproduced with permission of Lippincott Williams & Wilkins.

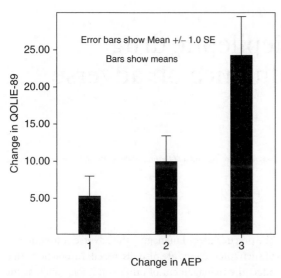

Figure 8.9 Bar graph illustrating the mean change in Quality of Life in Epilepsy-89 (QOLIE-89) scores with the change in mean Adverse Event Profile (AEP) scores. Change in AEP as defined by the total scores for the patients who completed the study (1 = ≤0, 2 = 0–15, 3 = ≥15 point change). Source: Gilliam et al., 2004 [10]. Reproduced with permission of Lippincott Williams & Wilkins.

References

1 Pearce JMS: Bromide, the first effective antiepileptic agent. *J Neurol Neurosurg Psychiatry* 2002; **72(3)**:412.

2 Clancy CM, Eisenberg JM: Outcomes research: measuring the end results of health care. *Science* 1998; **282(5387)**: 245–246.

3 Baker GA, Camfield C, Camfield P et al.: Commission on outcome measurement in epilepsy, 1994–1997: final report. *Epilepsia* 1998; **39(2)**:213–231.

4 Cramer JA: A clinimetric approach to assessing quality of life in epilepsy. *Epilepsia* 1993; **34(Suppl. 4)**:S8–S13.

5 Novelly RA, Schwartz MM, Mattson RH, Cramer JA: Behavioral toxicity associated with antiepileptic drugs: concepts and methods of assessment. *Epilepsia* 1986; **27(4)**:331–340.

6 Gillham R, Baker G, Thompson P et al.: Standardisation of a self-report questionnaire for use in evaluating cognitive, affective and behavioural side-effects of anti-epileptic drug treatments. *Epilepsy Res* 1996; **24(1)**:47–55.

7 Mattson RH, Cramer JA, Collins JF et al.: Comparison of carbamazepine, phenobarbital, phenytoin, and primidone in partial and secondarily generalized tonic-clonic seizures. *N Engl J Med* 1985; **313(3)**:145–151.

8 Baker GA, Jacoby A, Buck D et al.: Quality of life of people with epilepsy: a European study. *Epilepsia* 1997; **38(3)**: 353–362.

9 Cramer JA, Fisher R, Ben-Menachem E et al.: New antiepileptic drugs: comparison of key clinical trials. *Epilepsia* 1999; **40(5)**:590–600.

10 Gilliam FG, Fessler AJ, Baker G et al.: Systematic screening allows reduction of adverse antiepileptic drug effects: a randomized trial. *Neurology* 2004; **62(1)**:23–27.

11 Gilliam FG, Barry JJ, Hermann BP et al.: Rapid detection of major depression in epilepsy: a multicentre study. *Lancet Neurol* 2006; **5(5)**:399–405.

12 Smith DB, Mattson RH, Cramer JA et al.: Results of a nationwide veterans administration cooperative study comparing the efficacy and toxicity of carbamazepine, phenobarbital, phenytoin, and primidone. *Epilepsia* 1987; **28(Suppl. 3)**: S50–S58.

13 Aldenkamp AP, Baker GA: The neurotoxicity scale – II. Results of a patient-based scale assessing neurotoxicity in patients with epilepsy. *Epilepsy Res* 1997; **27(3)**:165–173.

14 Baker GA, Frances P, Middleton E: Initial development, reliability, and validity of a patient-based adverse events scale. *Epilepsia* 1994; **35(Suppl. 7)**:80.

15 Perucca P, Carter J, Vahle V, Gilliam FG: Adverse antiepileptic drug effects: toward a clinically and neurobiologically relevant taxonomy. *Neurology* 2009; **72(14)**:1223–1229.

16 Gilliam F: Optimizing health outcomes in active epilepsy. *Neurology* 2002; **58(Suppl. 5)**:S9–S19.

CHAPTER 9

Clinically important antiepileptic drug interactions and their influence on adverse effects in epilepsy

Frank M.C. Besag[1] and Philip N. Patsalos[2]

[1] South Essex Partnership University NHS Foundation Trust, Twinwoods Health Resource Centre, Bedford and Institute of Psychiatry, UK

[2] Department of Clinical and Experimental Epilepsy, UCL Institute of Neurology, UK

Background

Major problems can arise from antiepileptic drug (AED) interactions. These interactions can either be between different AEDs or between AEDs and medications used to treat other conditions. There are several reasons why such interactions need to be considered, including the following: 1) although patients should be treated with AED monotherapy, if possible, AED combinations continue to be widely prescribed in patients who have not responded to a single drug; 2) the chronic nature of epilepsy in many patients necessitates concomitant treatment with other drugs for the management of associated or intercurrent conditions; 3) many AEDs are potent inducers or inhibitors of drug-metabolizing enzymes and are highly likely to modify the pharmacokinetics of concurrently administered AEDs or other drugs; 4) some AEDs are involved in clinically important pharmacodynamic interactions with concurrently administered AEDs; and 5) many AEDs have a narrow therapeutic index, implying that even modest changes in plasma drug concentration can result in seizure breakthrough or signs of toxicity.

During the past 20 years, our understanding of AED interactions has increased significantly. However, the sheer size of available data might discourage many clinicians from taking an effective approach to minimizing the adverse consequences that can result from these interactions. This chapter summarizes the key interactions that can affect the management of the epilepsy.

The practicalities of managing the adverse consequences of such interactions are also discussed. Interactions that affect the management of other conditions, such as the decrease in concentration of antineoplastic drugs with enzyme-inducing AEDs when epilepsy and cancer are treated concurrently, will be mentioned but will not be discussed in detail.

Epidemiology

Adverse drug reactions (ADRs) are a major problem in drug therapeutics. More than 2 million serious ADRs have been estimated to occur annually in the United States, leading to 100 000 deaths [1]. However, this point estimate for ADR mortality is based on data that are more than 20 years old and a more accurate figure might be approximately 25 000 deaths – still not an insignificant number [2]. The contribution of AEDs to ADRs and possible death is not known. Many AEDs can modify the pharmacokinetics and pharmacodynamics of concomitantly administered drugs, and vice versa, which may result in clinically significant ADRs. Avoiding such drug combinations might reduce the propensity for AED-related ADRs. Although the prevalence of potential drug–drug interactions between AEDs is not known, some data are available concerning the potential prevalence of such interactions between AEDs and other medications. In a pharmaceutical claims database of AED prescriptions for 11 188 patients, polytherapy

---

Epilepsy and the Interictal State: Co-Morbidities and Quality of Life, First Edition.
Edited by Erik K. St. Louis, David M. Ficker, and Terence J. O'Brien.
© 2015 John Wiley & Sons, Ltd. Published 2015 by John Wiley & Sons, Ltd.

occurred in every age group and generally increased with age in both men and women until age 64 years [3]. The mean number of concomitant medications ranged from 2.41 for men aged 18–34 years to 7.67 for men aged >85 years; these values are greater than in the general (non-epilepsy) population [4]. That the most frequently prescribed AEDs were phenytoin, carbamazepine, and valproic acid suggests that physicians are not selecting AEDs based on the likelihood of drug–drug interactions. Phenytoin and carbamazepine are hepatic enzyme inducers, while valproic acid is an enzyme inhibitor. All three are known to interact with the various drugs that were prescribed for comorbid disorders in the patient population studied, particularly cardiovascular disease, psychiatric disorders, and cancer [3]. Another study based on 4966 patient claims in a Medicaid database revealed that approximately 45% of patients receiving monotherapy with an older AED had a potential interaction, while only 3.9% of patients had such an interaction when prescribed a new AED [5]. In hospitalized psychiatric patients most ADR were attributable to AEDs and cardiovascular agents, and of the 19 preventable ADRs, lithium was the drug reported most frequently, followed by phenytoin [6]. With antineoplastic agents, despite a low prevalence of combination therapy with AEDs (0.64%), exposure to such combinations is usually over long periods so that significant ADRs can occur, leading to adverse clinical outcomes [7].

Pathophysiology/etiology

The more drugs a patient takes, the greater the likelihood that a drug interaction will occur. The elderly and the severely ill are at greatest risk of suffering clinically serious adverse interactions, since they are more likely to be on many drugs, and also because drug dosage requirements may be reduced due to renal or hepatic disease or to increased drug sensitivity.

Many interactions involving AEDs have been documented over the years but fortunately, in most situations, the clinical importance of these interactions is probably small. However, the significance of an interaction can vary greatly from patient to patient, depending on the relative dosage of the interacting drugs, previous drug exposure, and genetic constitution. Thus, an interaction resulting in a marked or even modest elevation of a low AED concentration (level) may result in improved seizure control, while a small elevation of a nearly toxic concentration may precipitate toxicity. Considering the end result in individual patients, and given that different individuals respond differently, an interaction might have a relatively small effect in one person but could have a large, clinically important effect in another.

Drug interactions can be divided into two types: pharmacokinetic and pharmacodynamic. Pharmacokinetic interactions involve a change in drug concentration, whereas pharmacodynamic interactions do not, but instead result from an alteration in effect on the receptor. Pharmacokinetic interactions depend on the processes by which drugs are absorbed, distributed, metabolized, and excreted. The key mechanism of interaction of AEDs relates to inhibition or induction of drug metabolism, principally via cytochrome P450 and uridine glucuronyl transferase (UGT) isoenzymes. Inhibition results from competition between drugs for the same active site on the enzyme and circulating concentrations of the inhibited drug increase to a new steady state after five half-lives. Consequently, pharmacological potentiation will occur quickly if drugs have a short half-life (e.g., rufinamide and valproic acid) but occur more slowly if drugs have a long half-life (e.g., phenytoin and phenobarbital) (Table 9.1). Toxicity or undesirable effects will occur if dosage reduction is not undertaken.

In contrast, induction involves the synthesis of a new enzyme, requiring protein synthesis over many days before completion. The consequent enhancement of metabolism usually results in decreased efficacy of standard doses of the affected drug. Generally, increasing drug dose can restore the pharmacological response of a drug after its plasma concentration has been reduced by enzyme induction. The process goes in reverse when the inducer is withdrawn, with an increase in plasma concentrations of the target drug and hence an increased potential for toxic side effects. However, toxicity can be avoided by an appropriate decrease in dose. Paradoxically, enzyme induction can be associated with a potentiation of therapeutic or toxic effects of a drug if pharmacologically active metabolites are present, which occurs with carbamazepine metabolism to carbamazepine-epoxide. The same principle applies to clobazam, which is metabolized to the active metabolite N-desmethylclobazam.

Table 9.1 Time to steady-state of the affected antiepileptic drug (AED) consequent to an inhibition of hepatic metabolism interaction.

Affected AED	Half-life (hours)[a]	Steady-state blood levels achieved after five half-lives (days)[b]
Carbamazepine	8–20	2–4
Clobazam	10–30	2–7 (7–10)[c]
Ethosuximide	40–60	8–12
Felbamate	16–22	3–5
Lamotrigine	15–35	3–7
Phenobarbital	70–140	15–29
Phenytoin	30–100	6–21
Rufinamide	6–10	1–2
Valproic acid	11–20	2–4

[a]Values are in the absence of interacting medication [12].
[b]Values are rounded up or down for clarity.
[c]Includes time to steady-state for pharmacologically active metabolite N-desmethylclobazam.

Pharmacodynamic interactions occur when the effects of one drug are changed by the presence of another at the site of action. Drugs may compete directly for a receptor (additive, synergistic, or antagonistic) but often the interaction will be more indirect, involving interference of physiological mechanisms.

While pharmacokinetic interactions are readily identifiable and their time course and characteristics easily quantified, pharmacodynamic interactions are more difficult to identify and are usually seen when an unexpected change in a patient's clinical status cannot be ascribed definitively to a pharmacokinetic interaction.

Diagnosis

Adverse drug interactions can present in a number of different ways. Typically, they involve signs of toxicity or seizure breakthrough. However, some interactions have less obvious signs; for example, a person with a disability and epilepsy might be unable to verbally express distress caused by double vision or dizziness resulting from a pharmacodynamic interaction between lamotrigine and carbamazepine, presenting instead as a "behavioral disturbance." A small reduction in

carbamazepine dose could resolve the effects of such an adverse interaction, with swift resolution of the "disturbance." Pharmacokinetic interactions should be relatively easy to identify and quantify because they are associated with a change in plasma drug concentration. In the absence of a change in blood concentration, the change in the clinical status of a patient will be the consequence of a pharmacodynamic interaction.

This section highlights key major drug interactions and resultant AED-associated adverse effects.

AED–AED interactions

There are many interactions that can occur between AEDs. Of particular clinical relevance, hepatic inhibition results in increased blood concentrations of the affected drug and concentration-dependent adverse effects. Conversely, hepatic induction causes decreased blood concentrations of the affected drug, sometimes resulting in a breakthrough seizure.

Interactions mediated by enzyme inhibition

The principal AEDs associated with inhibition of hepatic metabolism are valproic acid, topiramate, oxcarbazepine, stiripentol, and felbamate. These AEDs can elevate the plasma concentrations of other AEDs and cause adverse (toxic) effects. Valproic acid is the broadest ranging and most potent AED inhibitor of drug metabolism, while topiramate is a modest inhibitor, and oxcarbazepine a weak inhibitor. Stiripentol and felbamate are also potent inhibitors, resulting in clinically important interactions and adverse effects, but these AEDs are rarely used in epilepsy. Stiripentol has a limited license for the adjunctive treatment of seizures in children with severe myoclonic epilepsy in infancy (Dravet syndrome) and felbamate is associated with serious liver and bone marrow toxicity.

Valproic acid is associated with major inhibitory interactions with carbamazepine, phenobarbital, and lamotrigine and moderate inhibitory interactions with felbamate and rufinamide. The inhibition of the enzyme epoxide hydrolase by valproic acid results in an increase in plasma concentrations of the pharmacologically active metabolite of carbamazepine, carbamazepine-epoxide. This interaction can occur without any significant changes in plasma carbamazepine concentrations and can result in signs of carbamazepine toxicity [8].

Valproate interaction with phenobarbital results from inhibition of CYP2C9 and CYP2C19, causing a 30–50% increase in plasma phenobarbital concentration. A reduction in phenobarbital (or primidone) dosage by up to 80% may be required to avoid adverse effects, particularly sedation and cognitive impairment [9]. Inhibition of the UGT1A4 isoenzyme is responsible for the glucuronide conjugation of lamotrigine, resulting in an approximate twofold increase in plasma lamotrigine concentrations [10]. Valproic acid is a potent inhibitor of lamotrigine metabolism; plasma lamotrigine concentrations are already fully increased at relatively low valproate doses ($\geq$500 mg/day in an adult) [11].

Valproic acid may inhibit the metabolism of other AEDs, including ethosuximide, felbamate, phenytoin, and rufinamide. Valproate interaction with phenytoin is complex, involving inhibition of phenytoin metabolism and concurrent displacement of phenytoin from plasma protein binding sites, resulting in increased free plasma phenytoin concentrations, which may not be readily apparent when a patient is monitored by use of total phenytoin concentrations. Because of this, free phenytoin concentrations should be used to guide patient management in this situation [12].

Although oxcarbazepine is a weak inhibitor of CYP2C19, at high dosages (>1800 mg/day) oxcarbazepine may increase plasma phenytoin concentrations by up to 40% and may also increase plasma phenobarbital concentrations to a lesser extent [13]. Topiramate, in contrast, is a modest inhibitor of CYP2C19 and can increase plasma phenytoin concentrations in a small subset of patients by 25%. Rufinamide can decrease the clearance of phenobarbital and phenytoin by <20% and increase their plasma concentrations [14].

Stiripentol is a potent inhibitor of CYP1A2, CYP2C19, and CYP3A4 and consequently inhibits the metabolism of carbamazepine, clobazam, phenobarbital, phenytoin, primidone, and valproic acid, causing a rise in their plasma concentrations, with the possibility of toxicity [15]. Inhibition of clobazam metabolism is particularly profound given concurrent inhibition of the pharmacologically active metabolite, N-desmethylclobazam, resulting in increases in both clobazam and N-desmethylclobazam plasma concentrations by several-fold [16]. Felbamate increases plasma concentration of carbamazepine-epoxide, N-desmethylclobazam, phenobarbital, phenytoin, and valproic acid, consequent to inhibition of CYP2C19 and epoxide hydrolase [17].

Interactions mediated by enzyme induction

Carbamazepine, phenytoin, phenobarbital, and primidone are potent inducers of various CYP isoenzymes, UGTs, and epoxide hydrolases [17]. Consequently, these AEDs enhance the metabolism and decrease the plasma concentrations of numerous AEDs, including clobazam, clonazepam, ethosuximide, felbamate, lamotrigine, oxcarbazepine (and its active monohydroxy metabolite), rufinamide, stiripentol, tiagabine, topiramate, valproic acid, and zonisamide. Rufinamide can decrease plasma concentrations of carbamazepine and lamotrigine, probably via induction of hepatic metabolism [14]. In addition, phenobarbital, phenytoin, and primidone can markedly induce the metabolism of carbamazepine, decreasing mean plasma carbamazepine concentrations by 33, 44, and 25%, respectively [18]. Carbamazepine, phenobarbital, and phenytoin can decrease plasma valproic acid concentrations by an average of 66, 76, and 49%, respectively [19]. In addition, the metabolism of lamotrigine is significantly enhanced by oxcarbazepine [20] and methsuximide [21]. Methsuximide has also been shown to decrease mean valproic acid concentrations by 31% [22]. The common feature of all these interactions is a marked decrease in the steady-state plasma concentration of the affected drug, and this can impact adversely on seizure control.

AED–antimicrobial drug interactions
Antifungal agents

Many imidazole antifungals are potent inhibitors of CYP isoenzymes [23]. Ketoconazole and fluconazole are CYP3A4 inhibitors, increasing plasma carbamazepine concentration by about 30% and resulting in carbamazepine intoxication [24,25]. Similarly, the CYP2C9 inhibitors miconazole, fluconazole, and voriconazole can increase plasma phenytoin concentrations two- to fourfold [26,27].

Antituberculosis agents

Metabolism of numerous AEDs, including carbamazepine, ethosuximide, phenytoin, and valproic acid, is inhibited by isoniazid, resulting in elevated plasma concentrations and associated toxicity [28–31]. When isoniazid is administered in combination with rifampicin, the rifampicin counteracts the inhibiting effect of isoniazid on phenytoin metabolism [32].

Antiviral agents

Seizures occur in 11–15% of HIV-seropositive individuals. Since many antiviral agents are inducers or inhibitors of hepatic isoenzymes, interactions between anti-HIV medication and AEDs are important [33]. Antiviral agents such as nevirapine and efavirenz are inducers of CYP3A4, whereas indinavir, ritonavir, and delaverdine are inhibitors of CYP3A4 [34]. Thus, while efavirenz can decrease plasma carbamazepine concentrations by about 30%, ritonavir can cause a two- to threefold increase in plasma carbamazepine concentrations [35,36]. Atanazavir can enhance the metabolism of lamotrigine via an action on UGT1A4 and can decrease plasma lamotrigine concentrations by 12%. Ritonavir in combination with atanazavir or lopinavir can decrease plasma lamotrigine concentrations by 32 and 55%, respectively [37,38]. Indinavir, nelfinavir, ritonavir, and saquinavir inhibit the metabolism of phenytoin, probably via an action on CYP2C9, and can significantly increase plasma phenytoin concentrations.

Carbapenem antibiotics

Carbapenem antibiotics have a profound effect on plasma valproic acid concentration. Doripenem and meropenem can decrease plasma valproic acid concentrations by 69 and 82%, respectively. Interactions involving ertapenem, imipenem, and panipenem are particularly profound, decreasing plasma valproic acid concentrations by >99% [39,40]. Because of the magnitude of these interactions, the combination of carbapenems and valproic acid should be avoided.

Chloramphenicol

Chloramphenicol may precipitate signs of AED toxicity by increasing the plasma concentrations of phenytoin and phenobarbital [41].

Macrolides

Some macrolide antibiotics are potent inhibitors of CYP3A4, potentially increasing plasma carbamazepine concentrations [42,43]. Erythromycin, clarithromycin, josamycin, and troleandomycin are potent inhibitors of carbamazepine metabolism, increasing plasma carbamazepine concentrations between two- and fourfold

and potentially causing serious toxicity. Choosing azithromycin can avoid this problem.

Sulfonamides

Sulfonamides such as sulfaphenazole and sulfadiazine may inhibit phenytoin metabolism and increase plasma phenytoin concentrations, potentially leading to toxicity [44]. Some sulfonamides concurrently displace phenytoin from plasma protein binding sites. Therefore, measurement of total phenytoin concentration may underestimate an increased concentration of free, pharmacologically active drug. In this setting, free phenytoin concentrations should be monitored [12].

AED–antineoplastic drug interactions

Antineoplastic agents can both inhibit and induce drug metabolizing enzymes, affecting AED pharmacokinetics. For example, doxifluridine, tamoxifen, 5-fluorouracil, and UFT (a mixture of uracil and the 5-fluorouracil prodrug tegafur) may cause phenytoin intoxication by inhibiting phenytoin metabolism via CYP2C9 [45–47]. Tamoxifen can increase plasma phenytoin concentrations by 44%, while coadministration with 5-fluorouracil, tegafur, and doxifluridine can result in a fourfold increase in phenytoin plasma concentrations [48,49]. In contrast, significant decreases in plasma phenytoin concentrations can occur when carmustine is given alone or in combination with cisplatin and etoposide, requiring an approximate 50% increase in phenytoin dosage. The effect of cisplatin may occur via enzyme induction, while similar reductions in plasma phenytoin concentrations by vinblastine, methotrexate, and bleomycin may be a consequence of antineoplastic damage to the intestinal mucosa and impaired phenytoin absorption. Cisplatin can decrease plasma carbamazepine and valproic acid concentrations, while methotrexate can decrease valproic acid concentrations [50–54].

AED–cardioactive drug interactions

The antiarrhythmic amiodarone increases plasma phenytoin concentrations and may precipitate signs of toxicity if phenytoin dosage is not adjusted accordingly [55]. Likewise, the antihypertensive agents diltiazem and verapamil are inhibitors of carbamazepine metabolism, resulting in increased plasma concentrations of carbamazepine and potential toxicity [56,57]. In addition, diltiazem inhibits the metabolism of phenytoin, resulting in phenytoin intoxication [56]. Finally, the antiplatelet drug ticlopidine inhibits phenytoin metabolism via CYP2C19, increasing plasma phenytoin concentrations [58].

AED–psychotropic drug interactions

Concomitant administration of AEDs and psychotropic drugs is common given the high frequency of psychiatric disorders in patients with epilepsy. Numerous clinically important drug interactions have been described between these drug groups [59,60].

Antidepressants

The antidepressants fluoxetine, fluvoxamine, sertraline, trazodone, viloxazine, and possibly imipramine inhibit the metabolism of phenytoin and increase plasma phenytoin concentrations. Typical increases in plasma phenytoin concentrations vary from 37% (viloxazine) to threefold (fluoxetine). Similarly, fluoxetine, fluvoxamine, nefazodone, trazodone, and viloxazine inhibit the metabolism of carbamazepine and can increase plasma carbamazepine concentrations from 26 (trazodone) to 70% (fluvoxamine). Exceptionally, nefazodone increases plasma carbamazepine concentrations threefold. Plasma concentrations of valproic acid and lamotrigine are increased threefold and twofold, respectively, by sertraline [61,62].

Antipsychotics

Overall, antipsychotic drugs do not substantially alter AED plasma concentrations. Haloperidol and risperidone can increase plasma carbamazepine concentrations by 42 and 19%, respectively. Risperidone can also increase plasma phenytoin concentrations by 20%. While quetiapine does not affect plasma carbamazepine concentrations, plasma carbamazepine-epoxide concentrations may increase three- to fourfold [63].

Practical aspects and treatment

Table 9.2 summarizes the concentration-related adverse effects associated with various AEDs. Prevention of interactions and consequent adverse effects is certainly the best approach to management, implying that clinicians should be informed regarding common interactions and should warn their patients of possibilities of interactions and monitor their patients

carefully. If the prescriber has a good understanding of the basic principles, managing the situation should not be particularly difficult. In practice, knowledge of whether the addition of a drug is likely to increase or decrease plasma concentrations of existing drugs is crucial. Measuring baseline drug concentrations before adding the interacting drug can be valuable [12]. If, for example, sodium valproate is to be added to lamotrigine and the concentration of the latter AED is already high then dose reduction will almost certainly be required to avoid toxicity, whereas with very low concentrations, dose reduction might not be required. If an enzyme-inducing drug is to be added to an existing AED regimen, the situation may be more complex, and tailoring of the titration of the new and existing drugs may depend upon the clinical scenario. In patients whose chief priority is maintaining seizure freedom, very slow and cautious dose alterations may be indicated, whereas in refractory patients with ongoing seizures, a temporary, modest deterioration in seizure control might be acceptable.

In practice, if toxicity or seizure deterioration occurs after the addition of an enzyme-inducing drug then a trough blood concentration should be determined as soon as possible and the AED dose adjusted accordingly. If trough concentration results are unexpectedly high or low, AED doses do not necessarily need to be adjusted. In all cases, practitioners need to manage the patient's clinical status of seizure control or adverse effects, not just the AED blood concentration result. There appears to be widespread misunderstanding with regard to how reference ranges for AEDs should be interpreted. Carefully considered decisions should be made, taking full account of the clinical situation. This issue has been discussed in detail elsewhere [12].

Regarding pharmacodynamic interactions, emphasis should be on informing and monitoring the patient, such as in an example of the pharmacodynamic interaction between lamotrigine and carbamazepine [64]. If the baseline carbamazepine level is moderately high – around 7.5 mg/L – and lamotrigine is to be added, the patient should be warned that possible adverse effects of diplopia, dizziness, or lethargy may appear. If the patient is unaware of this pharmacodynamic interaction then the adverse effects might be attributed solely to lamotrigine and this drug might be discontinued, which would be an inappropriate course of action. If patients and their physicians are

Table 9.2 Concentration-related adverse effects of antiepileptic drugs (AEDs).

Antiepileptic drug	Most common adverse effect	Other adverse effects
Carbamazepine	Diplopia, dizziness, headache, nausea	Drowsiness, neutropenia, hyponatremia, hypocalcemia, orofacial dyskinesia, cardiac arrhythmia
Clobazam	Fatigue, drowsiness	Ataxia, dizziness, irritability, aggression, hypersalivation, bronchorrhea, weight gain, muscle weakness, psychosis
Clonazepam	Fatigue, sedation, drowsiness	Ataxia, dizziness, irritability, aggression (children), hyperkinesia (children), hypersalivation, bronchorrhea, psychosis
Eslicarbazepine acetate	Dizziness, somnolence, headache, diplopia, vertigo, nausea, vomiting, diarrhea, fatigue	Amnesia, nystagmus, dysarthria, tinnitus, nocturia
Ethosuximide	Nausea	Anorexia, vomiting, agitation, drowsiness, headache, lethargy
Gabapentin	Somnolence, dizziness, ataxia, fatigue	Diplopia, paresthesia, amnesia
Lacosamide	Nausea, dizziness, headache, lethargy, diplopia	Tremor, anxiety, insomnia
Lamotrigine	Drowsiness, diplopia, headache, ataxia, insomnia, tremor	Nausea, vomiting, aggression, irritability
Levetiracetam	Fatigue, headache	Ataxia, drowsiness, irritability
Oxcarbazepine	Fatigue, drowsiness, diplopia, dizziness, hyponatremia	Ataxia, nausea, nystagmus, tremor
Phenobarbital	Fatigue, listlessness, tiredness, depression, insomnia (children), distractibility (children), hyperkinesia (children)	Irritability (children), aggression, poor memory, decreased libido, impotence, folate deficiency, hypocalcemia, osteomalacia
Phenytoin	Ataxia, nystagmus	Anorexia, dyspepsia, nausea, vomiting, aggression, depression, drowsiness, headache, paradoxical seizures, megaloblastic anemia, hyperglycemia, hypocalcemia, osteomalacia
Pregabalin	Dizziness	Ataxia, drowsiness, diplopia, abnormal thinking, tremor, weight gain
Primidone	Fatigue, listlessness, tiredness, depression, psychosis, decreased libido, impotence, hyperkinesia (children)	Irritability (children), nausea vomiting, nystagmus, ataxia, folate efficiency, hypocalcemia, osteomalacia, megaloblastic anemia
Retigabine	Dizziness, somnolence, fatigue, weight gain, anxiety, amnesia, aphasia, vertigo, tremor, dysphasia, dysarthria, nausea	Hypokinesia, dysphagia, hyperhidrosis, nephrolithiasis
Rufinamide	Fatigue, vomiting, loss of appetite, somnolence, drowsiness, diplopia, nystagmus	Ataxia, dizziness
Stiripentol	Anorexia, weight loss, insomnia, drowsiness, ataxia, hypotonia, dystonia, hyperkinesias, nausea, vomiting	Diplopia, fatigue, urticaria
Valproate	Tremor, weight gain, hair loss	Anorexia, dyspepsia, nausea, vomiting, alopecia, peripheral edema, drowsiness, hyperammonemia, amenorrhea
Tiagabine	Dizziness, headache, tremor, difficulty concentrating, light-headedness, nervousness	Fatigue, abnormal thinking
Topiramate	Anorexia, weight gain, impaired concentration	Impaired speech, paresthesias, kidney stones, impaired memory, ataxia
Vigabatrin	Drowsiness, fatigue, headache, ataxia, nystagmus, diplopia, irritability, depression	Psychosis, aggression, weight gain, stupor, tremor, impaired concentration
Zonisamide	Ataxia, anorexia, agitation, confusion, concentration impairment, drowsiness, dizziness	Depression, memory impairment, word-finding difficulties

aware that adverse effects might appear then they will be less likely to become alarmed, and decreasing the carbamazepine dose by 100–200 mg might swiftly resolve the problem. Even well-documented pharmacodynamic interactions do not occur predictably in all patients, implying that a single, uniform approach to altering drug regimens is inappropriate. Clinicians should monitor each patient as an individual and respond appropriately.

Pearls

If certain basic principles are followed, the majority of adverse AED interactions can be avoided or minimized. These principles are summarized here, with a few examples of interactions that are either particularly important or easily missed.
- First, prevention is the best approach.
- Whenever a drug is prescribed, clinicians should consider possible adverse interactions and reactions that might arise.
- Interactions may be pharmacokinetic or pharmacodynamic.
- Pharmacokinetic interactions involve either a rise in drug concentration (with the possibility of toxicity) or a fall in drug concentration (with the possibility of a seizure exacerbation). Knowing which drugs are enzyme inhibitors that can raise drug concentrations and which are enzyme inducers that can decrease concentrations allows the clinician to avoid or minimize most interactions.
- Pharmacodynamic interactions do not involve altered drug concentrations and are generally not predictable. Warning patients of adverse effects that might arise from pharmacodynamic interactions when a new drug is prescribed and explaining what action should be taken can greatly minimize the impact of pharmacodynamic interactions.
- Powerful enzyme inducers include phenytoin and carbamazepine. When these drugs are prescribed, careful consideration should be given to how they might decrease concentrations of existing medication.
- Valproate has the widest range of enzyme inhibition. When this drug is prescribed, careful consideration of potential increases in the concentration of existing medications is necessary, especially with lamotrigine.

- Many drugs interact with AEDs. Macrolide antibiotic drugs such as erythromycin and clarithromycin are among the most frequently prescribed antibiotics. These are powerful enzyme inhibitors and can cause carbamazepine toxicity. Carbapenem antibiotics can decrease plasma valproic acid concentrations profoundly, suggesting that this drug combination should be avoided.
- AEDs with minimal or no interacting potential (gabapentin, lacosamide, levetiracetam, pregabalin, and vigabatrin) minimize the potential for ADRs resulting from drug–drug interactions in patients with epilepsy.

In summary, a thorough knowledge of the basic principles of AED interactions, access to a sound database of interactions, careful thought before prescribing any drug that might interact, and, above all, careful monitoring of the patient should help avoid most problems in clinical practice.

References

1 Lazarou J, Pomeranz BH, Corey PN: Incidence of adverse drug reactions in hospitalized patients: a meta-analysis of prospective studies. *JAMA* 1998; **279**:1200–1205.
2 Bates DW: Adverse drug reactions in hospitalized patients. *JAMA* 1998; **280**:1743–1744.
3 Gidal BE, French JA, Grossman P, Le Teuff G: Assessment of potential interactions in patients with epilepsy: impact of age and sex. *Neurology* 2009; **72**:419–425.
4 Kaufman DW, Kelly JP, Rosenberg L et al.: Recent patters of medication use in the ambulatory adult population of the United States: the Slone Survey. *JAMA* 2002; **287**:337–344.
5 Dickson M, Bramley TJ, Kozma C et al.: Potential drug-drug interactions with antiepileptic drugs in Medicaid recipients. *Am J Health Syst Pharm* 2008; **65**:1720–1726.
6 Thomas M, Boggs AA, Dipaula B, Siddiqi S: Adverse drug reactions in hospitalized psychiatric patients. *Ann Pharmacother* 2010; **44**:819–825.
7 Cheung YT, Yap KYL, Chui WK, Chan A: Drug-drug interactions between oral antiepileptics and oral anticancer drugs: Implications to clinicians. *Eur Neurol* 2010; **64**:88–94.
8 Pisani F, Fazio A, Oteri G et al.: Sodium valproate and valpromide: differential interactions with carbamazepine in epileptic patients. *Epilepsia* 1986; **27**:548–552.
9 Kapetanovic IM, Kupferberg HJ, Porter RJ et al.: Mechanism of valproate–phenobarbital interaction in epileptic patients. *Clin Pharmacol Ther* 1981; **29**:480–486.
10 Yuen AWC, Land G, Weatherley B, Peck AW: Sodium valproate inhibits lamotrigine metabolism. *Br J Clin Pharmacol* 1992; **33**:511–513.

11 Gidal BE, Anderson GD, Rutecki PR et al.: Lack of an effect of valproate concentration on lamotrigine pharmacokinetics in developmentally disabled patients with epilepsy. *Epilepsy Res* 2000; **42**:23–31.

12 Patsalos PN, Berry DJ, Bourgeois BFD et al.: Antiepileptic drugs – best practice guidelines for therapeutic drug monitoring: a position paper by the Subcommission on Therapeutic Drug Monitoring, ILAE Commission on Therapeutic Strategies. *Epilepsia* 2008; **49**:1239–1276.

13 Barcs G, Walker EB, Elger CE et al.: Oxcarbazepine placebo-controlled, dose-ranging trial in refractory partial epilepsy. *Epilepsia* 2000; **41**:1597–1607.

14 Perucca E, Cloyd J, Critchley D et al.: Clinical pharmacokinetics and concentration-response relationships in patients with epilepsy. *Epilepsia* 2008; **49**:1123–1141.

15 Chiron C. Stiripentol. *Neurotherapeutics* 2007; **4**:123–125.

16 Levy RH, Loiseau P, Guyot M et al.: Stiripentol kinetics in epilepsy: nonlinearity and interactions. *Clin Pharmacol Ther* 1984; **36**:661–669.

17 Patsalos PN, Perucca E: Clinically important interactions in epilepsy: general features and interactions between antiepileptic drugs. *Lancet Neurol* 2003; **2**:347–356.

18 Patsalos PN: *Anti-Epileptic Drug Interactions: A Clinical Guide*, 2 edn. Springer: London, 2013.

19 May T, Rambeck B: Serum concentrations of valproic acid: influence of dose and comedication. *Ther Drug Monit* 1985; **7**:387–390.

20 May TW, Rambeck B, Jurgens U: Serum concentrations of lamotrigine in epileptic patients: the influence of dose and comedication. *Ther Drug Monit* 1996; **18**:523–531.

21 Besag FMC, Berry DJ, Pool F: Methsuximide lowers lamotrigine blood levels: a pharmacokinetic antiepileptic drug interaction. *Epilepsia* 2000; **41**:624–627.

22 Besag FMC, Berry DJ, Vasey M: Methsuximide reduces valproic acid serum levels. *Ther Drug Monit* 2001; **23(6)**: 694–697.

23 Strolin Benedetti M, Bani M: Metabolism-based interactions involving oral azole antifungals in humans. *Drug Metab Rev* 1999; **31**:665–717.

24 Nair DR, Morris HH: Potential fluconazole-induced carbamazepine toxicity. *Ann Pharmacother* 1999; **33**:790–792.

25 Spina E, Arena D, Scordo MG et al.: Elevation of plasma carbamazepine concentrations by ketoconazole in patients with epilepsy. *Ther Drug Monit* 1997; **19**:535–538.

26 Rolan PE, Somogy AA, Drew MR et al.: Phenytoin intoxication during treatment with parenteral miconazole. *Br Med J* 1983; **287**:1760.

27 Cadle RM, Zenon GJ, Rodrigues-Barradas MC, Hamill RJ: Fluconazole induced symptomatic phenytoin toxicity. *Ann Pharmacother* 1994; **28**:191–195.

28 Valsalan VC, Cooper GL: Carbamazepine intoxication caused by interaction with isoniazid. *Br Med J* 1982; **285**:261–262.

29 Van Wieringen A, Vrijlandt CM: Ethosuximide intoxication caused by interaction with isoniazid. *Neurology* 1983; **33**: 1227–1228.

30 Miller RR, Porter R, Greenblatt DJ: Clinical importance of the interaction of phenytoin and isoniazid: a report from the Boston Collaborative Drug Surveillance Program. *Chest* 1979; **75**:356–358.

31 Jonville AP, Gauchez AS, Autret E et al.: Interaction between isoniazid and valproate: a case of valproate overdosage. *Eur J Clin Pharmacol* 1991; **40**:197–198.

32 Kay L, Kampmann JP, Svendsen TL et al.: Influence of rifampicin and isoniazid on the kinetics of phenytoin. *Br J Clin Pharmacol* 1985; **20**:323–326.

33 Wong MC, Suite NDA, Labar DR: Seizures in human immunodeficiency virus infection. *Arch Neurol* 1990; **47**: 640–642.

34 Joly V, Yeni P: Non nucleoside reverse transcriptase inhibitors. *AIDS Rev* 1999; **1**:37–44.

35 Garcia AB, Ibara AL, Etessam JP et al.: Protease inhibitor-induced carbamazepine toxicity. *Clin Neuropharmacol* 2000; **23**:216–218.

36 Ji P, Damle B, Xie J et al.: Pharmacokinetic interaction between efavirenz and carbamazepine after multiple-dose administration in healthy subjects. *J Clin Pharmacol* 2008; **48**: 948–956.

37 Burger DM, Huisman A, van Ewijk N et al.: The effect of atazanavir and atazanavir/ritonavir on UDP-glucuronosyl-trasferase using lamotrigine as a phenotypic probe. *Clin Pharmacol Ther* 2008; **84**:698–703.

38 Van der Lee MJ, Dawood L, ter Hofstede HJM et al.: Lopinavir/ritonavir reduces lamotrigine plasma concentrations in healthy volunteers. *Clin Pharmacol Ther* 2006; **80**: 159–168.

39 Haroutiunian S, Ratz Y, Rabinovich B et al.: Valproic acid plasma concentrations decreases in a dose-independent manner following administration or meropenem: a retrospective study. *J Clin Pharmacol* 2009; **49**:1363–1369.

40 Liao FF, Huang YB, Chen CY: Decrease in serum valproic acid levels during treatment with ertapenem. *Am J Health Syst Pharm* 2010; **67**:1260–1264.

41 Krasinski K, Kusmiesz H, Nielson JD: Pharmacologic interaction among chloramphenicol, phenytoin and phenobarbital. *Pediatr Infect Dis* 1982; **1**:232–235.

42 Babany G, Larrey D, Pessayre D: Macrolide antibiotics as inducers and inhibitors of cytochrome P450 in experimental animals and man. *Prog Drug Metab* 1988; **11**:61–98.

43 Pauwels O. Factors contributing to carbamazepine-macrolide interactions. *Pharmacol Res* 2002; **45**:291–298.

44 Hansen JM, Kampmann JP, Siersbaek-Nielsen K et al.: The effect of different sulfonamides on phenytoin metabolism in man. *Acta Medica Scandinavica Supplement* 1979; **624**:106–110.

45 Gilbar PJ, Brodribb TR: Phenytoin and fluorouracil interaction. *Ann Pharmacother* 2001; **35**:1367–1370.

46 Wakisaka S, Shimauchi K, Kaji Y: Acute phenytoin intoxication associated with the antineoplastic agent UFT. *Fukuoka Igaku Zasshi* 1990; **81**:192–196.

47 Rabinowicz AL, Hinton DR, Dyck P, Couldwell WT: High-dose tamoxifen in treatment of brain tumours: interaction with antiepileptic drugs. *Epilepsia* 1995; **36**: 513–515.

48 Konishi H, Morita K, Minouchi T et al.: Probable metabolic interaction of doxifluridine with phenytoin. *Ann Pharmacother* 2002; **36**:831–834.

49 Boruban MC, Yasar U, Babaoglu MO et al.: Tamoxifen inhibits cytochrome P450 2C9 activity in breast cancer patients. *J Chemother* 2006; **18**:421–424.

50 Gattis WA, May DB: Possible interaction involving phenytoin, dexamethasone, and antineoplastic agents: a case report and review. *Ann Pharmacother* 1996; **30**: 520–526.

51 Dofferhoff AS, Berendsen HH, vd Naalt J et al.: Decreased phenytoin level after carboplatin treatment. *Am J Med* 1990; **89**:247–248.

52 Fincham RW, Schottelius DD: Decreased phenytoin levels in antineoplastic therapy. *Ther Drug Monit* 1979; **1**:277–283.

53 Neef C, de Voogd-van der Straaten I: An interaction between cytostatic and anticonvulsant drugs. *Clin Pharmacol Ther* 1988; **43**:372–375.

54 Schroder H, Ostergaard JR: Interference of high-dose methotrexate in the metabolism of valproate? *Pediatr Hematol Oncol* 1994; **11**:445.

55 Nolan PE, Erstad BL, Hoyer GL et al.: Steady-state interaction between amiodarone and phenytoin in normal subjects. *Am J Cardiol* 1990; **65**:1252–1257.

56 Bahls FH, Ozuma J, Ritchie DE: Interactions between calcium channel blockers and the anticonvulsants carbamazepine and phenytoin. *Neurology* 1991; **41**:470-472.

57 Macphee GJ, McInnes GT, Thompson GG, Brodie MJ: Verapamil potentiates carbamazepine neurotoxicity: A clinically important inhibitory interaction. *Lancet* 1986; **1**:700–703.

58 Donahue SR, Flockhart DA, Abernethy DR, Ko JW: Ticlopidine inhibition of phenytoin metabolism by potent inhibition of CYP2C19. *Clin Pharmacol Ther* 1997; **62**:572–577.

59 Spina E, Perucca E: Clinical significance of pharmacokinetic interactions between antiepileptic and psychotropic drugs. *Epilepsia* 2002; **43(Suppl. 2)**:37–44.

60 Besag FM, Berry D: Interactions between antiepileptic and antipsychotic drugs. *Drug Saf* 2006; **29**:95–118.

61 Berigan TR, Harazin J: A sertraline/valproic acid drug interaction. *Int J Psychiat Clin Pract* 1999; **3**:287–288.

62 Kaufman KR, Gerner R: Lamotrigine toxicity secondary to sertraline. *Seizure* 1998; **7**:163–165.

63 Fitzgerald BJ, Okos AJ: Elevation of carbamazepine-10, 11-epoxide by quetiapine. *Pharmacotherapy* 2002; **22**: 1500–1503.

64 Besag FMC, Berry DJ, Pool F et al.: Carbamazepine toxicity with lamotrigine: pharmacokinetic or pharmacodynamic interaction? *Epilepsia* 1998; **39**:183–187.

CHAPTER 10

Minimizing the adverse effects of epilepsy therapies: principles and practice

Erik K. St. Louis

Department of Neurology, Mayo Clinic, USA

Introduction

Antiepileptic drugs (AEDs) remain the mainstay of epilepsy management but, due to incomplete efficacy or adverse effects, adjunctive treatment or conversions between AED treatments are often necessary. The adverse effects of AEDs are one of the principle factors leading to reduced quality of life (QOL) in persons with epilepsy and minimizing adverse effects, along with stopping seizures, is one of the central tenets of epilepsy care. However, little evidence is available concerning how best to carry out conversions between AED therapies. It is important to consider patient factors such as age, gender, comorbidities, and comedications when selecting and titrating new AED treatments. This chapter discusses practical strategies for minimizing adverse effects during transitional polytherapy in newly diagnosed and refractory epilepsy care. Successful AED treatment involves careful questioning concerning adverse effects and appropriate adjustment of AED therapies.

Adverse effects encountered during antiepileptic drug polytherapy

Initial AED monotherapy manages nearly half of epilepsy patients successfully [1,2]. However, polytherapy is often still necessary, especially for the management of refractory epilepsy patients, and minimizing AED adverse effects during adjunctive AED dosing remains a challenge during epilepsy treatment. Transitional polytherapy, involving conversion from initial AED monotherapy onto a second monotherapy, is necessary when patients experience continued seizures or persistent and intolerable adverse effects. Nearly all AEDs newly approved for use in the United States come to market under the indication for adjunctive treatment of focal seizures; most newer AEDs are initially used in polytherapy. Unfortunately, no evidence basis for AED conversion is available, so the AED conversion process of transitional polytherapy is based on recommended principles, logic, judgment, experience, and expert consensus opinions in different patients and scenarios.

QOL in epilepsy is determined by seizure burden, but even more so by the interictal state, with AED adverse effects and comorbid mood disorders being chief determinants [3,4]. AED adverse effects may occur during transitional polytherapy and strategies of AED titration can impact the occurrence of adverse effects, patient tolerability, and treatment success or failure [5]. Thus, maximizing patient QOL in epilepsy care is highly dependent on clinicians being vigilant toward AED adverse effect monitoring and appropriate adjustment of AED dosing. Clinicians must be aware of patient-dependent factors during AED selection, dosing, and conversion and employ effective strategies during the treatment of patients with inadequate seizure control and those developing dose-related or idiosyncratic adverse effects.

Epilepsy and the Interictal State: Co-Morbidities and Quality of Life, First Edition.
Edited by Erik K. St. Louis, David M. Ficker, and Terence J. O'Brien.
© 2015 John Wiley & Sons, Ltd. Published 2015 by John Wiley & Sons, Ltd.

Defining and identifying antiepileptic drug adverse effects

An AED adverse effect may be defined as a clinical symptom, sign, or laboratory abnormality that is undesired by the patient, the physician, or both. Unfortunately, adverse effects are common, being reported in 40–50% of epilepsy patients treated with AEDs [6,7]. Common dose-related adverse effects include sedation, fatigue, dizziness, blurred or double vision, concentration problems, incoordination, and headache.

Identification of adverse effects may be difficult as patients are often reluctant to report them, due to fear of having seizures if their medications are changed, and clinicians are often focused on ensuring seizure control, prioritizing satisfactory AED levels instead of clinical outcomes. Use of a screening tool such as the Adverse Events Profile (AEP) greatly aids in identification of adverse effects and helps treating physicians recognize when therapeutic change may be indicated [8].

General strategies for minimzing adverse effects

Adverse effects can be improved or eliminated in most patients by reducing the number or doses of an AED or by converting to a better-tolerated AED. AED monotherapy at the lowest effective dose is the preferred strategy in newly diagnosed epilepsy and remediable epilepsy syndromes [9]. When AED polytherapy proves necessary in refractory epilepsy, maintaining the lowest effective drug load can help minimize adverse effects [10–12]. Polytherapy may be necessary for seizure control but the lowest possible drug load (the lowest numbers and doses of AEDs) should be used. Patients with refractory epilepsy often require chronic polytherapy. All newer AEDs have class 1 evidence for adjunctive treatment of refractory focal seizures in adults, while lamotrigine, oxcarbazepine, and topiramate are effective for the treatment of refractory focal seizures in children [13,14]. An evidence basis for AED polytherapy combinations is lacking but rational polytherapy – the practice of adding an AED with a different or complementary presumed mechanism of action – is common [12]. A previous study illustrating this principle suggested that the combination of valproate and lamotrigine may be synergistic [15].

Minimizing pharmacodynamic and pharmacokinetic drug–drug interactions may lead to heightened adverse effects. Dose-related adverse effects of memory complaints and fatigue are most common overall, especially in patients receiving polytherapy [18,23].

Only about 3% of patients having refractory seizures during the initial two AED monotherapy trials become seizure-free during subsequent polytherapy [16]. AED treatment goals differ in refractory epilepsy care: while trying to achieve seizure freedom remains an important tent, clinicians should be aware that palliation of seizure burden is most likely and that preventing overtreatment and toxicity is equally if not more important than seizure reduction in the treatment of refractory epilepsy patients. Early consideration of drug-sparing, nonpharmacologic therapies that may enable reduction of the cumulative AED load – including epilepsy surgery, neurostimulation, and dietary therapies – is also crucial [16–18]. Patients with refractory epilepsy should be referred to comprehensive epilepsy centers offering intensive evaluation for drug-sparing nonpharmacological therapies [17–21]. The syndrome of mesial temporal-lobe epilepsy (TLE) benefits particularly from surgical resection and patients undergoing successful surgery usually enjoy improved QOL and decreased AED drug loads [17,19,21].

Drug selection principles for minimizing adverse effects

Patient characteristics are crucial when selecting and using AEDs. Factors such as age, gender, medical and psychiatric comorbidities, and coexisting medications must be considered when choosing an AED to optimize pharmacokinetic and phamacodynamic properties for a patient and prevent adverse effects from developing. Elderly patients are more vulnerable toward developing AED adverse effects, due to heightened sensitivity to dose-related adverse effects and altered drug absorption, volume of distribution, hepatic enzymatic metabolism, protein binding, and renal clearance. Newer AEDs, including lamotrigine and levetiracetam, are usually better tolerated than older AEDs in the elderly and non-enzyme-inducing AEDs limit the potential for drug–drug interactions. AED titration and tapering should begin with lower initial doses, with slower titration toward a lower initial target dose [22]. Choosing

AEDs with a low potential for drug–drug interactions is important in elderly patients receiving polypharmacy with other medications, particularly drugs inducible by cytochrome enzymes such as warfarin and certain antihypertensive drugs. Undesirable AED combinations occur frequently in institutionalized elderly, so careful review of current prescribed medications is especially necessary when selecting and titrating new adjunctive AEDs [23].

Gender also impacts AED selection. Women of child-bearing potential are at risk for two worrisome AED-related adverse effects: pregnancy due to oral contraceptive failure and AED-induced fetal teratogenesis. In women of child-bearing potential, several AEDs are associated with teratogenicity – particularly valproate – and enzyme-inducing AEDs such as carbamazepine, phenytoin, phenobarbital, and high-dose topiramate (>200 mg/day) may lower hormonal contraceptive concentrations and are best avoided. The newer non-enzyme-inducing AEDs, such as lamotrigine and levetiracetam, are increasingly favored [37,42]. Clinicians should instruct women of child-bearing potential to use double-barrier contraception when receiving enzyme-inducing AEDs. Before pregnancy planning, women who are seizure-free and at low risk of seizure recurrence should be weaned off AEDs or converted to AED monotherapy at the lowest effective dose, since polytherapy increases risk for teratogenesis. Valproate should be avoided unless it has resulted in complete seizure freedom. Women of child-bearing potential who are receiving an AED should be recommended to take folic acid 1 mg daily or a prenatal multivitamin.

While the cosmetic adverse effects of phenytoin are particularly concerning in women, given the possibility of coarsening of facial features, hirsuitism, and gingival hyperplasia, chronic phenytoin exposure is of potential concern in all epilepsy patients, given its potential for causing axonal polyneuropathy and cerebellar ataxia. Phenytoin use should preferably be limited to a few months to a year, after which time the patient can be offered the opportunity to transition to another AED if continued therapy is necessary.

Bone health is a particular concern in elderly patients and women. Patients on chronic AED therapy may be at risk for bone density loss and fractures. Enzyme-inducing AEDs (carbamazepine, phenytoin, phenobarbital, primidone, oxcarbazepine, and high-dose topiramate) can decrease bone density and even non-inducer AEDs (including valproate) have the possibility of doing so [24,25]. Patients receiving enzyme-inducing AEDs chronically should be counseled about bone density risks and should receive bone mineral densitometry measurement and supplemental calcium [24,25]. Seizure-free patients at low recurrence risk should be counseled about AED withdrawal or offered the opportunity to transition to a newer AED.

Patient comorbidities, such as obesity, also impact AED selection. Valproate, carbamazepine, gabapentin, and pregabalin may contribute to weight gain, while topiramate and zonisamide are frequently associated with weight loss. Certain comorbid disorders are often benefitted by medications with anti-pain or mood-stabilizing properties; for example, topiramate or valproate might be chosen in patients having both migraine and epilepsy, while patients with bipolar affective disorder and epilepsy could receive lamotrigine or valproate. Patients with hepatic or renal disorders may be vulnerable for development of hepatotoxicity from AEDs that impact liver function, including phenytoin, carbamazepine, and valproate, and may metabolize or clear AEDs and other drugs poorly, requiring cautious titration similar to that in elderly individuals (initial low doses, aiming for low targets and titrating slowly) [22].

Patients receiving polypharmacy might be at a heightened risk for adverse effects or consequences of drug–drug interactions. Therapeutic failure of inducible drugs, such as hormonal contraceptives, anticoagulants, lipid-lowering drugs, and antihypertensives, is a potential hazard when enzyme-inducing AEDs such as phenytoin, carbamazepine, or phenobarbital are prescribed [26–28].

Clinicians must also be aware of genetic polymorphisms that indicate vulnerability to idiosyncratic adverse effects. The HLA-B*1502 genotype in Asian patients, especially those of Han Chinese ancestry, is associated with higher risk for severe cutaneous reactions (including Stevens–Johnson syndrome) with several AEDs, including carbamazepine, phenytoin, and lamotrigine [29,30,50,51]. Screening for the HLA-B*1502 allele should be performed prior to initiating treatment with carbamazepine or other aromatic ring-structure AEDs in patients of Asian race.

AED monotherapy remains the preferred initial approach in newly diagnosed epilepsy, since the first or second monotherapy AED trial is effective and well tolerated in most patients [1,2,9,22]. The patient characteristics of age, gender, comorbidities, and comedications are important considerations when selecting and titrating an AED. The dosage goal should be moderate in most patients and AED levels should be monitored both to ensure a sufficiently protective serum concentration and to establish a "benchmark" level for individual patients who are free of seizures and adverse effects, once a steady-state dosage and concentration have been reached. Historical levels can be helpful to clinicians when determining whether a breakthrough seizure might be due to decreased adherence or drug interactions, but one should avoid "treating the level" per se, because arbitrary AED dose adjustment simply to achieve "therapeutic" ranges can lead to overtreatment, inadvertently inducing adverse effects [31]. Ensuring seizure freedom without adverse effects is the central tenet of AED therapy.

Practical approaches to minimizing adverse effects during antiepileptic drug polytherapy

When an initial AED monotherapy is ineffective or intolerable, AED conversion becomes necessary. Inadequate seizure control or intolerable adverse effects are the main reasons for AED conversion. Before committing to chronic polytherapy, which has a higher chance for adverse effects, additional AED monotherapy attempts may be desirable. Transitional polytherapy involves adding and titrating a new AED to a target dosage while maintaining an existing AED therapy until the new AED reaches a protective dosage and level, with the goal of converting to subsequent montherapy with the newly added AED. The existing AED (the previously failed first baseline AED) is then tapered and withdrawn [32]. One approach to transitional polytherapy favored by expert consensus recommends titrating a new adjunctive AED completely to its target dosage prior to tapering the existing baseline AED [22,32]. The existing baseline AED is held at its present dosage to reduce the chance of breakthrough seizure occurrence, the new adjunctive AED is titrated up to its presumably effective protective goal target dosage, and the baseline AED is then tapered and ultimate withdrawn. This approach is appropriately measured and must of course be individualized but it has the advantage of preventing breakthrough seizures due to abrupt discontinuance of an existing baseline AED. However, caution and individualization are necessary, given that each patient has differential vulnerability toward dose-related adverse effects, which are multiplied during the process of transitional polytherapy. Too rapid introduction of the new adjunctive AED may lead to intolerable adverse effects.

A flexible approach to reducing the existing baseline AED earlier may also be necessary [5,22,32]. The transitional polytherapy approach should be modified and the clinician should react appropriately when adverse effects occur during titration. When patients report intolerable, persistent adverse effects, the existing baseline AED can be tapered earlier and more rapidly, instead of abandoning the new adjunctive AED titration [22,32], as the common dose-related adverse effects of sedation, dizziness, and ataxia are caused by the combination of AEDs, not just the new AED alone. Unfortunately, new AEDs are frequently abandoned prematurely when patients develop dose-related adverse effects during titration. However, if patients are seizure-free and at risk for losing driving privileges or injury, the baseline AED should be tapered more slowly and in smaller amounts, to minimize the risk of breakthrough seizure occurrence.

Idiosyncratic adverse effects, including rash and hematologic or hepatic dyscrasias, may necessitate a more radical and acute intervention to stop an offending AED precipitously. The causative AED should then be either simply discontinued or rapidly tapered over a few days, during which time bridging therapy with a short-acting benzodiazepine or levetiracetam can provide seizure protection while another adjunctive AED is rapidly titrated to a presumably effective dosage. In this setting, it is sensible to select a newer AED that can be safely and rapidly titrated over a few days or even started and continued at a potentially efficacious dose in inpatients, such as levetiracetam, gabapentin, or oxcarbazepine [33–35]. Bridging therapy with an intravenous newer AED can also be considered when a new adjunctive AED requiring slow titration is being adjusted toward its target. Newer parenteral AEDs that are useful in acute inpatient seizure treatment and prophylaxis include levetiracetam, lacosamide, and valproate [36–38,59–61]. The traditional IV AEDs phenobarbital and phenytoin are less favorable choices when patients have an allergic drug rash or other acute idiosyncratic reactions, given their aromatic ring structures, which may crossreact and cause anticon-vulsant hypersensitivity syndrome [39], as well as the risk of idiosyncratic hematologic dyscrasias and hepatic failure.

When two AEDs with an appropriate spectrum of action against a patient's epilepsy type are either ineffective or poorly tolerated, patients are considered to have evolved refractory epilepsy [40]. Most patients with refractory epilepsy have already failed at least two monotherapy AED trials with different mechanisms of action and require chronic polytherapy. The general strategy for adding a second or subsequent adjunctive AED to a chronic polytherapy regimen is similar to the transitional polytherapy approach, except that (given the increasing cumulative drug load) reducing existing baseline AED doses at the same time as new adjunctive AEDs are titrated is often more successful and tolerable [22]. Clinicians should be familiar with pharmacoki-netic and pharmacodynamic AED interactions, in order to minimize adverse effect potential. Cytochrome P450 and protein-binding interactions are the most important considerations when initiating or tailoring polytherapy. Enzyme-inducing AEDs such as phenobarbital, pheny-toin, carbamazepine, and high-dose topiramate increase and accelerate the metabolism of inducible drugs such as lamotrigine, oxcarbazepine, topiramate, or tiagabine, reducing the serum concentration of inducible AEDs. "De-induction" of drugs in a polytherapy regimen occurs when enzyme-inducing AEDs are reduced, resulting in higher serum concentration of coadministered inducible AEDs, which may lead to optimized levels of inducible AEDs such as lamotrigine – sometimes with improved seizure control – or to hemorrhagic adverse effects if warfarin is the de-induced medication and its concentrations are inadvertently increased unchecked [41,42]. When valproate is given in combination with lamotrigine, the clearance of lamotrigine is greatly decreased (due to the inhibition of glucuronidation), which both increases lamotrigine concentrations and raises the risk of serious rash.

Adverse effects also result from pharmacodynamic interactions during AED polytherapy. Cognitive side effects are especially frequent and may be subtle and difficult to detect. While standard bedside mental-status assessments often show minimal change, neuropsycho-logical measures may show difficulties with attention, concentration, executive function, and memory [43,44]. Routine screening with a quantitative instrument such

as the AEP may help identify subtle adverse effects in patients with refractory epilepsy receiving AED poly-therapy and guide clinicians in adjusting medications appropriately [8].

Conclusion

AED adverse effects are common, particularly during dynamic AED titration or conversion, and can reduce QOL in epilepsy patients. Routine monitoring for adverse effects with a quantitative instrument such as the AEP can help physicians identify subtle adverse effects and lead to drug adjustments that improve patient QOL. AED conversions and sequencing of adjunctive AEDs in polytherapy are needed when patients have inadequate seizure control or experience intolerable adverse effects on their current treatment. When adding a new AED, expert consensus has sug-gested a general approach for monotherapy conversions: the new planned adjunctive AED is titrated while the existing baseline AED is held at a constant protective dose. However, flexibility is necessary: when patients report intolerable adverse effects, the primary baseline drug must be decreased as needed. In seizure-free patients, prevention of breakthrough seizures is the key goal during AED conversions and a more cau-tious strategy with slower drug tapering in smaller dosage amounts is necessary. Patient characteristics that influence AED selection and titration strategies include older age, female gender, mood, pain, and medical comorbidities, and concurrent medications. Clinicians should be familiar with pharmacodynamic and pharmacokinetic drug–drug interactions, so they can appropriately tailor AED treatment in specific situations. Transitional polytherapy requires careful monitoring for adverse effects, consideration of patient characteristics that impact drug selection and titration, anticipation of drug–drug interactions, and monitoring for seizures or adverse effects during the titration of new adjunctive AEDs and tapering of existing baseline AEDs.

References

1 Kwan P, Brodie MJ: Epilepsy after the first drug fails: sub-stitution or add-on? *Seizure* 2000; **9**:464–468.
2 Kwan P, Brodie MJ: Effectiveness of the first antiepileptic drug. *Epilepsia* 2001; **4**:1255–1260.

3 Gilliam F, Hecimovic H, Sheline Y: Psychiatric comorbidity, health, and function in epilepsy. *Epilepsy Behav* 2003; **4(Suppl. 4)**:S26–S30.

4 Gilliam FG, Mendiratta A, Pack AM, Bazil CW: Epilepsy and common comorbidities: improving the outpatient epilepsy encounter. *Epileptic Disord* 2005; **7(Suppl. 1)**:S27–S33.

5 Naritoku DK, Hulihan JF, Schwarzman LK et al.: Effect of cotherapy reduction on tolerability of epilepsy add-on therapy: a randomized controlled trial. *Annals of Pharmacotherapy* 2005; **39**:418–423.

6 Mattson RM, Cramer JA, Collins JF et al.: Comparison of phenobarbital, phenytoin, carbamazepine, and primidone in partial and secondary generalized tonic-clonic seizures. *NEJM* 1985; **313**:145–151.

7 Baker GA, Camfield C, Camfield P et al.: Commission on Outcome Measurement in Epilepsy, 1994–1997: final report. *Epilepsia* 1998; **39**:213–231.

8 Gilliam FG, Fessler AJ, Baker G et al.: Systematic screening allows reduction of adverse antiepileptic drug effects: a randomized trial. *Neurology* 2004; **62**:23–27.

9 St. Louis EK, Rosenfeld WE, Bramley T: Antiepileptic drug monotherapy: the initial approach in epilepsy management. *Curr Neuropharmacol* 2009; **7**:77–82.

10 St. Louis EK: Minimizing AED adverse effects: improving quality of life in the interictal state in epilepsy care. *Curr Neuropharmacol* 2009; **7**:106–114.

11 St. Louis EK: Truly "rational" polytherapy: maximizing efficacy and minimizing drug interactions, drug load, and adverse effects. *Curr Neuropharmacol* 2009; **7**:96–105.

12 Baulac M: Rational conversion from antiepileptic polytherapy to monotherapy. *Epileptic Disorders* 2003; **5**:125–132.

13 French JA, Kanner AM, Bautista J et al.: Efficacy and tolerability of the new antiepileptic drugs. II: Treatment of refractory epilepsy: report of the Therapeutics and Technology Assessment Subcommittee and Quality Standards Subcommittee of the American Academy of Neurology and the American Epilepsy Society. *Neurology* 2004; **62**: 1261–1273.

14 Reife R, Pledger G, Wu SC: Topiramate as add-on therapy: pooled analysis of randomized controlled trials in adults. *Epilepsia* 2000; **41(Suppl. 1)**:S66–S71.

15 Brodie MJ, Yuen AW: Lamotrigine substitution study: evidence for synergism with sodium valproate? 105 Study Group. *Epilepsy Res* 1997; **26**:423–432.

16 Kwan P, Brodie MJ: Early identification of refractory epilepsy. *NEJM* 2000; **342**:314–319.

17 Engel J Jr, Weibe S, French J et al.: Practice parameter: temporal lobe and localized neocortical resections for epilepsy: report of the Quality Standards Subcommittee of the American Academy of Neurology, in association with the American Epilepsy Society and the American Association of Neurological Surgeons. *Neurology* 2003; **60**:538–547.

18 Renfroe JB, Wheless JW: Earlier use of adjunctive vagus nerve stimulation therapy for refractory epilepsy. *Neurology* 2002; **59(6 Suppl. 4)**:S26–S30.

19 Wiebe S, Blume WT, Girvin JP, Eliasziw M: A randomized, controlled trial of surgery for temporal-lobe epilepsy. *NEJM* 2001; **345**:311–318.

20 Labar DR: Antiepileptic drug use during the first 12 months of vagus nerve stimulation therapy: a registry study. *Neurology* 2002; **59**:S38–S43.

21 St. Louis EK, Chang S, Granner MA et al.: Reduction of antiepileptic drug treatment following epilepsy surgery. *Epilepsia* 2007; **48**:150.

22 St. Louis EK, Gidal BE, Henry TR et al.: Conversions between monotherapies in epilepsy: expert consensus. *Epilepsy Behav* 2007; **11**:222–234.

23 Harms SL, Eberly LE, Garrard JM et al.: Prevalence of appropriate and problematic antiepileptic combination therapy in older people in the nursing home. *JAGS* 2005; **53**: 1023–1028.

24 Pack AM, Morrell MJ: Epilepsy and bone health in adults. *Epilepsy Behav* 2004; **5**:S24–S29.

25 Souverein PC, Webb DJ, Weil JG et al.: Use of antiepileptic drugs and risk of fractures: case-control study among patients with epilepsy. *Neurology* 2006; **66**:1318–1324.

26 Sheth RD: Metabolic concerns associated with antiepileptic medications. *Neurology* 2004; **63**:S24–S29.

27 Mintzer S: Metabolic consequences of antiepileptic drugs. *Curr Opin Neurol* 2010; **23**:164–169.

28 Mintzer S, Skidmore CT, Abidin CJ et al.: Effects of antiepileptic drugs on lipids, homocysteine, and C-reactive protein. *Ann Neurol* 2009; **65**:448–456.

29 Hung SI, Chung WH, Jee SH et al.: Genetic susceptibility to carbamazepine-induced cutaneous adverse drug reactions. *Pharmacogenet Genomics* 2006; **16(4)**:297–306.

30 Man CB, Kwan P, Baum L et al.: Association between HLA-B*1502 allele and antiepileptic drug-induced cutaneous reactions in Han Chinese. *Epilepsia* 2007; **48**: 1015–1018.

31 St. Louis EK: Monitoring antiepileptic drugs: a level-headed approach. *Curr Neuropharmacol* 2009; **7**:115–119.

32 Garnett WR, St Louis EK, Henry TR, Bramley T: Transitional polytherapy: tricks of the trade for monotherapy to monotherapy AED conversions. *Curr Neuropharmacol* 2009; **7**:83–95.

33 Fisher RS, Sachdeo RC, Pellock J et al.: Rapid initiation of gabapentin: a randomized, controlled trial. *Neurology* 2001; **56**:743–748.

34 French J, Arrigo C: Rapid onset of action of levetiracetam in refractory epilepsy patients. *Epilepsia* 2005; **46**:324–326.

35 Mauro AM, Bomprezzi C, Morresi S et al.: Prevention of early postoperative seizures in patients with primary brain tumors: preliminary experience with oxcarbazepine. *J Neurooncol* 2007; **81**:279–285.

36 Biton V, Rosenfeld WE, Whitesides J et al.: Intravenous lacosamide as replacement for oral lacosamide in patients with partial-onset seizures. *Epilepsia* 2008; **49**:418–424.

37 Gilad R, Izkovitz N, Dabby R et al.: Treatment of status epilepticus and acute repetitive seizures with i.v. valproic acid vs phenytoin. *Acta Neurol Scand.* 2008; **118**:296–300.

38 Szaflarski JP, Sangha KS, Lindsell CJ, Shutter LA: Prospective, randomized, single-blinded comparative trial of intravenous levetiracetam versus phenytoin for seizure prophylaxis. *Neurocrit Care* 2010; **12**:165–172.

39 Bohan KH, Mansuri TF, Wilson NM: Anticonvulsant hypersensitivity syndrome: implications for pharmaceutical care. *Pharmacotherapy* 2007; **27**:1425–1439.

40 Kwan P, Arzimanoglou A, Berg AT et al.: Definition of drug resistant epilepsy: consensus proposal by the ad hoc Task Force of the ILAE Commission on Therapeutic Strategies. *Epilepsia* 2010; **51**:1069–1077.

41 Patsalos PN, Froscher W, Pisani F, van Rijn CM: The importance of drug interactions in epilepsy therapy. *Epilepsia* 2002; **43**:365–385.

42 Anderson GD, Gidal BE, Messenheimer JA, Gilliam FG: Time course of lamotrigine de-induction: impact of stepwise withdrawal of carbamazepine or phenytoin. *Epilepsy Re.* 2002; **49**:211–217.

43 Meador KJ. Cognitive outcomes and predictive factors in epilepsy. *Neurology* 2002; **58**:S21–S26.

44 Rahmann A, Stodieck S, Husstedt IW, Evers S: Pre-attentive cognitive processing in epilepsy: a pilot study on the impact of epilepsy type and anti-epileptic treatment. *European Neurology* 2002; **48**:146–152.

CHAPTER 11

Idiosyncratic adverse side effects of antiepileptic drugs: risk, prevention, and counseling

Mary L. Zupanc and Lily H. Tran

Department of Pediatrics and Neurology, University of California at Irvine and Children's Hospital of Orange County, USA

Introduction

When counseling patients about the side effects of antiepileptic medications, the perspective of a risk/benefit ratio should be a primary consideration. In young infants and children, for example, risks of continued seizures in the developing brain are high – sometimes catastrophic – often outweighing the risks of antiepileptic drug (AED) therapy. Risk/benefit ratios are often a difficult concept for parents to understand, given societal concerns about the risks of "foreign substances" with potential toxicities, such as the controversies regarding vaccinations and autism, which illustrate the tenacity of belief systems that have been debunked in the scientific world. The Internet has become the main source of information for patients and families. Physicians must counsel patients and parents wisely, listen to their concerns in a nonjudgmental fashion, and address each concern carefully, with facts and information. For most, this is very helpful, but for a rare few, the belief system supersedes logic. In these difficult cases, the physician has to decide whether they can continue to care for the patient. Allowing concomitant use of "natural" substances along with antiepileptic medication is sometimes a necessary practice. There are a few epilepsy syndromes, however, that must be treated quickly and appropriately, before windows of developmental opportunity disappear. This chapter first considers the balance between appropriately aggressive and directed therapies for patients with catastrophic epilepsy syndromes and the idiosyncratic adverse effects

associated with those AED therapies, then looks at the range of idiosyncratic adverse effects associated with the most commonly utilized AEDs in both children and adults. A summary of idiosyncratic AED adverse effects is shown in Table 11.1.

Therapeutic considerations and idiosyncratic adverse drug reactions in infantile spasms treatment

Infantile spasms is a catastrophic epilepsy syndrome. Once infantile spasms occur, along with the signature of electroencephalographic hypsarrhythmia – characterized by high-amplitude polymorphic delta activity and frequent, multifocal spike, polyspike, and slow wave discharge pattern – there is a 4–6 week treatment window. The longer infantile spasms and hysparrhythmia persist, the more difficult this syndrome is to treat [1]. Brain cells that "fire together, wire together" (seize together, network together). Both treatment of the infantile spasms and elimination of hypsarrhythmia pattern are necessary treatment goals. ACTH (adrenocorticotrophin hormone) is the treatment of choice. When this option is presented to families, it is often met with fear and skepticism, especially given the need for repeated injections for the child. In addition, the long list of side effects of ACTH is daunting to parents, including immunosuppression, hypertension, bleeding/hemorrhage, gastritis, irritability, diabetes,

Epilepsy and the Interictal State: Co-Morbidities and Quality of Life, First Edition.
Edited by Erik K. St. Louis, David M. Ficker, and Terence J. O'Brien.
© 2015 John Wiley & Sons, Ltd. Published 2015 by John Wiley & Sons, Ltd.

Table 11.1 Idiosyncratic adverse effects of antiepileptic drugs (AEDs).

Antiepileptic drug/therapy	Idiosyncratic reaction
Ketogenic diet	Cardiac complications: QT prolongation, impaired myocardial function
Felbamate	Aplastic anemia, hepatic toxicity
Topiramate	Ocular dysfunction: abnormal vision, acute secondary angle-closure glaucoma, acute myopia, suprachoroidal effusion, metabolic acidosis
Lamotrigine	Allergic rash
Valproate	Hepatotoxicity, hyperammonemia, pancreatitis
Phenytoin	Allergic rash and hypersensitivity syndrome (lymphadenopathy, fever, cytopenias) cerebellar ataxia, gingival hyperplasia, hepatotoxicity, hirsutism, peripheral neruopathy, purple-glove syndrome (intravenous phenytoin only)
Ethosuximide	Allergic rash
Carbamazepine	Hyponatremia, allergic rash - especially in patients of Asian ancestry possessing HLA-B*1502 genetic allele
Oxcarbazepine	Hyponatremia
Zonisamide	Oligohidrosis, metabolic acidosis, psychosis
Rufinamide	Short QT interval
Ezogabine	Skin discoloration, retinal pigment changes

femoral necrosis, increased appetite, and weight gain. Physicians need to discuss the important risks and consequences of nontreatment as well as the benefits of therapy [1,2]. Clinical studies have shown that the use of ACTH therapy in short treatment bursts, without prolonged therapy, rarely causes significant side effects [1–3]. When ACTH therapy is sustained for months, children may have significant consequences. Hence, the treatment paradigm should be for high-dose therapy, short term, over 6–8 weeks maximum. For patients with tuberous sclerosis and infantile spasms, the treatment of choice is probably vigabatrin, which now has orphan drug status in the United States. This drug can produce peripheral visual deficits. In adults, the earliest finding of the first abnormal visual field exam is after 9 months of treatment (11 months in children) [4]. The incidence of peripheral visual constriction is about 10–40% [2], a complication that is difficult to test for in children. However, it does not appear to be clinically significant in the majority of patients. In addition, infantile spasms is an age-dependent epileptic encephalopathy and it is rarely necessary to treat the infant/child with vigabatrin for longer than 6–8 months. Often, a single course lasting 4 months suffices

for successful treatment of infantile spasms in children with tuberous sclerosis. When considering the risks of an ongoing epileptic encephalopathy compared with either ACTH or vigabatrin, the risks posed by continued seizures to healthy brain development are much greater. Continued infantile spasms and hypsarrhythmia evolve into Lennox–Gastaut syndrome (LGS) in approximately 80–90% of patients, with a generalized spike and slow wave discharge pattern, multiple seizure types, and psychomotor maldevelopment.

Therapeutic considerations and idiosyncratic adverse drug reactions in Lennox–Gastaut syndrome treatment

LGS is often the result of continued seizures from infancy. As a child grows older, seizure types and epilepsy syndromes evolve as infantile spasms disappear. LGS is characterized by the triad of multiple seizure types (including tonic, atonic, atypical absence, myoclonic, and generalized tonic–clonic seizures), EEG findings of generalized slow spike-and-wave discharges at 2.0–2.5 Hz, and cognitive impairments. LGS is very difficult to treat and patients frequently have recurrent episodes of status epilepticus.

AEDs can be quite effective in treating LGS. When counseling parents about choices of drugs, they may be reluctant to try medications that could cause impairments in their child. Typically, parents may have already learned that their child's epilepsy syndrome is difficult to treat. Most often, children with LGS require polytherapy with multiple antiepileptic medications, which frequently cause sedation. Even with toxic AED polytherapy, refractory daily seizures usually persist in LGS patients. Understandably, parents often fear or resist addition of further antiepileptic medications and, given desperation to achieve improved seizure control and improved alertness, the ketogenic diet is highly appealing to many families of LGS patients.

Approved AEDs for LGS include topiramate, felbamate, lamotrigine, rufinamide, and clobazam. Valproate carries Food and Drug Administration (FDA) approval for complex partial seizures with secondary generalization and for generalized seizures, including absence seizures, but is one of the initial drugs used by clinicians for LGS, despite its lacking evidence for this use from prospective, double-blind trials [5]. The ketogenic diet has also been shown to be effective for multiple seizure types but does not carry a specific indication limited to LGS and instead may be used in a wide variety of refractory epilepsy syndromes.

When counseling patients and parents about AED choices in LGS, the most important consideration should again be the risk/benefit ratio. In current practice, parents have often heard about the ketogenic diet, popularized recently in the United States following a television movie entitled *Do No Harm* [6]. The idea of a dietary approach is often appealing to patients and their families, as it seems to be "natural" and does not pose some of the risks and side effects of AEDs. Physicians and dieticians should emphasize that the ketogenic diet is in reality not natural and produces important changes in bodily metabolism, including metabolic derangements, gastrointestinal symptoms, carnitine deficiency, renal calculi, hypercholesteremia, and slowed growth [7]. In addition, severe side effects include impaired myocardial function and QT prolongation [8]. Two children treated with the ketogenic diet for refractory epilepsy were found to have selenium deficiency and suffered sudden cardiac death from QT prolongation and torsades de

pointes [9]. Children who are oral feeders are at risk for severe dehydration when they are sick or when they refuse to eat the meticulously calculated meals. In addition, for children who have defects in fatty acid oxidation or inborn errors of metabolism, the ketogenic diet produces a high risk for vomiting, encephalopathy, and even death [7]. The metabolic adaptation to the ketogenic diet involves shifting the primary energy source from carbohydrates to lipid. Thus, patients with fatty acid oxidation defects or inborn errors of metabolism cannot adjust to this change appropriately and suffer devastating catabolic crisis.

Streamlining polytherapy AED regimens is an important goal in LGS therapy as it allows adverse effects and drug–drug interactions to be avoided through judicious tapering of medications that have proven ineffective or that have possibly even exacerbated seizures. Carbamazepine (CBZ) frequently exacerbates some seizures of LGS, particularly tonic and astatic seizure types [10]. Phenobarbital and phenytoin are both sedating medications causing chronic drowsiness, which may in turn produce nearly continuous generalized slow spike-and-wave discharges [11].

Felbamate is one of the best antiepileptic medications for LGS. Felbamate was initially approved by the FDA in 1993, and at the time was the first antiepileptic medication to be approved in over 10 years. Clinical trials had been very encouraging with respect to seizure control. Felbamate was given to many patients with refractory epilepsy, particularly those with LGS. Clinical trials of felbamate had involved over 7000 patients and showed no sign of significant idiosyncratic risk, giving it the initial appearance of being a very safe medication, so routine blood work was often not performed. In the first year following approval of felbamate, there were 34 cases of aplastic anemia and 18 cases of liver toxicity, and the drug was almost pulled off the market [12]. However, experience of felbamate efficacy in the pediatric population, particularly in patients with LGS, was compelling [12]. Therefore, due to an active parent voice and with the help of the Child Neurology Society, the FDA allowed felbamate to stay on the market, with a specific indication for medically refractory epilepsy and for patients over 4 years of age with LGS [13]. Subsequently, risk factors for aplastic anemia have been identified, including female gender, AED polytherapy, history of cytopenia, postpubertal status, antinuclear antibody (ANA) titer, and autoimmune disease [12,14].

In patients with two or more of these risk factors, the relative risk of developing aplastic anemia is quadrupled [14]. Risk factors for liver toxicity have not been successfully identified. However, of all patients on felbamate who developed liver toxicity, all were on polytherapy, most also received valproate, and most were female [12,14]. Since 1994, there have been over 50 000 additional exposures to felbamate, many of them children [12]. There has been only one case of aplastic anemia – in a 45-year-old woman with autoimmune disease [12]. There have been no further cases of liver toxicity. The FDA has recommended rigorous, frequent screening of hematological and liver function parameters, particularly in the first 6 months following felbamate initiation, given that the idiosyncratic, adverse side effects of felbamate, including aplastic anemia and liver failure, are most frequent during the first 6 months of therapy. Following 6 months of use, these side effects have been only rarely reported [12,14].

Parents should be counseled that the risks of continued seizures with LGS include a risk of continued cognitive decline, since this type of epilepsy is considered by most to involve progressive cognitive dysfunction [4]. Many patients with LGS, as they age, develop cerebral atrophy [4]. As adults, seizure types in LGS may change, and EEG demonstrates less frequent generalized slow spike-and-wave discharges with more multifocal discharges and persistence of diffuse fast rhythms in non-REM sleep [15]. Sudden unexpected death in epilepsy (SUDEP) is a catastrophic complication with an incidence rate of up to 9 per 1000 patient years in patients with intractable epilepsy. Risk factors include male sex, young age at epilepsy onset, symptomatic etiology, long duration of epilepsy, frequent convulsive seizures, and polytherapy [16]. Physicians, patients, and parents again need to weigh the risks versus benefits of AED compared with the risks of continued seizures. All risks considered, initiation of felbamate is usually worth considering. In a retrospective study of felbamate in LGS, 75% of patients had a greater than 50% reduction in tonic and atonic seizure frequency. In addition, felbamate is a relatively alerting medication that typically does not cause drowsiness, with common side effects of insomnia, agitation, and anorexia. Insomnia can be avoided by "front-loading" the medication – giving a higher dosage in the morning – while melatonin can help with sleep induction and cyproheptadine with sleep and appetite stimulation.

Topiramate is also used for the treatment of LGS but can induce drowsiness and cognitive slowing. In a retrospective case series, ocular adverse effects were reported in 150 patients receiving topiramate, including abnormal vision, acute secondary angle-closure glaucoma, acute myopia, and suprachoroidal effusions [17]. All ocular conditions are reversible with discontinuation of topiramate. In patients with only mild cognitive impairments, trying alternative medications first such as lamotrigine, valproate, or felbamate may be worthwhile.

Idiosyncratic allergic rash risk associated with antiepileptic drug therapies

Lamotrigine is also used for LGS and has been shown to be effective for the treatment of the tonic and atonic generalized tonic–clonic and atypical absence seizures. Lamotrigine carries a black-box warning for severe allergic rash. Allergic rash is found as a particular risk in antiepileptic medications that contain a benzene ring, including phenobarbital, phenytoin, CBZ, oxcarbazepine (OXC), lamotrigine, and felbamate. Cross-reactivity may occur, so if a rash occurs with one of these AEDs, the others are relatively contraindicated. The risk of a severe allergic rash – such as Stevens–Johnson syndrome – for these medications varies. For lamotrigine, according to the German Registry for Serious Cutaneous Reactions, the risk of a severe allergic rash in the pediatric population is approximately 0.8% [18]. In comparison to phenobarbital, phenytoin, and CBZ, the rate of serious rash for lamotrigine is similar, and in adolescence and adulthood, the severe rash risk for lamotrigine drops further to 0.3% [19]. Rash most often occurs 7–10 days following medication initiation, but at the latest usually within the first 6 weeks of therapy. Risk for severe rash is highest in those having HLA-B*1502 genotype, especially for rash with CBZ. The HLA-B*1502 allele is most common in patients of Han Chinese ethnicity and other South East Asian populations and can be assessed by a blood test. Therefore, it is important to advise patients and families who are of South East Asian descent that they may be at risk for the development of a severe allergic rash, especially with CBZ, and to arrange for a test of the HLA-B*1502 allele in at-risk patients prior to consideration of initiating CBZ or other aromatic-ring-structure AEDs such as phenytoin, OXC, or lamotrigine [20]. Phenytoin may also manifest a unique hypersensitivity syndrome characterized by fever, a severe morbilliform skin eruption accompanied by follicular papules and pustules, lymphadenopathy, hepatitis, and variable additional systemic manifestations, which may include anemia and other cytopenias, pharyngitis, diarrhea, or nephritis [21,22]. Other non-allergic chronic idiosyncratic adverse reactions of oral phenytoin may include gingival hyperplasia, hirsuitism, facial coarsening, peripheral neuropathy, cerebellar ataxia, and bone density loss, and extravasation of intravenous phenytoin may lead to the dreaded purple glove syndrome (a risk that does not occur with the safer intravenous prodrug fosphenytoin) [22]. The threshold for stopping an antiepileptic medication suspected of causing an allergic rash or severe systemic allergic reaction should be low. Patients being started on antiepileptic medications should be carefully counseled about the risks of rash, including severe rash, especially when they have reported a history of allergic rash with other medications.

Idiosyncratic adverse effects associated with valproate and ethosuximide

Valproate poses a risk of hepatotoxicity. When it was first released in the late 1970s, this risk was not appreciated. In the early 1980s, 78 cases of fatal hepatotoxicity due to valproate were reported [23]. Risk for valproate hepatotoxicity was estimated to be $1:500$ and was highest in children under 2 years of age, those with hypotonia and developmental delays, those receiving AED polytherapy, and children suspected of having an inborn error of metabolism. Valproate, being a fatty acid metabolized in the mitochondria, is suspected of "derailing" the metabolism of the mitochondria. As our knowledge of mitochondrial disorders has improved over the past 25 years, we now know that patients with the POLG1 mutation may be at highest risk for fatal hepatotoxicity [24]. Recently, it has been recommended that all young patients be screened for POLG1 before considering initiation of valproate [24]. POLG1 mutations can produce a broad spectrum of clinical symptoms [25]. Previously, POLG1 mutation

was associated with severe neurological symptoms, including hypotonia, severe cognitive impairments, and intractable epilepsy (Alpers–Huttenlocher syndrome). However, the mutation can also be found in patients who have mild neurological problems or cognitive impairments and intractable epilepsy [19].

Valproate can also cause an encephalopathy due to hyperammonemia. Patients who become drowsy and/or stuporous on valproate should have blood drawn for an ammonia level, liver function studies, lactate, pyruvate, carnitine, acylcarnitine profile, and amino acid profile and have urine collected for organic acids to screen for mitochondrial dysfunction and defects in fatty acid oxidation. High-dose carnitine rescue can be used in patients with acute liver toxicity and encephalopathy. Carnitine rescue dosage should be 100–200 mg/kg/h intravenously, until the liver function tests and/or ammonia start to decline [10].

Valproate also contains a black-box warning for pancreatitis. Pancreatitis occurs more often in children but may occur at any age [26]. If there is a previous history of pancreatitis or a family history of pancreatitis, valproate should not be used. Careful screening of the family history is imperative prior to valproate prescription.

In patients with other idiopathic/symptomatic generalized epilepsies, such as childhood absence epilepsy (CAE), drug choices include valproate and ethosuximide. Ethosuximide remains the drug of choice for CAE that is not associated with concomitant generalized tonic–clonic seizures [27]. Ethosuximide can produce an allergic rash and idiosyncratic reactions of aplastic anemia and liver toxicity.

Idiosyncratic adverse effects associated with carbamazepine and oxcarbazepine

CBZ is a narrow-spectrum AED with efficacy for partial-onset seizures that has some important limitations that must be considered during both initiation and chronic administration, including autoinduction and chronic hepatic induction, which can produce drug–drug interactions. The chief metabolite of CBZ, carbamazepine-10,11-epoxide provides both antiepileptic efficacy and clinical toxicity. OXC is a 10-keto analogue of CBZ that is chemically similar to CBZ but has an improved side-effect profile. Several studies have emerged reporting a higher risk of developing hyponatremia in patients treated with OXC compared to CBZ [6,28,29]. Hyponatremia is an electrolyte disturbance that is usually clinically asymptomatic but can sometimes lead to serious complications when overlooked or not treated appropriately. Mild hyponatremia (Na+ ≤134 mEq/L) occurs in 29.9% of OXC- and 13.5% of CBZ-treated adult patients, while severe hyponatremia (Na+ ≤128 mEq/L) is seen in 12.4% of OXC- and 2.8% of CBZ-treated patients [28]. During a multicenter drug surveillance program in which severe or new adverse drug reactions were assessed during psychopharmacological treatment in adult psychiatric inpatients, the rate of hyponatremia was highest with OXC. The report involved 80 psychiatric hospitals in Germany, Switzerland, and Austria and showed the rate of hyponatremia to be 0.10% with CBZ and 1.29% with OXC [30]. The exact mechanism underlying hyponatremia is unknown but proposed mechanisms include altered sensitivity to serum osmolality of the hypothalamic osmoreceptors and increased sensitivity of the renal tubules to circulating ADH. CBZ has also been associated with syndrome of inappropriate antidiuretic hormone (SIADH). Hyponatremia related to OXC is due not to SIADH but rather to a direct effect of OXC on the renal collecting tubules or an enhancement of the responsiveness of renal collecting tubules to circulating antidiuretic hormone [29]. Risk factors for developing hyponatremia in patients with epilepsy treated with OXC include higher dosages [31], polypharmacy [31], and advanced age [28]. One study reported that an increase of 1 mg in the dosage of OXC increased the risk of hyponatremia by 0.2% [31]. In 72 children treated with OXC for epilepsy, the rate of hyponatremia (Na+ ≤134 mEq/L) without clinical symptoms was 26.6%, while that of severe hyponatremia was 2.6% (Na+ ≤128 mEq/L). Clinically relevant hyponatremia occurred in one child (1.3%) [32]. In the same study, CBZ was directly replaced with OXC in a subgroup of 27 children and hyponatremia without symptoms was found in one child with CBZ (3.7%) and six children with OXC (22.2%) [32]. No predictive value was found for the development of hyponatremia when examining dosage of OXC, serum levels of active metabolite of OXC, antiepileptic comedication, age, or gender.

Taken together, the risk for hyponatremia appears to be higher with OXC compared to CBZ, with higher dosages of OXC and antiepileptic polypharmacy

increasing the potential for OXC-induced hyponatremia. In patients who have renal disease and those taking medication which may lower serum sodium levels, such as diuretics, baseline serum sodium level measurement should be considered and monitored periodically, especially if symptoms of hyponatremia develop [33]. In otherwise healthy individuals, as higher dosages of CBZ or OXC are attained, serum sodium levels should be measured if the patient becomes symptomatic with headache, general malaise, gait disturbance, and somnolence. If symptomatic hyponatremia is encountered or if serum sodium concentration falls under 125 mEq/L, options may include free water restriction to less than 1 L daily, salt tablet supplementation, decrease of the dosage of OXC or CBZ, and discontinuation of the offending drug with substitution for an AED with a similar major mechanism of action (such as lamotrigine or valproate) that does not have a significant sodium-lowering profile or substitution for eslicarbamazepine, which appears to be associated with a lower frequency of hyponatremia [34].

Idiosyncratic adverse effects associated with topiramate and zonisamide

Zonisamide is a sulfonamide anticonvulsant. It was first synthesized in Japan in 1972 [35] and later approved in the United Sates as adjunctive therapy for partial-onset seizures in 2000. Oligohidrosis has been reported in a small number of patients treated with zonisamide [7]. In a proportion of these patients – mostly children in the summer months – hyperthermia has occurred [36]. The exact mechanism for oligohydrosis associated with zonisamide is not fully known but it has been proposed that carbonic anhydrase inhibition influences pH dynamics, hydrogen ion concentration, and available calcium transients and that functionality of the eccrine glands is subsequently impeded [7,36]. Thus, patients receiving zonisamide should stay well hydrated during hot-weather months to minimize the potential for hyperthermia from oligohidrosis.

Both topiramate and zonisamide have been reported to cause metabolic acidosis, with more frequent reports for topiramate [12]. This is probably due to impairment in the normal reabsorption of filtered bicarbonate by the proximal renal tubule and excretion of hydrogen by the distal renal tubule, resulting in mixed renal tubular acidosis, which can lead to acute illness, nephrolithiasis, osteoporosis, and growth retardation in the pediatric population [12]. Evidence on when to monitor serum bicarbonate levels is lacking, so monitoring should be done on an individualized basis. The adverse effect of metabolic acidosis is not determined by drug dose or treatment duration; one report suggests that genetic polymorphisms in the gene for carbonic anhydrase type XII are a potential cause [25]. Thus, in counseling patients who are to receive topiramate or zonisamide, sufficient hydration should be emphasized, to prevent nephrolithiasis. In patients with a known history of kidney stones, other AEDs should be considered before initiating either of these medications.

Idiosyncratic adverse effects associated with rufinamide

Rufinamide is a triazole derivative that is structurally different from other AEDs and has been approved as an adjuvant therapy for LGS. In a randomized, double-blind control study consisting of adults and children with LGS, rufinamide was shown to significantly decrease drop attacks and total seizures [37].While the precise antiepileptic mechanism is unknown, *in vitro* studies suggest rufinamide modulates sodium channel activity and prolongs its inactive state [38]. Rufinamide can shorten the QT interval, mostly in the higher dosage range of 2400–4800 mg/day, and is contraindicated in patients with familial short QT syndrome [39]. Short QT syndrome can lead to episodes of syncope, ventricular arrhythmia, and potential death. Thus, caution should be exercised in patients with a known familial short QT syndrome, and a careful family cardiac history is beneficial. Screening EKG should be considered before use of rufinamide in patients who may be at risk.

Idiosyncratic adverse effects associated with ezogabine

Ezogabine was approved by the European Union in March 2011 and by the FDA in June 2011 as an adjunctive therapy to partial-onset seizures in adults. Ezogabine was formerly known as retigabine. In one randomized, double-blind, placebo-controlled trial in

partial epilepsy, ezogabine was shown to be effective as an add-on therapy for reducing seizure frequency in patients with drug-resistant partial-onset seizures [13]. Another multicenter, randomized, double-blind, placebo-controlled trial in adults demonstrated titration of ezogabine to 600–900 mg/day over 4 weeks was generally well tolerated and effective [40]. Both studies provided class II evidence that adjunctive therapy with ezogabine is effective in the treatment of partial-onset seizures. Ezogabine is the first neuronal potassium channel opener, making it a unique AED and a novel approach to the treatment of epilepsy. The main mechanism of action of ezogabine involves acting as a positive allosteric modulator of KCNQ2-5 (Kv7.2-7.5) ion channels [5].

Since being introduced to the market in April 2012 through February 2013, approximately 2900 patients have received ezogabine prescription [41]. Retinal abnormalities and skin discoloration have been reported only in patients who were originally enrolled in clinical trials and have taken the drug for long periods of time. The skin discoloration typically involves blue or blue-gray pigmentation occurring around the lips or in the nail beds of the fingers and toes. There are also reports of similar changes involving the face and legs. Skin and retinal discoloration have occurred in approximately 6.3% of the patients followed in the clinical trial, with the mean time of occurrence of skin discoloration being 4.04 years (median 4.1 years) following exposure to the drug [41]. Most of these patients have been taking the drug for at least 2 years [41]. The nature of this clinical consequence, whether these changes can be reversed, and the mechanism of action underlining pigment changes are still unknown at this time.

To date, there are 89 patients still remaining in ongoing studies with ezogabine, of which 36 have had eye exams. Of these, 11 have been found to have retinal pigment abnormalities; all have been on the drug for at least 3 years. Five of these patients have worse than 20/20 visual acuity: one has 20/160 visual acuity in one eye and four have visual acuity of 20/25 to 20/40 in one or both eyes. However, no baseline visual acuity data are available, so it remains unknown whether decreased visual acuity could be related to the retinal pigment changes from exposure to ezogabine. There is one patient who has shown findings consistent with retinal dystrophy. About one-third of patients who have had eye exams have been found to have retinal pigment changes, and approximately one-third of these have no skin discoloration [41]. Again, information regarding the consequences, reversibility, pathophysiology, rate of progression, and time to onset of the retinal changes is incomplete or unknown. At this point, the FDA recommends that all patients who receive ezogabine obtain baseline and periodic eye exams involving visual acuity testing, dilated fundus photography, and optional fluorescein angiograms, ocular coherence tomography, perimetry, and electroretinograms (ERGs).

Several of the older and newer AEDs have other idiosyncratic risks that are most relevant to the adult patient population, including cognitive adverse effects, teratogenic risk, and risk of bone density loss. These topics will be discussed in other chapters of this book, including those on cognition (Chapter 4), AED adverse effects (Chapter 9), epilepsy in the elderly (Chapter 18), and epilepsy and bone health (Chapter 20).

Conclusion

In conclusion, patients and families should be counseled about each drug within an AED regimen, highlighting the reasons for AED selection, the risk/benefit ratio of initiation, potential side-effect profile, and the necessity of baseline blood draws and frequent repeat surveillance monitoring. The risk/benefit ratio should be discussed between the physician and the patient and/or family members, including the perils of persistent seizures on a developing brain, weighed against the possible occurrence of rare idiosyncratic AED reactions. Families want to be informed and to know that they are making an informed decision concerning their child's care. They should be reminded that their child's safety is of utmost importance and that the goal of treatment is to control seizures to maximize the patient's quality of life. Collaboration between health care providers, the patient, and family members/caretakers is paramount in the ongoing management and care of epilepsy. Mutual understanding that each party in this team has the patient's best interests at heart allows for a successful collaboration.

References

1 Pellock JM, Hrachovy R, Shinnar S et al.: Infantile spasms: A US consensus report. *Epilepsia* 2010; **51**:2175–2189.

2 MacKay MT, Weiss SK, Adams-Webber T et al.: Practice parameter: medical treatment of infantile spasms: report of the American Academy of Neurology and the Child Neurology Society. *Neurology* 2004; **62**:1668–1681.

3 Arya R, Shinnar S, Glauser TA: Corticosteroids for the treatment of infantile spasms: a systematic review. *J Child Neurol* 2012; **27**:1284–1288.

4 Willmore LJ, Abelson MB, Ben-Menchem E et al.: Vigabatrin: 2008 update. *Epilepsia* 2009; **50**:163–173.

5 Gunthrope MJ, Large CH, Sankar R: The mechanism of action of retigazine (ezogabine), a first-in-class K+ channel opener for the treatment of epilepsy. *Epilepsia* 2012; **53**: 412–424.

6 VanAmelsvoort Th, Bakshi R, Devaux CB, Schwabe S: Hyponatremia associated with carbamazepine and oxcarbazepine therapy: a review. *Epilepsia* 1994; **35**:181–188.

7 Knudsen JF, Thambi LR, Kapcala LP, Racoosin JA: Oligohydrosis and fever in pediatric patients treated with zonisamide. *Pediatr Neurol* 2003; **28(3)**:184–189.

8 Best TH, Franz DN, Gilbert DL et al.: Cardiac complications in pediatric patients on the ketogenic diet. *Neurology* 2000; **54**:2328–2330.

9 Bank IM, Shemie SD, Rosenblatt B et al.: Sudden cardiac death in association with the ketogenic diet. *Pediatr Neurol* 2008; **39**:429–431.

10 Perrott J, Murphy NG, Zed PJ: L-carnitine for acute valproic acid overdose: a systematic review of published cases. *Ann Pharmacother* 2010; **44**:1287–1293.

11 Panday VA, Rhee DJ: Review of sulfonamide-induced acute myopia and acute bilateral angle-closure glaucoma. *Compr Ophthalmol Update* 2007; **8(5)**:271–276.

12 Zaccara G, Franciotta D, Perucca E: Idiosyncratic adverse reactions to antiepileptic drugs. *Epilepsia* 2007; **48(7)**: 1223–1244.

13 French JA, Abou-Khalil BW, Leroy RF et al.: Randomized, double-blind, placebo-controlled trial of ezogabine (retigabine) in partial epilepsy. *Neurology* 2011; **76**:1555–1563.

14 Pellock JM: Felbamate. *Epilepsia* 1999; **40(Suppl. 5)**: S57–S62.

15 Astencio AMG, Machado RA, Merayo Y et al.: Electroclinical features of Lennox–Gastaut syndrome in adulthood and adolescence. *J Neurol Neurophysiol* 2013; **S2**:008.

16 Stafstrom CE, Grippon S, Kirkpatrick P: Ezogabine (retigabine). *Nat Rev* 2011; **10**:729–730.

17 Ferrell PB Jr,, McLeod HL. Carbamazepine, HLA-B*1502 and risk of Stevens-Johnson syndrome and toxic epidermal necrolysis: US FDA recommendations. *Pharmacogenomics* 2008; **10**:1543–1546.

18 Mockenhaupt M, Messenheimer J, Teenis P, Schlingmann J: Risk of Stevens–Johnson syndrome and toxic epidermal necrolysis in new users of antiepileptics. *Neurology* 2005; **12**:1134–1138.

19 Isohanni P, Hakonen AH, Euro L et al.: POLG1 manifestations in childhood. *Neurology* 2011; **76**:811–815.

20 Hung SI, Chung WH, Liu ZS et al.: Common risk allele in aromatic antiepileptic-drug induced Stevens–Johnson syndrome and toxic epidermal necrolysis in Han Chinese. *Pharmacogenomics* 2010; **11(3)**:349–356.

21 Tomsick RS. The phenytoin syndrome. *Cutis* 1983; **32(6)**: 535–541.

22 Scheinfeld N. Impact of phenytoin therapy on the skin and skin disease. *Expert Opin Drug Saf* 2004; **3(6)**:655–665.

23 Bryant A, Dreifuss FE: Valproic acid hepatic fatalities. III: US experience since 1986. *Neurology* 1996; **46(2)**:465–469.

24 Saneto RP, Lee IC, Koenig MK et al.: POLG DNA testing as an emerging standard of care before instituting valproic acid therapy for pediatric seizure disorders. *Seizure* 2010; **19**:140–146.

25 Mirza NS, Alfirevic A, Jorgensen A et al.: Metabolic acidosis with topiramate and zonisamide: an assessment of its severity and predictors. *Pharmacogenet Genomics* 2011; **21**: 2997–2302.

26 Asconape JJ, Penry JK, Dreifuss FE et al.: Valproate-associated pancreatitis. *Epilepsia* 1999; **34**:177–184.

27 Glauser TA, Cnaan A, Shinnar S et al.: Ethosuximide, valproic acid, and lamotrigine in childhood absence epilepsy: initial monotherapy outcomes at 12 months. *Epilepsia* 2013; **54(1)**:141–155.

28 Dong Z, Leppik IE, White J, Rarick J: Hyponatremia froom oxcarbazepine and carbamazepine. *Neurology* 2005; **65**: 1976–1978.

29 Sachdeo RC, Wasserstein A, Mesenbrink PJ, D'Souza J: Effects of oxcarbazepine on sodium concentration and water handling. *Ann Neurol* 2002; **51**:613–620.

30 Letmaier M, Painold A, Holl AK et al.: Hyponatraemia during psychopharmacological treatment: results of a drug surveillance programme. *Int J Neuropsychopharmacol* 2012; **15**:739–748.

31 Lin CH, Lu CH, Wang FJ et al.: Risk factors of oxcarbazepine-induced hyponatremia in patients with epilepsy. *Clin Neuropharmacol* 2010; **33**:293–296.

32 Holtmann M, Krause M, Opp J et al.: Oxcarbazepine-induced hyponatremia and the regulation of serum sodium after replacing carbamazepine with oxcarbazepine in children. *Neuropediatrics* 2002; **33**:298–300.

33 Schmidt D, Arroyo S, Baulac M et al.: Recommendations on the clinical use of oxcarbazepine in the treatment of epilepsy: a consensus view. *Acta Neurol Scand* 2001; **104**: 167–170.

34 Singh RP, Asconapé JJ: A review of eslicarbazepine acetate for the adjunctive treatment of partial-onset epilepsy. *J Cent Nerv Syst Dis* 2011; **3**:179–187.

35 Leppik IE: Zonisamide. *Epilepsia* 1999; **40(Suppl. 5)**: S23–S29.

36 Low PA, James S, Peschel T et al.: Zonisamide and associated oligohidrosis and hyperthermia. *Epilepsy Res* 2004; **62(1)**:27–34.

37 Kluger G, Bauer B: Role of rufinamide in the management of Lennox–Gastaut syndrome (childhood epileptic encephalopathy). *Neuropsychiatr Dis Treat* 2007; **3**:3–11.

38 Hsieh DT, Thiele EA: Efficacy and safety of rufinamide in pediatric epilepsy. *Ther Adv Neurol Disord* 2013; **6(3)**: 189–198.

39 Wheless JW, Vazquez B: Rufinamide: a novel broad-spectrum antiepileptic drug. *Epilepsy Currents* 2010; **10**:1–6.

40 Brodie MJ, Lerche H, Gil-Nagal A et al.: Efficacy and safety of adjunctive exogabine (retigabine) in refractory partial epilepsy. *Neurology* 2010; **75(20)**:1817–1824.

41 US Food and Drug Administration. FDA Drug Safety Communication: anti-seizure drug Potiga (ezogabine) linked to etinal abnormalities and blue skin discoloration. April 26, 2013. http://www.fda.gov/Drugs/DrugSafety/ucm349538.htm (last accessed July 15, 2014).

CHAPTER 12

Antiepileptic drug therapy and fetal development

Frank J.E. Vajda

Department of Medicine and Neuroscience, University of Melbourne, Royal Melbourne Hospital, Australia

Introduction

Antiepileptic drugs (AEDs) in pregnancy are associated with an increased risk of fetal malformations (FMs). This has been documented by studies dating from the 1970s related to the traditional AEDs and more recently from prospective studies. Due to lack of prospective data and a lack of adequate numbers, not enough is known as yet concerning the new AEDs but it appears that they are no more teratogenic than the traditional ones. A significant period of time – perhaps a decade – must elapse before any long-term adverse effects become apparent.

Minimum numbers are required before robust statistical assessments of the risk associated with each AED in monotherapy can be arrived at. Polytherapy data are too complex to allow accurate assessment to be based on the teratogenic risk, as innumerable combinations exist. Seizure freedom for 12 months or more before conception is a useful marker of the course of pregnancy, delivery, and seizure occurrence during this time. Seizures are relevant as they may harm the baby. Prospective studies are essential to clarify the effect of confounding factors. Comparative outcomes in groups of pregnant women not exposed to AEDs are valuable in dissecting the role of AEDs. Pregnancy registers are a major advance, as pregnant women cannot participate in controlled clinical trials.

The burden of epilepsy

Risk of seizures and resultant injuries, restrictions on driving and alcohol, and employment discrimination are all important to the patient with epilepsy, but for the parent with an unborn child, the greatest concern is usually for the child's safety. Three questions are often posed:
1 Will the baby inherit epilepsy?
2 Will the baby be physically normal?
3 Will the baby be normal in terms of mental and emotional development?

The third question is particularly complex. Answers to the first two may emerge from prospective studies.

The inheritance of epilepsy is complex. Counseling is available and should be utilized to obtain an estimate of the risk, which may be quite favorable for a normal outcome. Inheritance is not generally regarded as subject to influence by drug therapies, but AEDs may have a role in genetic mutation. After an initial uncertainty about the etiological role of the epileptic condition in causing malformations, the relationship between fetal exposure to AEDs and an increased incidence of birth defects has become well recognized [1–6]. Despite this, AEDs are continued throughout pregnancy in the majority of affected women, because of the increased risk of mortality and morbidity to both fetus and mother – especially from convulsive seizures, sudden unexpected death in epilepsy (SUDEP), and mood disorders – if treatment is withheld. Safer alternatives are thus sought for women of child-bearing potential within neurology and psychiatry, resulting in the emergence of the second generation of AEDs.

Study of the effect of AEDs on various aspects of cognition poses difficulties. Small children are not generally accepted as suitable subjects for testing, cognitive studies are costly and logistically difficult, and

Epilepsy and the Interictal State: Co-Morbidities and Quality of Life, First Edition.
Edited by Erik K. St. Louis, David M. Ficker, and Terence J. O'Brien.
© 2015 John Wiley & Sons, Ltd. Published 2015 by John Wiley & Sons, Ltd.

prospective studies are needed, ideally in conjunction with studies designed to look at physical malformations. Numerous studies indicate that multiple drug therapy is an added risk [2,7–9].

Seizures themselves may pose a hazard, but comparative figures are difficult to obtain [10–12]. All studies have different designs and generally small numbers. None of the new antiepileptics have been systematically studied for their effects on babies. No specific drug has yet been linked to a single defect.

In terms of physical malformations, it has been suspected since 1979 that valproate (VPA) is significantly more hazardous than other drugs, but prospective studies were lacking, although VPA has been confirmed to be teratogenic [13–17].

Epidemiology

The role of AEDs is to minimize seizures, which in addition to threatening the health of the expectant mother also pose a risk to the unborn child. The most effective drug discovered to date against primary generalized epilepsy (PGE), VPA, also appears to be the most teratogenic, in a dose-related manner. A dilemma thus exists in treating women effectively while protecting the baby.

About 90% of women with epilepsy receive treatment against seizures, but many choose not to avail themselves of the therapeutic option. Untreated women with epilepsy may serve as a control group versus those receiving treatment.

From the 1960s onwards, case reports and open uncontrolled studies began to emerge on the hazards of AED and FMs. Retrospective studies suffered from the shortcomings of disparate study formats, with specific types of epilepsy treated with different drugs, often focusing on specific malformations and providing little comparability between AEDs.

Although the frequency of major malformations, growth retardation, and hypoplasia of the midface and fingers (known as anticonvulsant embryopathy) is increased in infants exposed to anticonvulsant drugs *in utero*, whether these abnormalities are caused by the maternal epilepsy or by exposure to AEDs has long been questioned [18]. In a landmark paper, Holmes et al. [8] screened 128 049 pregnant women at delivery to identify three groups of infants:

1 Those exposed to anticonvulsant drugs.
2 Those unexposed to anticonvulsant drugs but with a maternal history of seizures.
3 Those unexposed to anticonvulsant drugs with no maternal history of seizures (control group).

The combined frequency of anticonvulsant embryopathy was higher in 223 infants exposed to one anticonvulsant drug than in 508 control infants (20.6 versus 8.5%, odds ratio (OR) 2.8, 95% CI 1.1–9.7). The frequency was also higher in 93 infants exposed to two or more anticonvulsant drugs than in the controls (28.0 versus 8.5%, OR 4.2, 95% CI 1.1–5.1). The 98 infants whose mothers had a history of epilepsy but took no anticonvulsant drugs during the pregnancy did not have a higher frequency of those abnormalities than the control infants. A distinctive pattern of FMs in infants of women with epilepsy was thus shown to be associated with the use of AEDs during pregnancy, rather than with epilepsy itself.

Pregnancy registers

Registers were established in the late 1990s in order to allow observational studies based on Ethics Committee approval, informed consent, and voluntary participation. Their ethical basis has been soundly affirmed by Julain Savulescu [19].

Registers comprise the North American, European International (EURAP), Danish, British, and Australian registers, which collaborate closely. Their similarities and differences have been published [20–24]. International and national registers evaluate all enrolled pregnancies and follow comprehensive protocols, recording family, medical, social, epilepsy, and treatment history; frequency, severity, and type of seizures; medical conditions; and substance and alcohol abuse. Attention is paid to prior pregnancies.

Pharmaceutical company registers focus on their own product, so the data are limited. These efforts are a form of post-marketing surveillance.

Initially envisaged to report on teratogenicity, registers serve as a resource for studying the efficacy and adverse effects of drugs. Malformations rates can be expressed in terms of pregnancies studied, of live births, or of total number of fetuses, including or excluding abortions.

Registers may not be representative of the total population of women with epilepsy; it is estimated that in most countries they include only 10–15% of all women with epilepsy who become pregnant [25].

The question of controls is difficult. It is possible to compare each drug exposure with exposure to other drugs, as in EURAP. Historical controls may be employed from population-based studies. Attempts by the Australian Register to use women treated with AEDs for pain or psychiatric disorders as controls have proved unsuccessful. Using untreated women with epilepsy as controls is feasible and justifiable. A comparison of 10 factors related to their epilepsy between treated and untreated women with epilepsy revealed no significant differences in their characteristics [26].

Polytherapy considerations

Despite conservative teaching on the merits of monotherapy in the treatment of epilepsy, about 25% of patients report exposure to more than one AED.

The number of combinations possible with AEDs is high, so exploration of the teratogenicy of AED combinations has been undertaken only infrequently [7] and remains a fertile field for study.

The concept that polytherapy is inherently more teratogenic than monotherapy has been challenged by recent reports, which suggest that it is the content of the multidrug combinations and the dose of valproic acid (valproate, VPA) that is likely to determine teratogenicity [27].

Folate

It is advised on less than perfect evidence that folic acid is beneficial, especially for prevention of neural tube defects [28–30].

Results emerging from studies of AED exposure in pregnancy

Data from one prospective study [31] show the following results:
- Normal births, no defect: 91%.
- Live birth with defect: 3.9%.
- Spontaneous abortion: 2.4%.
- Induced abortion, death *in utero*: 1%.
- Induced abortion with defect: 1%.

- Stillbirth: 1%.
- Lost to follow-up: 1%.

These outcomes indicate a favorable result for the overwhelming proportion of women with epilepsy.

From the mothers' seizure point of view, the outcome is also highly favorable: of 1480 women with epilepsy studied over their entire pregnancy, 1369 had no seizures during this period, 28 suffered seizures, and 83 were uncertain (due to the factors of abortion, stillbirth, and other medical conditions); 1% of the original group was lost to follow-up.

Teratogenicity of individual AEDs

Focus on individual AEDS and FMs has been the subject of an excellent review by Eadie [35] (see Tables 12.1 and 12.2).

Phenobarbitone

A number of authors reported FMs in relation to this drug as early as 1963. Subsequently, a case–control study of the use of the prodrug methyl-phenobarbitone showed further association with oral clefts and cardiac malformations. Five studies with a total of 2200 patients reported a malformation rate of 1.50–5.35% in association with phenobarbitone. Two of these used untreated women with epilepsy as controls [1,2,35]. An important report by Holmes et al. [8] confirmed a statistically significant increase in FMs associated with phenobarbital.

Phenytoin

Phenytoin was the major AED for treatment of convulsive seizures in the 1940s and for many subsequent decades. Speidel and Meadow [5] first raised the question of FMs caused by this drug, but further studies failed to convincingly demonstrate that phenytoin in monotherapy was an important teratogen. Although a fetal hydantoin syndrome has been described involving facial appearance and terminal digit changes, these are not considered specific or major malformations. No specific pattern arose. The significance of phenytoin as a major teratogen is considered not proven [35].

Carbamazepine

Carbamazepine (CBZ) was initially favored over phenytoin as posing a lesser teratogenic hazard. Subsequently, it became known that this drug was associated with an increase in FM rate in seven out of nine studies, and a

Table 12.1 Effect of AED therapy on unborn fetuses [32].

AED	Mono	No. of FMs	% of FMs	Poly	No. of FMs	% of FMs
VPA	245	27	11%	157	9	5.7%
CBZ	323	8	2.5%	113	6	5.3%
PHT	38	1	2.6%	37	1	2.7%
LTG	262	5	1.9%	196	5	2.6%
TPM	35	1	2.9%	57	3	5.3%
LEV	42	0	0	61	2	3.3%
GBP	14	0	0	16	0	0
NO MEDS	135	5	3.7%			

VPA, valproic acid; CBZ, carbamazepine; PHT, phenytoin; LTG, lamotrigine; TPM, topiramate; LEV, levetiracetam; GBP, gabapentin.

Table 12.2 Types of malformation: list of fetal abnormalities found in 37 outcomes. Data obtained from a prospective study on women with epilepsy treated with AEDs [33]. Classification based on Victorian Birth Register [60].

System	Abnormality	Times detected
Central nervous	Aanencephaly	2
	Spina bifida ± hydrocephalus	6
	Arnold Chiari malformaction	1
	Danny Walker syndrome	2
	Micropolygyria	1
	Holoprosencephaly	1
	Bulbus cordis and various septal defects	15
	Patent ductus arteriosus	3
	Hypoplastic left heart	2
	Airway narrowing	1
	Nasal narrowing	1
Alimentary	Cleft palate	5
	Anal atresia	1
Urogenital	Hypospadias	8
	Renal pelvis dilation	3
	Extra/deformed digits	5
	Absent thumb	1
	Talipes	3
Skull	Various sutural abnormalities	2
Face	Retrognathism	1
	Dysmorphism	1
Viscera	Situs inversus	1

meta-analysis by Matalon et al. [36] showed a statistically significant association of CBZ with FMs.

Valproate

VPA was introduced in Europe in 1962 and appeared to be well tolerated. It was used in a dose that controlled most generalized seizures and all other manifestations of PGE. However, the dose was probably higher than necessary: doses over 700 mg/day are currently regarded as unacceptably teratogenic, as shown by a profusion of studies [37–41]. Several reports of the most serious major malformations (e.g., spina bifida)

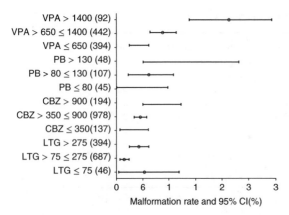

Figure 12.1   Malformation rate at 1 year after birth for monotherapy exposures to carbamazepine (CBZ), phenobarbital (PB), valproic acid (VPA), and lamotrigine (LTG), by dose.

were recorded in France. An almost 20% FM rate was reported in a *Lancet* editorial related to VPA use in mono- and polytherapy. This figure exceeds most of the results published since. Lindhout and Schmidt [6] also reported an increase in incidence of spina bifida in a rigorously conducted study.

As Eadie [35] observed, genetic factors play a part in the susceptibility of the fetus, as shown by a family of six infants with major malformations following exposure to VPA.

Eight of ten major studies on VPA reported malformations in excess of 3%, the usual upper limit for normal populations. VPA remains a significant teratogen, although the effect has become increasingly clearly dose-related. The initially suggested upper limit of VPA

dose was 1400 mg/day; this was subsequently lowered to 1100, 760, and later 600 mg/day by more extensive studies [14,16,17]. In most studies, doses that resulted in FMs were significantly higher than those that produced no FMs, although this has not been fully demonstrated as yet with regard to cognitive development.

Figure 12.1 shows FM rate determined after 1 year in relation to dose categories of AEDs. This indicates a comparable teratogenicty for the major AEDs, with the exception of phenobarbital and valproate. At doses up to 650 mg/day day, the risk of VPA teratogenicity is not significantly higher, statistically, than that of other AEDs.

Figure 12.2 [30] indicates the cumulative rates of occurrence of pregnancies with FMs below VPA threshold daily doses in monotherapy. Figure 12.3 shows data related to combined mono- and polytherapy. Dose categories were delineated to enable analyses to be performed on dose relationships to fetal malformation rates.

A recent major study evaluating the use of VPA monotherapy in the first trimester was associated with significantly increased risks of several congenital malformations, as compared with children unexposed to AEDs and with use of other AEDs [42].

Data from cohort studies were combined to identify VPA-related malformations among offspring exposed during the first trimester. A population-based, case–control study was conducted using the database established by European Surveillance of Congenital Anomalies (EUROCAT). It did not address dose issues related to VPA, however [43].

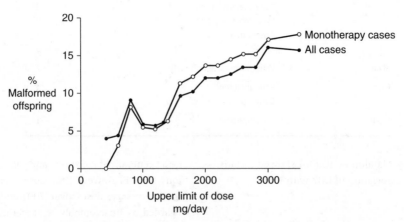

Figure 12.2 Cumulative rates of occurrence of pregnancies with malformations below various threshold daily valproate doses. Source: Eadie & Vajda, 2005 [17]. Reproduced with permission of Dove Medical Press.

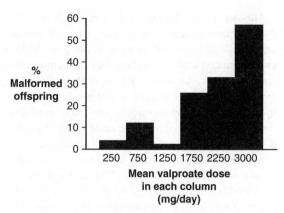

Figure 12.3 Rates of occurrence of pregnancies with malformations at various daily valproate doses Source: Eadie & Vajda, 2005 [17]. Reproduced with permission of Dove Medical Press.

Ethosuximide

Ethosuximide is specifically used to treat absences, mainly in children, and rarely as monotherapy. Information derived from prospective studies on its teratogenocity is not available.

Zonisamide

This drug was originally trialed in Australia in the late 1980s, but was withdrawn due to concerns over renal stones. These proved not to be a problem in Japan and the United States, where it has been widely used. Kondo et al. [44] described 2 FMs in 26 pregnancies but none in monotherapy.

Benzodiazepines

Clonazepam and diazepam are not considered to be major teratogens. Wide et al. [41] reported on 48 pregnancies exposed to clonazepam that produced 3 fetuses with FM but in a case–control study of diazepam exposure the OR for FM was not statistically significantly increased.

New (second-generation) AEDS

All new drugs were designed initially to treat partial epilepsy. Effective and specific drugs for the treatment of PGI are sadly lacking. Over time, the approvals for lamotrogine, topiramate (TPM), and levarecetam have been extended to include PGE.

Data on their use in monotherapy are less robust for these drugs than for the traditional ones, as they are used mainly as add-ons in many countries. Among live-born infants in Denmark, first-trimester exposure to lamotrigine (LTG), oxcarbazepine (OXC), TPM, gabapentin (GBP), or levetiracetam (LEV), compared with no drug exposure, was not associated with an increased risk of major birth defects [45]. These results are in line with those from Australia [46].

Lamotrigine

This appeared to be the ideal drug for use in pregnancy when it was first introduced, with minimal teratogenic effects recorded: a report from GlaxoSmithKline's LTG-related company register showed a lower than expected FM rate with LTG monotherapy [47]. This report was questioned, however, and in a major analysis of high-quality data in 2006, Morrow et al. [48] showed a dose-related teratogenic effect for LTG. However, GlaxoSmithKline's data on LTG-related malformations show that if LTG is a teratogen, it is not a potent one [49].

One of the major limitations of LTG in pregnancy, apart from its lower convulsive seizure efficacy than VPA or CBZ, is the problem of induction by sex homones, which makes management difficult [50].

Vigabatrin

This potent antie pileptic drug, now largely in disuse because of its effect of visual acuity, has no prospective data relating to its teratogenicty.

Topiramate

Morrison et al. [51] reported an FM rate of 7.1% in pregnancies exposed to TPM monotherapy and in 2011 the FDA issued a warning about the use of TPM in pregnancy, based on the North American Registry's data. Infants exposed to TPM in the first trimester had a 1.4% prevalence of oral clefts, compared to 0.38–0.55% of infants exposed to other AEDs [52]. However, a Danish population-based study failed to note this trend in association with TPM [45]. The matter is not resolved.

Oxcarbazepine

OXC has become widely used in Scandinavia and North America. There have been retrospective reports of malformations in association with this drug in monothearpy. Artama et al. [53], reported an FM incidence of 11.1%, in comparison to 0.8% in women not exposed to OXC.

Gabapentin

This drug is remarkably free of interactions and seems relatively free of any reports of associated malformations. Montouris [54] reported one case of malformation in 31 pregnancies receiving GBP monotherapy.

Levetiracetam

In preclinical studies, LEV has been shown to be the safest of all AEDs in terms of adverse effects. The Australian Register of Antiepileptic Drugs in Pregnancy (APR) has no information on LEV-related teratogenicity in monotherapy in 60 women treated prospectively, and only one case in polytherapy. Other reports in the literature also appear to attest to its apparent safety in pregnancy [53,54].

Tiagabin

Little information is available on this drug, which has not enjoyed a wide acceptance for the treatment of partial epilepsy, largely because of poor tolerability.

Lacosamide

This drug has been released only recently. No specific information is available about its teratogenic potential in clinical practice.

Felbamate

Felbamate is a last-resort drug, largely abandoned. No information is available on its teratogenicty but it is unlikely pregnant women would be prescribed this drug in significant numbers, due to occasionally fatal hepatic and hematological toxicity.

Cognitive developmental defects and AED exposure

The collaborative Neurodevelopmental Effects of Antiepileptic Drugs (NEAD) study represents a major landmark initiative, reporting prospective results from extensive investigations into children exposed to AEDs in pregnancy [57]. Its key findings are very important, implying that neurodevelopmental dysfunction may be even more devastating than many of the physical malformations resulting from AED exposure *in utero* [57]. The findings of this study are a cause for concern and are quoted in detail here.

After adjustment for maternal IQ, maternal age, AED dose, gestational age at birth, and maternal preconception use of folate, the mean IQ at age 3 of children exposed to LTG was 101, of those exposed to phenytoin was 99, of those exposed to CBZ was 98, and of those exposed to VPA was 92. The association between VPA use and IQ was dose-dependent. The question of dose needs to be considered in future studies, as VPA at high doses is clearly a neurodevelopmental teratogen.

A recent prospective study evaluated the cognitive impact of prenatal exposure to VPA and polytherapy in school-aged children. Children exposed to VPA monotherapy (n = 57), polytherapy with VPA (n = 515), or polytherapy without VPA (n = 519) were assessed using the Wechsler Intelligence Scale for Children. Verbal Comprehension and Working Memory scores in all groups fell significantly below the standardized test mean, but Perceptual Reasoning and Processing Speed scores were relatively intact, suggesting that VPA has a dose-dependent negative impact on verbal intellectual abilities [58].

The language skills of 102 AED-exposed children were assessed using the Clinical Evaluation of Language Fundamentals – Assessments. Language scores of children exposed to sodium VPA in monotherapy were significantly below the standardized test mean, but those scores of children exposed to CBZ or LTG monotherapy or to polytherapy without sodium VPA were not significantly different from normal [59].

Conclusion

- Prospective studies are needed to obtain valid data on fetal exposure to AEDs.
- Pregnancy registers can be used to study aspects besides the teratogenicy of AEDs.
- All AEDS are teratogenic, to a variable degree among untreated women with epilepsy.
- Dose issues are important, particularly for VPA, as high doses are responsible for both physical FMs and cognitive defects, affecting IQ, language, and possibly development of autism. A suggested upper VPA dose limit is on the order of 400–700 mg/day in divided doses, but this value is changing over time.
- Genetic factors play a part in teratogenicity. In children, cognitive testing is not possible under 2–3 years of age.

- Physical malformations may be missed at birth, especially if minor or occult. Classification of FMs is difficult and complex.
- Traditional drugs have yielded more evaluable data. New AEDs appear less teratogenic than the older ones, but they were introduced as add-ons, so monotherapy data are not as robust.
- Polytherapy appears to be no more teratogenic than monotherapy, but this depends on its content, particularly of VPA. No drug has yet been fully linked with a single malformation.
- Folate supplementation has not produced the expected benefit.

Acknowledgments

I wish to thank my colleagues, M.J. Eadie, T.J. O'Brien, C.M. Lander, A. Wood, and the coordinators of the Australian Pregnancy Register: J. Graham, A. Hitchcock, and A Roten; thanks also to T. Tomson and the EURAP Central Project Commission: D. Battino, E. Bonizzoni, J. Craig. D. Lindhout, E.Perucca, and A. Sabers.

References

1 Kaneko S, Battino D, Andermann E et al.: Congenital malformations due to antiepileptic drugs. *Epilepsy Res* 1999; **33**:145–158.

2 Samren EB, Van Duijn CM , Koch S et al.: Maternal use of antiepileptic drugs and the risk of major congenital malformations: a joint European propective study of human teratogenesis associated with maternal epilepsy. *Epilepsia* 1997; **38**:98990.

3 Matalon S, SchermanS, Goldzweig G, Ornoy A: The teratogenic effect of carbamazepine: a meta-analysis of 1255. *Reprod Toxicol* 2002; **16(1)**:9–17.

4 Dalens B, Reynaud EJ, Gaulme J: Teratogenicity of valproic acid. *J Paediatr* 1981; **97**:332–333.

5 Speidel BD, Meadow SR Maternal epilepsy and abnormalities of the fetus and newborn. *Lancet* 1972; **2**:839–843.

6 Lindhout D, Schmidt D: In utero exposure to valproate and neural tue defects. *Lancet* 1986; **ii**:1392–1393.

7 Lindhout D, Hoppener RJEA, Mainardi H: Teratogeniciy of drug combinations with special emphasis on epoxidation of carbamazepine. *Epilepsia* 1984; **25**:77–83.

8 Holmes LB, Harvey EA, Coull BA et al.: The teratogenicity of anticonvulsant drugs. *N Engl J Med* 2001; **344**:1132–1138.

9 Morrow J, Russell A, Guthrie E et al.: Malformation risks of anti-epileptic drugs in pregnancy: a prospective study from the UK Epilepsy and Pregnancy Register. *J Neurol Neurosurg Psychiatry* 2006; **71**:193–198.

10 Vajda FJ, Hitchcock A, Graham J et al.: Foetal malformations and seizure control: 52 months data of the Australian Pregnancy Register. *Eur J Neurol* 2006; **13(6)**:645–654.

11 F Vajda, Hitchcock A, Graham J et al.: Seizure control in antiepileptic drug-treated pregnancy. *Epilepsia* 2008; **49(1)**:172–175.

12 Somerville ER, Cook MJ, O'Brien TJ: Pregnancy treatment guidelines: throwing the baby out with the bathwater. *Epilepsia* 2009; **50(9)**:2167.

13 Wyszynski DF Nambisan M, Surve T et al.: Increased rate of major malformations in offspring exposed to valproate during pregnancy. *Neurology* 2005; **64(6)**:961–965.

14 Tomson T, Battino D, Bonizzoni E et al.: Dose-dependent risk of malformations with antiepileptic drugs: an analysis of data from the EURAP epilepsy and pregnancy registry. *Lancet Neurol* 2011; **10(7)**:609–617.

15 EURAP Study Group: Drug Utilization. European Epilepsy Congress, July 2010, Rhodes.

16 Vajda FJ, O'Brien TJ, Hitchcock A et al.: Critical relationship between sodium valproate dose and human teratogenicity: results of the Australian Register of Anti-Epileptic Drugs in Pregnancy. *J Clin Neurosci* 2004; **11(8)**:854–858.

17 Eadie MJ, Vajda FJE: Should valproate be taken during pregnancy? *Therap Clin Risk Manage* 2005; **1(1)**:21–26.

18 Dean JCS, Hailey H, Moore SJ et al.: Long term health and neurodevelopment in children exposed to antiepileptic drugs before birth. *J Med Genet* 2002; **39**:251–259.

19 Sevulescu J: personal communication, 1999.

20 Beghi E, Annegers JF, Collaborative Group for the Pregnancy Registries in Epilepsy: Pregnancy registries in epilepsy. *Epilepsia* 2001; **42(11)**:1422–1425.

21 Holmes LB, Wyszynski DF, Leberman E, AED Pregnancy Registry: A 6 year experience. *Arch Neurol* 2004; **61**: 673–678.

22 Meador KJ, Pennell PB, Harden GL et al.: Pregnancy registries in epiepsy: a consensus statement on health outcomes. *Neurology* 2008; **71**:1109–1117.

23 Meador K, Reynolds MW, Crean S et al.: Pregnancy outcomes in women with epilepsy: a systematic review and meta-analysis of published pregnancy registries and cohorts. *Epilepsy Res* 2008; **81(1)**:1–13.

24 Tomson T, Battino D, Hernandez-Diaz S et al.: Pregnancy registries: differences, similarities and possible harmonization. *Epilepsia* 2010; **51(5)**:909–915.

25 Vajda FJ, O'Brien T, Hitchcock A et al.: The Australian antiepileptic drug in pregnancy register: aspects of data collection and analysis. *J Clin Neurosci* 2007; **14(10)**:936–942.

26 Vajda FJ, O'Brien T, Hitchcock A et al.: The internal control group in a register of antiepileptic drug use in pregnancy. *J Clin Neurosci* 2008; **15(1)**:29–35.

27 Vajda FJ, Hitchcock AA, Graham J et al.: The teratogenic risk of antiepileptic drug polytherapy. *Epilepsia* 2010; **51(5)**: 805–810.

28 MRC Vitamin Study Research Group: Prevention of neural tube defects: results of the Medical Research Council Vitamin Study. *Lancet* 1991; **338(8760)**:131–137.

29 Czeizel AE, Dudas I: Prevention of the first occurrence of neural tube defects by periconceptual vitamin supplementation. *N Engl J Med* 1992; **327**:1832–1835.

30 Craig J, Morrison P, Morrow J et al.: Failure of periconceptual folic acid to prevent a neural tube defect in the offspring of a mother taking sodium valproate. *Seizure* 1999; **8**:253–254.

31 Vajda F, Graham J, Hitchcock A et al.: Malformation outcome data from the Australian Pregnancy Register. World Congress of Obstetrics Medicine, Melbourne, 2010 [abstract]. Table 1, outcome references.

32 Vajda F, Graham J, Hitchcock A et al.: Relative teratogenicity of individual antiepileptic drugs. Epilepsy Society of Australia, Annual Scientific Meeting, 2009. Table 2, relative teratogenicty.

33 Vajda F, Graham J, Hitchcock A et al.: Malformation outcome data from the Australian Pregnancy Register. World Congress of Obstetrics Medicine, Melbourne, 2010 [abstract]. Table 3, types of FM.

34 Vajda FJ: Dose related teratogenicity of valproate. 5th International Congress, Controversies in Neurology platform presentation, October 2010, Barcelona, Spain. Figure 2, VPA dose-related risk of FM.

35 Eadie MJ: Antiepileptic drugs as human teratogens. *Expert Opin Drug Saf* 2008; **7(2)**:195–209.

36 Matalon S, Scherman S, Goldzweig G, Ornoy A: The teratogenic effect of carbamazepine: a meta analysis of 1255 exposures. *Reprod Toxicol* 2002; **16**:9–17.

37 Dalens B, Reynaud EJ, Gaulme J: Teratogenicity of valproic acid. *J Paediatr* 1981; **97**:332–333.

38 Clay SA, McVie R, Chen H: Possible teratogenici effect of valproic acid. *J Paediatr* 1981; **99**:828.

39 Robert B, Gibaud P: Maternal valproic acid use and congenital neural tube defects. *Lancet* 1982; **ii**;937.

40 Editorial: Valproate and malformations. *Lancet* 1986; **ii**: 1313–1314.

41 Wide K, Windbladh B, Kallen B: Major malformations in infants exposed to antiepileptic drugs in utero, with emphasis on carbamazepine and valproic acid: a nationwide, population-based register study. *Acta Paediatr Scand* 2004; **93**:174–176.

42 Jentink J, Loane MA, Dolk H et al.: Valproic acid monotherapy on pregnancy and major congenital malformations. *New Eng J Med* 2010; **362**:218–293.

43 Vajda FJE, O'Brien TJ: Valproic acid use in pregnancy and congenital malformations. *New Engl J Med* 2011; **362**:1771.

44 Kondo T, Kaneko S, Amano Y, Egawa Y: Preliminary report on teratogenic effects of zonisamide in the offsrping of tretaed women with epilepsy. *Epilepsia* 1996; **37**:1242–1244.

45 Mølgaard-Nielsen D, Hviid A: Newer-generation antiepileptic drugs and the risk of major birth defects. *JAMA* 2011; **305(19)**:1996–2002.

46 Vajda FJ, Graham J, Roten A et al.: Second generation of antiepileptic drugs. Report from the Australian Pregnancy Register. Epilepsy World Congress, Rome, August 28–September 2, 2011 [abstract].

47 Cunnington M, Tennis P: Lamotrigine and the risk of malformations in pregnancy. *Neurology* 2005; **64**:955–969.

48 Morrow J, Russell A, Guthrie E et al.: Malformation risks of anti-epileptic drugs in pregnancy: a prospective study from the UK Epilepsy and Pregnancy Register. *J Neurol Neurosurg Psych* 2006; **71**:193–198.

49 Vajda FJ, Graham J, Hitchcock AA et al.: Is lamotrigine a significant human teratogen? Observations from the Australian Pregnancy Register. *Seizure* 2010; **19(9)**:558–561.

50 Sabers A, Buchholz JM, Udall P, Hansen EL: Lamotrigine plasma levels reduced by oral contraceptives. *Epilepsy Res* 2001; **47(1–2)**:151–154.

51 Morrison PJ, Morrow J, Craig J: Topiramate in pregnancy: preliminary experience from the UK Epilepsy and Pregnancy Register. *Neurology* 2008; **71**:272–276.

52 FDA: Risk of oral birth defects in children born to mothers taking topiramate. March 4, 2011. Available from: http://www.fda.gov/newsevents/newsroom/pressannouncements/ucm245594.htm (last accessed July 15, 2014).

53 Artama M, Auvinen A, Raudaskovski T et al.: Antiepileptic drug use of women with epilepsy and congenital malformations in the offspring. *Neurology* 2005; **64**:1874–1878.

54 Montouris G: Safety of the newer antiepileptc drug oxcarbazepine during pregnancy. *Curr Med Res Opin* 2005; **21**:693–701.

55 Long L. Levetiracetam monotherapy during pregnancy: case series. *Epilepsy Behav* 2003; **4**:447–448.

56 Hunt S, Craig J, Russell A et al.: Levetiracetam in pregnancy: preliminary experience from the UK Epilepsy and Pregnancy Register. *Neurology* 2006; **67**:1876–1879.

57 Meador KJ, Baker GA, Browning N et al.: Cognitive function at 3 years of age after fetal exposure to antiepileptic drugs. *N Engl J Med* 2009; **360(16)**:1597–1605.

58 Nadebaum C, Anderson V, Vajda F et al.: The Australian Brain and Cognition and Antiepileptic Drugs Study: IQ in school-aged children exposed to sodium valproate and polytherapy. *J Inter Neuropsychol Soc* 2011; **17**:133–142.

59 Nadebaum C, Anderson VA, Vajda F et al.: Language skills of school-aged children prenatally exposed to antiepileptic drugs. *Neurology* 2011; **76**:719–726.

60 Riley M, Halliday J: Birth defects in Victoria 1983–1998, Perinatal Data Collection Unit, Victorian Government Department of Human Services. Victorian Government Department of Human Services, Melbourne, 2000.

SECTION IV
Mood state, psychiatric comorbidity, and epilepsy

CHAPTER 13

Mood state, anxiety, and psychosis in epilepsy

Michael Salzberg

Department of Psychiatry, St. Vincent's Hospital, University of Melbourne, Australia

Introduction

The psychiatric comorbidities of epilepsy are common and distressing, add to disability and impaired quality of life (QOL), and contribute to an elevated suicide rate. In most places, specialist psychiatric care is unavailable, and even where it is available, it is poorly integrated with neurological care. Thus, psychiatric comorbidities often remain poorly diagnosed and managed, although there are some excellent models of integrated care and much research progress. Interest has intensified in causal processes shared by the two sets of disorders and the likelihood that comorbid psychiatric disorder may exacerbate the course of some epilepsies. Thinking about comorbidity has become more sophisticated, research gradually revealing a complex interplay of genetics, neurobiology, life stress, and psychosocial milieu. Alas, clinical practice lags, as does organization of services.

The brief of this chapter is to review recent developments concerning mood and anxiety disorders and the psychoses. It focuses on key publications in the last 5 years concerning epilepsy in adult populations (for childhood epilepsy, note recent reviews [1–3]). Concerns about suicidality triggered by antiepileptic drugs (AEDs) have been well reviewed elsewhere [4].

Mood disorders and epilepsy

Recent years have seen a burgeoning literature on mood disorders, with an expert consensus statement [5] and advances on several fronts: better descriptive clinical [6] and epidemiological studies [7–11]; clarification of the considerable impact of depression on subjective cognition [12–15], QOL [16–18], reported AED side effects [19], and adherence; new evidence that depression predicts treatment resistance [20,21] and poorer seizure outcome following epilepsy surgery [22,23]; and even evidence that depression may be a risk factor for SUDEP [24] and that, in an animal model, antidepressant treatment reduces risk [25]. Debate continues about interictal dysphoric disorder (IDD), as to whether it is a distinct disorder or a form of dysthymia [26]. From human and animal studies there is greater appreciation of bidirectional and shared causal interconnections between epilepsy and depression [27,28]. Innovative psychological treatment studies have appeared [29–32] but medication trials remain rare. The underrecognition and undertreatment of depression by physicians have long been known: recent studies probe the reasons [33] and explore patients' preferences regarding depression care [34]. Mood disorders help cause metabolic syndrome, obesity, diabetes, and vascular disease, disorders prevalent in epilepsy populations [35,36], but this link has largely been overlooked. This section will focus on depression (for bipolar disorder in epilepsy, see [37]).

Epidemiology

Recent studies sharpen earlier epidemiological work on estimates of depression rates in epilepsy [7,9,38]. For example, a Canadian general-population survey reported a rate of major depression in the prior 12 months in epilepsy patients of 13%, versus 7% in those without epilepsy [8]. Higher odds ratios (OR) were found with female gender, non-white minority status, older age, and poverty. Of the depressed, 38% had had no contact with a mental health professional in the prior year [8]. In an Australian study, "psychological

Epilepsy and the Interictal State: Co-Morbidities and Quality of Life, First Edition.
Edited by Erik K. St. Louis, David M. Ficker, and Terence J. O'Brien.
© 2015 John Wiley & Sons, Ltd. Published 2015 by John Wiley & Sons, Ltd.

distress" also predicted higher rates of health service utilization [39].

Depression may be a risk factor for subsequent epilepsy onset [40]; if this is true, there are both neurobiological and preventive implications. The finding that depression may be a risk factor for post-traumatic epilepsy supports this idea [41].

Rates of suicidal thoughts and actions and completed suicide are markedly elevated in epilepsy over general population rates [42,43]. Depression is not the only psychiatric pathway to suicide, but it is a potent and prevalent one [44].

Etiologies and pathophysiology

Human studies of depression in epilepsy tend to be psychosocial or neurobiological in nature, with few spanning both domains. Psychosocial studies employ combinations of psychological constructs (optimism, helplessness, perceived control, self-efficacy, coping style, personality traits, life stress, illness representations) and social and cultural factors, such as social support, employment status, experienced stigma, and social disadvantage [45–54], sometimes augmented with routine neurological data, which are often available for subjects.

Neurobiologically oriented studies have employed structural [55–61] or functional imaging [62–67], or both [68], and, where available, excised temporal lobe [69]. The most consistent findings have been in mesial temporal-lobe epilepsy (TLE), with suggestions of enlarged amygdalae, diminished hippocampal and neocortical volumes (both temporal and extratemporal cortex), diminished 5HT1A receptor binding in the hippocampus (and possibly raphe nuclei, insula, and cingulate gyrus) [66], and a correlation between depression and degree of hippocampal abnormality on ^{1}H-magnetic resonance spectroscopy imaging (^{1}H-MRSI) [64]. Most such studies are cross-sectional, and are thus unable to determine causality, but the association of depression with diminished extratemporal cortical thickness [60] is important, as such thinning is found in both ordinary (non-epilepsy-associated) depression and mesial TLE [58].

Other studies have explored epilepsy-related variables, such as seizure type, severity, and frequency [70], either as clues to neurobiological mechanisms or as pointers to the psychological impact of seizures. In most studies, AEDs are an important confound, given their often potent positive or negative effects on mood [71].

Most of these approaches have some partial explanatory value (reviewed recently in [27,38,72–74]). Much depression research in the epilepsy field is "either/or" – either psychosocial or neurobiological – and lacks a longitudinal perspective. Present-day general (non-epilepsy) depression research is biopsychosocial in nature (integrating insights from genetics, epidemiology, psychology, and neurobiology), operates within a stress–diathesis framework [38], and adopts a lifespan perspective. The causation of depression is a multistage process with origins in early life (as is the case for many epilepsies [75]). After onset of the disorder, there is very high chance of recurrence throughout the lifespan [76]. The many parallels between epilepsy and mood disorder in this regard were highlighted by Post [77]. Recently, there have been calls for these perspectives to be adopted more fully in the epilepsy field [78,79].

Animal epilepsy models reinforce these points vividly. Depression-like behaviors are typically present in genetic or acquired models, such as GAERS and GEPR rats, or following electrical kindling or status epilepticus. Early life stress, presumably via effects on neurodevelopment and neuroendocrine "programming," creates enduring vulnerability to later limbic epilepsy, and environmental enrichment is protective [80]. Effects of early exposures are seen at many levels, from genes to ion channels, cells, and micro- and macrocircuits [80,81]. Animal studies can disentangle the bidirectional and shared causal pathways underlying comorbidity [27]. In translating these insights to humans, one vital underutilized methodology is the prospective cohort study. But even small, idiographic studies can provide vivid insights into the interplay of psychology and neurobiology: for example, in a study of early postoperative depression in temporal lobectomy patients, marital conflict was an important triggering factor [47].

Diagnosis/evaluation

An important development is depression screening. The Neurological Disorders Depression Inventory for Epilepsy (NDDI-E) is a six-item scale for use in epilepsy populations [82–84]. Validated in tertiary epilepsy centers, its properties are as yet unknown in community-based samples with lower depression prevalence. Obviously, screening needs to be embedded within a system – or pathway – of care, and does not obviate the need for psychological probes in the clinical interview, if only because clinicians need to be alert to "false negatives."

Treatment

In many settings, psychological treatments are difficult to access or unavailable; antidepressant medication becomes the default. This is unfortunate because of good evidence for the efficacy of psychotherapies in depression, with probable superiority to antidepressants in reducing relapse. There is also growing evidence specifically for depression in epilepsy [29,30,85,86]. In neuroimaging studies of depressed non-epilepsy patients, psychotherapy alters brain structures known to be affected in the depression of epilepsy; perhaps this neurobiological argument strengthens the case for psychotherapy in depression of epilepsy [87]. Psychosocial interventions to promote more effective coping and self-management with epilepsy [88,89] do not focus on frank psychiatric comorbidity *per se*, but by enhancing self-efficacy and resilience are likely also to mitigate mental-illness risk.

Antidepressant use in epilepsy has been extensively discussed [38,90] but clinical trials are scarce and many clinicians remain reluctant to prescribe, ostensibly because of perceived seizure risk [33]. Evidence mounts against this perception; both human and animal studies [91,92] show that in general "second-generation" antidepressants (selective serotonin reuptake inhibitors (SSRIs), serotonin–norepinephrine reuptake inhibitors (SNRIs)) raise seizure threshold and reduce seizure risk, prompting the proposal they be trialed as antiepileptic therapy [93]. However, other biological effects of antidepressants, such as on neurogenesis [94], have not yet been evaluated in this regard.

Prognosis

Major depression (like bipolar disorder) tends to be a long-term, relapsing–remitting illness [76]. Thus, from the outset, the treatment plan needs to address relapse prevention – preferably by psychological means – and rehabilitation. Achieving remission is vital but insufficient.

Practical advice/pearls

- Depression is common, with pervasive effects on patient well-being and possibly on the course of epilepsy itself. Its detection, diagnosis, and care need to be "built in" to routine epilepsy care.

- Screening instruments (e.g., NDDI-E) are effective and worthwhile. Physicians need to prepare to deal with the many "positive" patients that result from implementing screening and be alert to possible "false negatives." Screening does not abolish the need for depression questions during the clinical interview.
- For most episodes of mild–moderate depression, psychotherapy is effective. Wherever possible, epileptologists and epilepsy services should try to make psychotherapy available to their patients.
- Second-generation antidepressants do not in general lower seizure threshold and trigger seizures: animal and human data suggest the reverse.

Anxiety disorders and epilepsy

Key issues concerning anxiety in epilepsy include: the high prevalence of anxiety symptoms and disorders, rates often exceeding those of depression, which has received more attention [95]; the associations with impaired QOL [96,97], suicide [44], experience of adverse effects of AEDs, and greater health care utilization and costs; the diagnostic difficulties in differentiating panic disorder from ictal fear [98]; and the pressing need for better detection and management (note the comprehensive review in [99]). As with depression, explanatory models tend to be "either/or": anxiety is either an understandable reaction to the stresses of living with epilepsy or a neurobiological epiphenomenon of the epileptic brain; integrative hypotheses are rare. As with depression and psychosis, shared and bidirectional causation between anxiety disorder and epilepsy is a key insight.

Epidemiology

Given the dominance of studies based on subjects from tertiary centers (e.g., [100–102]), two recent population-based studies are welcome [10,103]. The first shows an approximate doubling of lifetime anxiety disorders and of panic disorder with agoraphobia compared to the general population [10]. In the second, 20.5% scored above the cut-off for "caseness" on an anxiety screening scale [103]. Predictors of "caseness" included current depression, reported AED side effects, low education, chronic health problems, female gender, and unemployment.

This last finding raises the issue of the interconnections between anxiety and depression [104]. There are overlaps in symptomatology, including diagnostic criteria (e.g., sleep disturbance, difficulty concentrating). Anxiety disorders are potent risk factors for subsequent depression, and to a lesser extent the reverse is true. There are many overlaps in both causation (life stress, personality traits, and neurobiology) and treatments (e.g., the efficacy of SSRIs in both sets of disorders). This interconnection of anxiety and depression has been little examined in epilepsy research [104,105].

Pathophysiology and etiology

Psychosocial, neurochemical, and neuroanatomical studies have emerged in recent years (reviewed in [99,106,107]). Velissaris et al. [45], using qualitative and quantitative methods, prospectively examined the adjustment process after a first seizure. Their subjects fell into two groups: those with a limited and those with a pervasive sense of loss of control following the first seizure. The "pervasive" group showed higher anxiety and depression scores. Interestingly, higher score at 1 month was associated with subsequent seizure recurrence. This last finding accords with several studies suggesting that psychopathology predicts treatment resistance, including postsurgical seizure outcome [20–22,108]. This in turn suggests more widespread brain pathology, leading both to psychiatric disturbance and to more severe and treatment-resistant epilepsy.

Most animal epilepsy models show affective disturbance, including anxiety-like behaviors [109–111]. The shared anatomical circuitry involved in anxiety [112] and epilepsy helps explain this. This shared circuitry is very clear for limbic epilepsy, given the role of the amygdala, but extratemporal structures are increasingly recognized as being affected in TLE [113] and anxiety circuitry is increasingly recognized as extending to nonlimbic structures, such as orbitofrontal, medial prefrontal, and anterior cingulate cortices [112,114]. The idea of a particular link between TLE and affective disturbance has progressively weakened, with increasing appreciation of anxiety and mood disturbance in extratemporal focal [115] and generalized epilepsies [116].

One of the few imaging studies with data specifically regarding anxiety is an MRS study of refractory partial epilepsy, showing relative preservation of amygdala and hippocampus in those with anxiety compared to those without [117], an effect most noticeable in the right,

nondominant hemisphere. These suggestive results have not been followed up, although one study of temporal-lobe-surgery patients found that resection or deafferentation of an amygdala within the normal range of volume was associated with greater postoperative anxiety [118]. In TLE, experimental studies show impaired emotion recognition (discussed in [119]) and altered emotional memory encoding [120]. Curiously, such methods have not been used to gain insight into the pathogenesis of anxiety and mood disorder in epilepsy, to which they seem highly relevant. An exception is a study of temporal lobectomy patients with hippocampal sclerosis who underwent fMRI to gauge amygdala activation in response to fearful faces [62]: preoperatively, in right TLE patients, amygdala activation correlated with anxiety and depression scores; greater preoperative activation was associated with worsening of anxiety and depression scores postoperatively in the same group.

The obvious neurochemical and neuroendocrine commonalities between anxiety and epilepsy are often discussed, notably the roles of GABA, serotonin, noradrenalin, dopamine, neurosteroids, calcium channels, corticotropin-releasing hormone (CRH), and the hypothalamic–pituitary–adrenal (HPA) axis [99,106,107]. However, progress remains slow, especially in human studies.

Diagnosis/evaluation

As with depression, there is much informal evidence that anxiety disorders in epilepsy patients are underrecognized and undertreated – just as in non-epilepsy populations. The reasons have not themselves been a focus of research.

Once suspected by the clinician, assessment of anxiety symptoms can be complex and may require referral to a psychiatrist. In addition to a syndromic diagnosis (panic disorder, generalized anxiety disorder (GAD), etc.), a formulation is needed, namely an understanding of why this anxiety disorder has emerged in this individual patient at this time. Similar-appearing panic disorders in two different epilepsy patients may have very different geneses, with different consequences for management. Typically, formulations are biopsychosocial and encompass predisposing, precipitating, and perpetuating factors. Relevant factors may include the nature of the epilepsy itself, AEDs, and the patient's personality, culture, developmental history, and current life stressors and circumstances.

Differential diagnoses of anxiety disorders need to be considered, including other psychiatric disorders (notably depression, alcohol abuse) and organic disorders (such as hyperthyroidism, pheochromocytoma).

AEDs can exacerbate or moderate anxiety, both with exposure and on withdrawal, and may do so by pharmacodynamic or pharmacokinetic mechanisms. Some AEDs induce enzymes that metabolize psychotropic drugs, thus lowering blood levels [99,121,122]. Excellent discussions have appeared recently on panic [98,123] and obsessive–compulsive disorder (OCD) [124,125] in epilepsy, both of which present substantial diagnostic and management challenges. In contrast to depression [84], no screening instrument validated for use in epilepsy has been developed, although the PHQ-GAD7 has been proposed [104].

Treatment

Ideally, management is guided by the individualized formulation just mentioned. It may entail reconsideration of the AED regime, efforts to achieve better seizure control, and psychotherapy and psychotropic medication. Effective psychotherapies, principally one-to-one cognitive behavioral therapy (CBT), exist for all the main forms of anxiety disorder (social phobia, GAD, panic, OCD, post-traumatic stress disorder (PTSD), etc). Virtually none has been trialed in epilepsy populations, but they are likely to have utility and should be employed [126]. Psychotherapies probably have greater efficacy than medication in preventing relapse and their combination with medication is synergistic. Given the limited availability of psychotherapy in many places, group-based psychotherapies have been piloted [31].

For more severe anxiety disorders, or where psychotherapy proves ineffective, psychotropic medications are indicated, principally SSRIs and SNRIs; the evidence base in epilepsy patients is slender but use of these medications is justified given the risk/benefit ratio [98,99,106,121,122]. SSRIs and SNRIs can cause some agitation initially and take 4–6 weeks to have noticeable benefit, so it is important to inform patients fully, monitor regularly, commence with low doses, and usually to temporarily prescribe a benzodiazepine, such as alprazolam.

Prognosis

It is essential that the clinician looks beyond the short-term achievement of remission. Anxiety disorders tend to be long-term, relapsing–remitting illnesses, so thought needs to be given to relapse prevention and rehabilitation. In addition, they constitute a risk factor for depression.

Practical advice/pearls

- Anxiety disorders in epilepsy patients are common but underrecognized and undertreated.
- Just as for other comorbidities of epilepsy, such as osteoporosis, clinicians need to be alert to the possibility of anxiety disorder, know how to elicit its symptoms, and ideally have established links with psychiatric and/or psychological care.
- First-line treatment is usually psychotherapy, such as CBT. When psychotherapy is ineffective or unavailable, SSRIs or SNRIs are indicated. These can cause agitation initially and take 4–6 weeks to have noticeable effect, so it is vital to inform patients, monitor regularly, commence with low doses, and usually to temporarily prescribe a benzodiazepine, such as alprazolam.

Psychoses and epilepsy

Recent advances concerning psychoses of epilepsy (POE) involve pathogenesis and the interrelationships of subtypes, with few developments regarding clinical practice, as highlighted by a Cochrane review showing a near absence of randomized controlled treatment trials [127] (for recent reviews, see [128–131]).

Epidemiology

Population-based studies of POE prevalence are uncommon compared to studies emanating from tertiary centers, which makes a large Danish national register-based study especially important [132]. This showed an increased risk of schizophrenia (rate ratio (RR) ~2.5) and of the broader category of schizophrenia-like psychosis (RR ~2.9) in people with a history of epilepsy. Both family history of epilepsy and family history of psychosis conferred greater risk, suggesting roles for both genetic and environmental factors in the causation of POE. There was no significant association with type of epilepsy.

Most discussions of POE grapple with the subtypes and their interconnections. These are ictal psychosis; postictal psychosis (PIP); acute, brief interictal psychosis (AIP, in contrast to PIP, defined either by its occurrence after diminution or cessation of seizures (often termed "alternate psychosis") or by its lack of relationship to a prior seizure cluster or intensification); and chronic interictal psychosis (CIP).

Two recent findings concern PIP. First, a variant PIP was described [133], which often lacked a lucid interval and was more common than classical, "nuclear" PIP, defined by the now conventional Logsdail and Toone criteria [134]. Complex partial seizures may occur episodes of this variant PIP episodes and the authors speculated that it might be caused by "limbic status epilepticus." Whether this variant should be included under the rubric of PIP could be debated. Second, an 8-year follow-up of PIP in focal epilepsy patients confirmed prior reports that progression from PIP to CIP occurs in a substantial minority of patients [135].

A relatively neglected issue is the similarities and differences between the POEs and functional psychoses [128], a basic issue in approaching the question of pathogenesis [136,137]. A further problem is the preponderance of studies in focal epilepsies. This may reflect not so much a lack of association of POE with generalized epilepsies as an understandable dominance in tertiary epilepsy centers of focal epilepsy cases.

Pathogenesis

Only halting progress has been made, mainly in the painstaking accrual of a range of risk factors for the various POEs, together with only very general hypotheses about pathogenesis [128,138].

For CIP, the evidence remains inconclusive regarding epilepsy-related factors such as type (generalized versus focal; if focal, whether temporal or extratemporal; if temporal, whether left- or right-sided), age of onset, seizure severity and frequency, and so on. The most consistent findings are of onset of CIP some 10–15 years after onset of epilepsy, an association with family history of psychosis, and *distributed* cerebral pathology, as revealed by structural or functional imaging, EEG, or neuropathology (see discussion in Mellers [130], pp. 344–347). This suggests combined contributions from genetic diathesis, brain structural and functional abnormalities underlying the seizure disorder (abnormalities which themselves probably evolve over time), and the cumulative effect of seizures [139].

A similar picture is supported for PIP by two recent studies of focal epilepsy in video-EEG patients [140,141]. The first showed associations between occurrence of PIP and four domains of risk: ambiguous or extratemporal localization, family history of psychiatric disorder and/or epilepsy, abnormal interictal EEG, and past history of encephalitis [140]. The authors concluded that PIP in focal epilepsy is associated with involvement of broad, bilateral brain networks, genetic diathesis, and encephalitis. Consistent with this, the second study showed a strong association between PIP and the presence of bilateral ictal foci [141]. Several imaging and neuropsychological studies reinforce this picture [142–144], suggesting commonalities in the pathogenesis of CIP and PIP and of functional psychosis.

Etiology

A crucially important development is the discovery of genetic mutations that may contribute to both epilepsy and psychosis [145–147].

The most common clinical situation in which a single etiological agent appears to trigger POE involves AEDs. Whether particular AEDs have a greater or lesser propensity to induce psychosis is often difficult to ascertain, due to confounding by epilepsy severity, coexisting brain pathology, and other factors [90,148].

Diagnosis/evaluation

The imperative and sometimes difficult issue is to differentiate POE, especially PIP, from nonconvulsive status epilepticus (NCS). NCS subsumes absence status, as well as simple and complex partial status. It can present with psychotic phenomena, including hallucinations, delusions, and bizarre and disorganized behavior, and even catatonia. The EEG may be normal. In contrast to POE, NCS patients may retain insight, but typically (by definition, in complex partial status) show impaired consciousness. Although little new research has emerged in recent years, awareness of NCS and its diverse manifestations has risen [129,130].

Treatment

As suggested earlier, there has been little advance in pharmacological or psychosocial treatment of POE [127] and almost no attention has been given to prevention.

Prevention – including relapse prevention – of functional psychotic disorders is a thriving area within psychiatry.

For PIP, better seizure control is imperative, utilizing AEDs and, where feasible, epilepsy surgery. Given the association of PIP with bilateral temporal foci, presurgical assessment needs to be thorough. Most PIP episodes can be controlled with short-term use of benzodiazepines. Patients and their families can learn to recognize occasions with high risk of PIP, institute benzodiazepine therapy early, and often prevent development of an episode. In some places, antipsychotics are used instead of benzodiazepines. The evidence base for both types of medication is slender: largely reports of cases or small series.

For CIP, antipsychotic therapy is usually necessary, necessitating use of medications with low impact on seizure threshold, such as risperidone, sulpiride, trifluoperazine, or haloperidol [129]. There has been little discussion of psychosocial modalities of management widely employed for functional psychoses, including CBT and other therapies, family therapies, and cognitive remediation.

Prognosis

For this question too, few new data have emerged. PIP episodes tend to recur unless there is improved seizure control and/or timely intervention to prevent individual episodes. As already mentioned, in a substantial minority of focal epilepsy patients, CIP emerges. PIP is associated with considerable risk of inadvertent harm due to impaired judgment and disturbed behavior stemming from delusions and other psychotic experiences, as well as risks of self-harm and suicide and occasionally harm to others. There is as yet no clear evidence of whether prevention of PIP lowers risk of subsequent CIP. The prognosis for CIP, like that for schizophrenia, is variable, although in general the severity of CIP is less than that of demographically comparable schizophrenia.

When epilepsy surgery succeeds in alleviating seizures, PIP ceases (see [129], p. 202 ff.). The effects of surgery on preexisting CIP are highly variable and unpredictable. It is also clear that there are *de novo* cases of psychosis that emerge after epilepsy surgery, both when it has succeeded and when it has not. Reported rates vary from 3 to 10% of anterior temporal-lobectomy patients. Only fragmentary information is available regarding possible risk factors, which

include: family history of psychosis, ganglioglioma, or DNET, older age at surgery, and right-sided seizure focus.

Practical advice/pearls

- NCS can mimic psychosis. It is often unrecognized or slow to be recognized. The EEG may be normal or nondiagnostic. Look for abnormal movements, which may be fleeting, and impaired consciousness. Consider benzodiazepine treatment.
- PIP patients may have bilateral temporal foci and thus need thorough assessment prior to epilepsy surgery.
- Educate PIP patients and their families about PIP, its early recognition, and treatment. Many episodes of PIP can be averted.
- Psychosis is a real – albeit low-frequency – risk of epilepsy surgery and of add-on AED therapy. Inform patients.
- If your own service cannot provide psychosocial care for CIP, establish a link with services that can do so.

Conclusion

The themes that emerge from this brief review apply to both research and clinical domains. In research on comorbidities, there has been an intensified, interdisciplinary rethinking of the causal relationships between epilepsy and psychiatric disorder. Shared factors, especially in neurodevelopment, may contribute to both; each may affect the other. Genetic mutations that give rise to both epilepsy and psychosis are one example [145,146]. Another is the many well-established effects of stress on ion channels, neurocircuitry, gene expression, and neurochemical systems relevant to both epilepsy and psychiatric disturbance [75,80,81].

The counterpart to this research shift is the need for clinicians to adopt a patient-centered [149], biopsychosocial and lifespan approach. Many clinicians already practice in this spirit without naming it as such, but often care is oriented to short-term goals and is thus episodic and fragmented. Both epilepsy and the psychiatric comorbidities tend to be life-long, relapsing–remitting illnesses, each with psychosocial impacts that can affect the course of illness and accompanied by further comorbidities, such as obesity. Thus, health services caring for epilepsy patients require integrated psychiatric care wherever possible, preferably onsite and as part of the multidisciplinary team. Unfortunately, psychotherapy trials remain rare in epilepsy populations, with a Cochrane review concluding "no evidence" [150]. Psychotherapy research is challenging and expensive, but should be a priority. Psychosocial programs to improve self-management and coping in epilepsy [89,151] are also likely to buffer patients against psychiatric disorder [86], an aspect deserving study. Some interventions, notably physical activity [152], may benefit other serious comorbidities of epilepsy, such as obesity and osteoporosis, as well as mental health, cognition, and possibly epilepsy itself. Hopefully, as evidence accrues, comprehensive epilepsy care, like comprehensive cardiovascular, diabetes, or cancer care, will come routinely to encompass all these dimensions.

References

1 Jones JE, Austin JK, Caplan R et al.: Psychiatric disorders in children and adolescents who have epilepsy. *Pediatr Rev* 2008; **29(2)**:e9–14.

2 Ekinci O, Titus JB, Rodopman AA et al.: Depression and anxiety in children and adolescents with epilepsy: prevalence, risk factors, and treatment. *Epilepsy Behav* 2009; **14(1)**:8–18.

3 Bujoreanu IS, Ibeziako P, DeMaso DR: Psychiatric concerns in pediatric epilepsy. *Child Adolesc Psychiatr Clin N Am* 2010; **19(2)**:371–386, x.

4 Hesdorffer DC, Kanner AM: The FDA alert on suicidality and antiepileptic drugs: fire or false alarm? *Epilepsia* 2009; **50(5)**:978–986.

5 Barry JJ, Ettinger AB, Friel P et al.: Consensus statement: the evaluation and treatment of people with epilepsy and affective disorders. *Epilepsy Behav* 2008; **13(Suppl. 1)**: S1–S29.

6 Kanner AM, Trimble M, Schmitz B: Postictal affective episodes. *Epilepsy Behav* 2010; **19(2)**:156–158.

7 Hesdorffer DC, Krishnamoorthy E: Neuropsychiatric disorders in epilepsy: epidemiology and classification. In: Trimble M, Schmitz B (eds): *The Neuropsychiatry of Epilepsy*, 2 edn. Cambridge University Press, Cambridge, 2011, pp. 3–13.

8 Fuller-Thomson E, Brennenstuhl S: The association between depression and epilepsy in a nationally representative sample. *Epilepsia* 2009; **50(5)**:1051–1058.

9 Tellez-Zenteno JF, Wiebe S: Prevalence of psychiatric disorders in patients with epilepsy: what we think we know and what we know. In: Kanner AM, Schachter S (eds): *Psychiatric Controversies in Epilepsy*. Academic Press, Amsterdam, 2008, pp. 1–18.

10 Tellez-Zenteno JF, Patten SB, Jette N et al.: Psychiatric comorbidity in epilepsy: a population-based analysis. *Epilepsia* 2007; **48(12)**:2336–2344.

11 McLaughlin DP, Pachana NA, McFarland K: Depression in a community-dwelling sample of older adults with late-onset or lifetime epilepsy. *Epilepsy Behav* 2008; **12(2)**:281–285.

12 Velissaris SL, Wilson SJ, Newton MR et al.: Cognitive complaints after a first seizure in adulthood: Influence of psychological adjustment. *Epilepsia* 2009; **50(5)**:1012–1021.

13 Salas-Puig J, Gil-Nagel A, Serratosa JM et al.: Self-reported memory problems in everyday activities in patients with epilepsy treated with antiepileptic drugs. *Epilepsy Behav* 2009; **14(4)**:622–627.

14 Marino SE, Meador KJ, Loring DW et al.: Subjective perception of cognition is related to mood and not performance. *Epilepsy Behav* 2009; **14(3)**:459–464.

15 Rayner G, Wrench JM, Wilson SJ: Differential contributions of objective memory and mood to subjective memory complaints in refractory focal epilepsy. *Epilepsy Behav* 2010; **19(3)**:359–364.

16 McLaughlin DP, Pachana NA, McFarland K: The impact of depression, seizure variables and locus of control on health related quality of life in a community dwelling sample of older adults. *Seizure* 2010; **19(4)**:232–236.

17 Kanner AM, Barry JJ, Gilliam F et al.: Anxiety disorders, subsyndromic depressive episodes, and major depressive episodes: do they differ on their impact on the quality of life of patients with epilepsy? *Epilepsia* 2010; **51(7)**:1152–1158.

18 Canuet L, Ishii R, Iwase M et al.: Factors associated with impaired quality of life in younger and older adults with epilepsy. *Epilepsy Res* 2009; **83(1)**:58–65.

19 Panelli RJ, Kilpatrick C, Moore SM et al.: The Liverpool Adverse Events Profile: relation to AED use and mood. *Epilepsia* 2007; **48(3)**:456–463.

20 Hitiris N, Mohanraj R, Norrie J et al.: Predictors of pharmacoresistant epilepsy. *Epilepsy Res* 2007; **75(2–3)**:192–196.

21 Petrovski S, Szoeke CEI, Jones NC et al.: Neuropsychiatric symptomatology predicts seizure recurrence in newly treated patients. *Neurology* 2010; **75(11)**:1015–1021.

22 Kanner AM, Byrne R, Chicharro A et al.: A lifetime psychiatric history predicts a worse seizure outcome following temporal lobectomy. *Neurology* 2009; **72(9)**:793–799.

23 Metternich B, Wagner K, Brandt A et al.: Preoperative depressive symptoms predict postoperative seizure outcome in temporal and frontal lobe epilepsy. *Epilepsy Behav* 2009; **16(4)**:622–628.

24 Ridsdale L, Charlton J, Ashworth M et al.: Epilepsy mortality and risk factors for death in epilepsy: a population-based study. *Br J Gen Pract* 2011; **61(586)**:e271–e278.

25 Faingold CL, Tupal S, Randall M: Prevention of seizure-induced sudden death in a chronic SUDEP model by semichronic administration of a selective serotonin reuptake inhibitor. *Epilepsy Behav* 2011; **22(2)**:186–190.

26 Mula M, Jauch R, Cavanna A et al.: Interictal dysphoric disorder and periictal dysphoric symptoms in patients with epilepsy. *Epilepsia* 2010; **51(7)**:1139–1145.

27 Kanner AM: Depression and epilepsy: a bidirectional relation? *Epilepsia* 2011; **52(Suppl. 1)**:21–27.

28 Ettinger AB, Copeland LA, Zeber JE et al.: Are psychiatric disorders independent risk factors for new-onset epilepsy in older individuals? *Epilepsy Behav* 2010; **17(1)**:70–74.

29 Thompson NJ, Walker ER, Obolensky N et al.: Distance delivery of mindfulness-based cognitive therapy for depression: project UPLIFT. *Epilepsy Behav* 2010; **19(3)**:247–254.

30 Ciechanowski P, Chaytor N, Miller J et al.: PEARLS depression treatment for individuals with epilepsy: a randomized controlled trial. *Epilepsy Behav* 2010; **19(3)**:225–231.

31 Macrodimitris S, Wershler J, Hatfield M et al.: Group cognitive-behavioral therapy for patients with epilepsy and comorbid depression and anxiety. *Epilepsy Behav* 2011; **20(1)**:83–88.

32 McLaughlin DP, McFarland K: A randomized trial of a group based cognitive behavior therapy program for older adults with epilepsy: the impact on seizure frequency, depression and psychosocial well-being. *J Behav Med* 2011; **34(3)**:201–207.

33 Cotterman-Hart S. Depression in epilepsy: why aren't we treating? *Epilepsy Behav* 2010; **19(3)**:419–421.

34 Margrove KL, Thapar AK, Mensah SA, Kerr MP: Help-seeking and treatment preferences for depression in epilepsy. *Epilepsy Behav* 2011; **22(4)**:740–744.

35 Daniels ZS, Nick TG, Liu C et al.: Obesity is a common comorbidity for pediatric patients with untreated, newly diagnosed epilepsy. *Neurology* 2009; **73(9)**:658–664.

36 Hinnell C, Williams J, Metcalfe A et al.: Health status and health-related behaviors in epilepsy compared to other chronic conditions – a national population-based study. *Epilepsia* 2010; **51(5)**:853–861.

37 Mula M, Marotta AE, Monaco F: Epilepsy and bipolar disorders. *Expert Rev Neurother* 2010; **10(1)**:13–23.

38 Hoppe C, Elger CE: Depression in epilepsy: a critical review from a clinical perspective. *Nat Rev Neurol* 2011; **7(8)**:462–472.

39 Lacey CJ, Salzberg MR, Roberts H et al.: Psychiatric comorbidity and impact on health service utilization in a community sample of patients with epilepsy. *Epilepsia* 2009; **50(8)**:1991–1994.

40 Hesdorffer DC, Hauser WA, Olafsson E et al.: Depression and suicide attempt as risk factors for incident unprovoked seizures. *Ann Neurol* 2006; **59(1)**:35–41.

41 Ferguson PL, Smith GM, Wannamaker BB et al.: A population-based study of risk of epilepsy after hospitalization for traumatic brain injury. *Epilepsia* 2010; **51(5)**:891–898.

42 Stefanello S, Marin-Leon L, Fernandes PT et al.: Psychiatric comorbidity and suicidal behavior in epilepsy: a community-based case-control study. *Epilepsia* 2010; **51(7)**:1120–1125.

43 Stefanello S, Marin-Leon L, Fernandes PT et al.: Suicidal thoughts in epilepsy: a community-based study in Brazil. *Epilepsy Behav* 2010; **17(4)**:483–488.

44 Christensen J, Vestergaard M, Mortensen PB et al.: Epilepsy and risk of suicide: a population-based case-control study. *Lancet Neurol* 2007; **6(8)**:693–698.

45 Velissaris SL, Wilson SJ, Saling MM et al.: The psychological impact of a newly diagnosed seizure: losing and restoring perceived control. *Epilepsy Behav* 2007; **10(2)**:223–233.

46 Thapar A, Kerr M, Harold G: Stress, anxiety, depression, and epilepsy: investigating the relationship between psychological factors and seizures. *Epilepsy Behav* 2009; **14(1)**:134–140.

47 Wrench JM, Wilson SJ, O'Shea MF, Reutens DC: Characterising de novo depression after epilepsy surgery. *Epilepsy Res* 2009; **83(1)**:81–88.

48 Reisinger EL, DiIorio C: Individual, seizure-related, and psychosocial predictors of depressive symptoms among people with epilepsy over six months. *Epilepsy Behav* 2009; **15(2)**:196–201.

49 Hesdorffer DC, Lee P: Health, wealth, and culture as predominant factors in psychosocial morbidity. *Epilepsy Behav* 2009; **15(Suppl. 1)**:S36–S40.

50 Lee S-A, Lee S-M, No Y-J: Factors contributing to depression in patients with epilepsy. *Epilepsia* 2010; **51(7)**:1305–1308.

51 Goldstein LH, Holland L, Soteriou H, Mellers JD: Illness representations, coping styles and mood in adults with epilepsy. *Epilepsy Res* 2005; **67(1–2)**:1–11.

52 Wagner JL, Smith G, Ferguson PL et al.: A hopelessness model of depressive symptoms in youth with epilepsy. *J Pediatr Psychol* 2009; **34(1)**:89–96.

53 Donnelly KM, Schefft BK, Howe SR et al.: Moderating effect of optimism on emotional distress and seizure control in adults with temporal lobe epilepsy. *Epilepsy Behav* 2010; **18(4)**:374–380.

54 Wilson SJ, Wrench JM, McIntosh AM et al.: Profiles of psychosocial outcome after epilepsy surgery: the role of personality. *Epilepsia* 2010; **51(7)**:1133–1138.

55 Briellmann RS, Hopwood MJ, Jackson GD: Major depression in temporal lobe epilepsy with hippocampal sclerosis: clinical and imaging correlates. *J Neurol Neurosurg Psychiatry* 2007; **78(11)**:1226–1230.

56 Elst LT, Groffmann M, Ebert D, Schulze-Bonhage A: Amygdala volume loss in patients with dysphoric disorder of epilepsy. *Epilepsy Behav* 2009; **16(1)**:105–112.

57 Finegersh A, Avedissian C, Shamim S et al.: Bilateral hippocampal atrophy in temporal lobe epilepsy: effect of depressive symptoms and febrile seizures. *Epilepsia* 2011; **52(4)**:689–697.

58 Labate A, Cerasa A, Aguglia U et al.: Neocortical thinning in "benign" mesial temporal lobe epilepsy. *Epilepsia* 2011; **52(4)**:712–717.

59 Paparrigopoulos T, Ferentinos P, Brierley B et al.: Relationship between post-operative depression/anxiety and hippocampal/amygdala volumes in temporal lobectomy for epilepsy. *Epilepsy Res* 2008; **81(1)**:30–35.

60 Salgado PC, Yasuda CL, Cendes F: Neuroimaging changes in mesial temporal lobe epilepsy are magnified in the presence of depression. *Epilepsy Behav* 2010; **19(3)**:422–427.

61 Shamim S, Hasler G, Liew C et al.: Temporal lobe epilepsy, depression, and hippocampal volume. *Epilepsia* 2009; **50(5)**:1067–1071.

62 Bonelli SB, Powell R, Yogarajah M et al.: Preoperative amygdala fMRI in temporal lobe epilepsy. *Epilepsia* 2009; **50(2)**:217–227.

63 Assem-Hilger E, Lanzenberger R, Savli M et al.: Central serotonin 1A receptor binding in temporal lobe epilepsy: a [carbonyl-(11)C]WAY-100635 PET study. *Epilepsy Behav* 2010; **19(3)**:467–473.

64 Gilliam FG, Maton BM, Martin RC et al.: Hippocampal 1H-MRSI correlates with severity of depression symptoms in temporal lobe epilepsy. *Neurology* 2007; **68(5)**:364–368.

65 Hasler G, Bonwetsch R, Giovacchini G et al.: 5-HT1A receptor binding in temporal lobe epilepsy patients with and without major depression. *Biol Psychiatry* 2007; **62(11)**:1258–1264.

66 Lothe A, Didelot A, Hammers A et al.: Comorbidity between temporal lobe epilepsy and depression: a 18F MPPF PET study. *Brain* 2008; **131(Pt 10)**:2765–2782.

67 Theodore WH, Hasler G, Giovacchini G et al.: Reduced hippocampal 5HT1A PET receptor binding and depression in temporal lobe epilepsy. *Epilepsia* 2007; **48(8)**:1526–1530.

68 Richardson EJ, Griffith HR, Martin RC et al.: Structural and functional neuroimaging correlates of depression in temporal lobe epilepsy. *Epilepsy Behav* 2007; **10(2)**:242–249.

69 Frisch C, Hanke J, Kleineruschkamp S et al.: Positive correlation between the density of neuropeptide y positive neurons in the amygdala and parameters of self-reported anxiety and depression in mesiotemporal lobe epilepsy patients. *Biol Psychiatry* 2009; **66(5)**:433–440.

70 Dias R, Bateman LM, Farias ST et al.: Depression in epilepsy is associated with lack of seizure control. *Epilepsy Behav* 2010; **19(3)**:445–447.

71 Mula M, Monaco F: Antiepileptic drugs and psychopathology of epilepsy: an update. *Epileptic Disord* 2009; **11(1)**:1–9.

72 Kanner AM: Depression and epilepsy: do glucocorticoids and glutamate explain their relationship? *Curr Neurol Neurosci Rep* 2009; **9(4)**:307–312.

73 Kanner AM: Depression and epilepsy: a review of multiple facets of their close relation. *Neurol Clin* 2009; **27(4)**:865–880.

74 Dhir A: Novel discoveries in understanding the complexities of epilepsy and major depression. *Expert Opin Ther Targets* 2010; **14(1)**:109–115.

75 Salzberg M: Neurobiological links between epilepsy and mood disorders. *Neurology Asia* 2011; **16(Suppl. 1)**:37–40.

76 Colman I, Ataullahjan A: Life course perspectives on the epidemiology of depression. *Can J Psychiatry* 2010; **55(10)**:622–632.

77 Post RM, Weiss SR: Convergences in course of illness and treatments of the epilepsies and recurrent affective disorders. *Clin EEG Neurosci* 2004; **35(1)**:14–24.

78 Hermann B, Seidenberg M, Jones J: The neurobehavioural comorbidities of epilepsy: can a natural history be developed? *Lancet Neurol* 2008; **7(2)**:151–160.

79 Hermann B, Jacoby A: The psychosocial impact of epilepsy in adults. *Epilepsy Behav* 2009; **15(Suppl. 1)**:S11–S16.

80 Koe AS, Jones NC, Salzberg MR: Early life stress as an influence on limbic epilepsy: an hypothesis whose time has come? *Front Behav Neurosci* 2009; **3**:24.

81 Ali I, Salzberg MR, French C, Jones NC: Electrophysiological insights into the enduring effects of early life stress on the brain. *Psychopharmacology (Berl)* 2011; **214(1)**:155–173.

82 Cole AJ: New screening tool for identifying major depression in patients with epilepsy. *Nat Clin Pract Neurol* 2006; **2(12)**:656–657.

83 Friedman DE, Kung DH, Laowattana S et al.: Identifying depression in epilepsy in a busy clinical setting is enhanced with systematic screening. *Seizure* 2009; **18(6)**:429–433.

84 Gilliam FG, Barry JJ, Hermann BP et al.: Rapid detection of major depression in epilepsy: a multicentre study. *Lancet Neurol* 2006; **5(5)**:399–405.

85 Walker ER, Obolensky N, Dini S, Thompson NJ: Formative and process evaluations of a cognitive-behavioral therapy and mindfulness intervention for people with epilepsy and depression. *Epilepsy Behav* 2010; **19(3)**:239–246.

86 Martinovic Z, Simonovic P, Djokic R: Preventing depression in adolescents with epilepsy. *Epilepsy Behav* 2006; **9(4)**:619–624.

87 Charyton C, Elliott JO, Moore JL, Klatte ET: Is it time to consider cognitive behavioral therapy for persons with epilepsy? Clues from pathophysiology, treatment and functional neuroimaging. *Expert Rev Neurother* 2010; **10(12)**:1911–1927.

88 Wagner JL, Smith G, Ferguson P et al.: Pilot study of an integrated cognitive-behavioral and self-management intervention for youth with epilepsy and caregivers: Coping Openly and Personally with Epilepsy (COPE). *Epilepsy Behav* 2010; **18(3)**:280–285.

89 Mittan RJ: Psychosocial treatment programs in epilepsy: a review. *Epilepsy Behav* 2009; **16(3)**:371–380.

90 Perr J, Ettinger A: Psychiatric illness and psychotropic medication use in epilepsy. In: Trimble M, Schmitz B (eds): *The Neuropsychiatry of Epilepsy*, 2 edn. Cambridge University Press, Cambridge, 2011, pp. 165–195.

91 Alper K: Do antidepressants improve or worsen seizures in patients with epilepsy? In: Kanner AM, Schachter S (eds): *Psychiatric Controversies in Epilepsy*. Academic Press, Amsterdam, 2008, pp. 255–268.

92 Alper K, Schwartz KA, Kolts RL, Khan A: Seizure incidence in psychopharmacological clinical trials: an analysis of Food

and Drug Administration (FDA) summary basis of approval reports. *Biol Psychiatry* 2007; **62(4)**:345–354.

93 Kanner A: Should antidepressant drugs be tested as antiepileptic agents? *ILAE, Rome*, August 29, 2011.

94 Danzer SC: Depression, stress, epilepsy and adult neurogenesis. *Exp Neurol* 2011; **233(1)**:22–32.

95 Kanner AM: Anxiety disorders in epilepsy: the forgotten psychiatric comorbidity. *Epilepsy Curr* 2011; **11(3)**:90–91.

96 Kwan P, Yu E, Leung H et al.: Association of subjective anxiety, depression, and sleep disturbance with quality-of-life ratings in adults with epilepsy. *Epilepsia* 2009; **50(5)**:1059–1066.

97 Park S-P, Song H-S, Hwang Y-H et al.: Differential effects of seizure control and affective symptoms on quality of life in people with epilepsy. *Epilepsy Behav* 2010; **18(4)**:455–459.

98 Kanner AM: Ictal panic and interictal panic attacks: diagnostic and therapeutic principles. *Neurol Clin* 2011; **29(1)**:163–175, ix.

99 Kanner A, Ettinger A: Anxiety disorders. In: Engel J, Pedley T (eds): *Epilepsy: A Comprehensive Textbook*, 2 edn. Lippincott Williams & Wilkins, Philadelphia, PA, 2008.

100 Brandt C, Schoendienst M, Trentowska M et al.: Prevalence of anxiety disorders in patients with refractory focal epilepsy – a prospective clinic based survey. *Epilepsy Behav* 2010; **17(2)**:259–263.

101 Desai SD, Shukla G, Goyal V et al.: Study of DSM-IV Axis I psychiatric disorders in patients with refractory complex partial seizures using a short structured clinical interview. *Epilepsy Behav* 2010; **19(3)**:301–305.

102 Jones JE, Bell B, Fine J et al.: A controlled prospective investigation of psychiatric comorbidity in temporal lobe epilepsy. *Epilepsia* 2007; **48(12)**:2357–2360.

103 Mensah SA, Beavis JM, Thapar AK, Kerr MP: A community study of the presence of anxiety disorder in people with epilepsy. *Epilepsy Behav* 2007; **11(1)**:118–124.

104 Kanner AM: Psychiatric issues in epilepsy: the complex relation of mood, anxiety disorders, and epilepsy. *Epilepsy Behav* 2009; **15(1)**:83–87.

105 Jones JE: Are anxiety and depression two sides of the same coin? In: Kanner AM, Schachter S (eds): *Psychiatric Controversies in Epilepsy*. Academic Press, Amsterdam, 2008, pp. 89–110.

106 Beyenburg S, Mitchell AJ, Schmidt D et al.: Anxiety in patients with epilepsy: systematic review and suggestions for clinical management. *Epilepsy Behav* 2005; **7(2)**:161–171.

107 Hamid H, Ettinger AB, Mula M: Anxiety symptoms in epilepsy: salient issues for future research. *Epilepsy Behav* 2011; **22(1)**:63–68.

108 Kanner AM: Is depression a risk factor of worse response to therapy in epilepsy? *Epilepsy Curr* 2011; **11(2)**:50–51.

109 Bouilleret V, Hogan RE, Velakoulis D et al.: Morphometric abnormalities and hyperanxiety in genetically epileptic rats: a model of psychiatric comorbidity? *Neuroimage* 2009; **45(2)**:267–274.

110 Jones NC, Salzberg MR, Kumar G et al.: Elevated anxiety and depressive-like behavior in a rat model of genetic generalized epilepsy suggesting common causation. *Exp Neurol* 2008; **209(1)**:254–260.

111 Kalynchuk LE, Pinel JPJ, Meaney MJ: Serotonin receptor binding and mRNA expression in the hippocampus of fearful amygdala-kindled rats. *Neurosci Lett* 2006; **396(1)**:38–43.

112 Kim MJ, Loucks RA, Palmer AL et al.: The structural and functional connectivity of the amygdala: from normal emotion to pathological anxiety. *Behav Brain Res* 2011; **223(2)**:403–410.

113 Bernasconi N, Duchesne S, Janke A et al.: Whole-brain voxel-based statistical analysis of gray matter and white matter in temporal lobe epilepsy. *Neuroimage* 2004; **23(2)**:717–723.

114 Pessoa L, Adolphs R: Emotion processing and the amygdala: from a "low road" to "many roads" of evaluating biological significance. *Nat Rev Neurosci* 2010; **11(11)**:773–783.

115 Adams SJ, O'Brien TJ, Lloyd J et al.: Neuropsychiatric morbidity in focal epilepsy. *Br J Psychiatry* 2008; **192(6)**:464–469.

116 Akanuma N, Hara E, Adachi N et al.: Psychiatric comorbidity in adult patients with idiopathic generalized epilepsy. *Epilepsy Behav* 2008; **13(1)**:248–251.

117 Satishchandra P, Krishnamoorthy ES, van Elst LT et al.: Mesial temporal structures and comorbid anxiety in refractory partial epilepsy. *J Neuropsychiatry Clin Neurosci* 2003; **15(4)**:450–452.

118 Halley SA, Wrench JM, Reutens DC, Wilson SJ: The amygdala and anxiety after epilepsy surgery. *Epilepsy Behav* 2010; **18(4)**:431–436.

119 Bonora A, Benuzzi F, Monti G et al.: Recognition of emotions from faces and voices in medial temporal lobe epilepsy. *Epilepsy Behav* 2011; **20(4)**:648–654.

120 Richardson MP, Strange BA, Dolan RJ: Encoding of emotional memories depends on amygdala and hippocampus and their interactions. *Nat Neurosci* 2004; **7(3)**:278–285.

121 Kanner AM: The use of psychotropic drugs in epilepsy: what every neurologist should know. *Semin Neurol* 2008; **28(3)**:379–388.

122 Kanner AM, Gidal BE: Pharmacodynamic and pharmacokinetic interactions of psychotropic drugs with antiepileptic drugs. *Int Rev Neurobiol* 2008; **83**:397–416.

123 Deutsch SI, Rosse RB, Sud IM, Burket JA: Temporal lobe epilepsy confused with panic disorder: implications for treatment. *Clin Neuropharmacol* 2009; **32(3)**:160–162.

124 Kaplan PW: Obsessive-compulsive disorder in chronic epilepsy. *Epilepsy Behav* 2011; **22(3)**:428–432.

125 Roth RM, Jobst BC, Thadani VM et al.: New-onset obsessive-compulsive disorder following neurosurgery for medication-refractory seizure disorder. *Epilepsy Behav* 2009; **14(4)**:677–680.

126 Kerr MP, Mensah S, Besag F et al.: International consensus clinical practice statements for the treatment of neuropsychiatric conditions associated with epilepsy. *Epilepsia* 2011; **52(11)**:2133–2138.

127 Farooq S, Sherin A: Interventions for psychotic symptoms concomitant with epilepsy. *Cochrane Database Syst Rev* 2008; **4**:CD006118.

128 Kanemoto K, Tadokoro Y, Oshima T: Does psychosis of epilepsy differ from primary psychotic disorders? In: Kanner AM, Schachter S (eds): *Psychiatric Controversies in Epilepsy*. Academic Press, Amsterdam, 2008, pp. 111–128.

129 Kanner AM: Psychosis of epilepsy. In: Shorvon S, Pedley T (eds): *The Epilepsies 3*. Saunders, Philadelphia, PA, 2008, pp. 194–210.

130 Mellers J. Epilepsy. In: David AS, Fleminger S, Kopelman MD et al (eds): *Lishman's Organic Psychiatry*, 4 edn. Wiley-Blackwell, Oxford, 2009, pp. 309–395.

131 Trimble M, Kanner A, Schmitz B: Postictal psychosis. *Epilepsy Behav* 2010; **19(2)**:159–161.

132 Qin P, Xu H, Laursen TM et al.: Risk for schizophrenia and schizophrenia-like psychosis among patients with epilepsy: population based cohort study. *BMJ* 2005; **331(7507)**:23.

133 Oshima T, Tadokoro Y, Kanemoto K: A prospective study of postictal psychoses with emphasis on the periictal type. *Epilepsia* 2006; **47(12)**:2131–2134.

134 Logsdail SJ, Toone BK: Post-ictal psychoses: a clinical and phenomenological description. *Br J Psychiatry* 1988; **152**:246–252.

135 Kanner AM, Ostrovskaya A: Long-term significance of postictal psychotic episodes: II. Are they predictive of interictal psychotic episodes? *Epilepsy Behav* 2008; **12(1)**:154–156.

136 Elliott B, Joyce E, Shorvon S: Delusions, illusions and hallucinations in epilepsy: 2. *Complex phenomena and psychosis. Epilepsy Res* 2009; **85(2–3)**:172–186.

137 Elliott B, Joyce E, Shorvon S: Delusions, illusions and hallucinations in epilepsy: 1. *Elementary phenomena. Epilepsy Res* 2009; **85(2–3)**:162–171.

138 Sachdev P: Schizophrenia-like psychosis and epilepsy. In: Sachdev P, Keshavan M (eds): *Secondary Schizophrenia*. Cambridge University Press, Cambridge, 2010, pp. 79–102.

139 Adachi N, Akanuma N, Ito M et al.: Epileptic, organic and genetic vulnerabilities for timing of the development of interictal psychosis. *Br J Psychiatry* 2010; **196**:212–216.

140 Alper K, Kuzniecky R, Carlson C et al.: Postictal psychosis in partial epilepsy: a case-control study. *Ann Neurol* 2008; **63(5)**:602–610.

141 Kanner AM, Ostrovskaya A: Long-term significance of postictal psychotic episodes: I. Are they predictive of bilateral ictal foci? *Epilepsy Behav* 2008; **12(1)**:150–153.

142 Canuet L, Ishii R, Iwase M et al.: Working memory abnormalities in chronic interictal epileptic psychosis and schizophrenia revealed by magnetoencephalography. *Epilepsy Behav* 2010; **17(1)**:109–119.

143 DuBois JM, Devinsky O, Carlson C et al.: Abnormalities of cortical thickness in postictal psychosis. *Epilepsy Behav* 2011; **21(2)**:132–136.

144 Fukao K, Inoue Y, Yagi K: Magnetoencephalographic characteristics of psychosis in temporal lobe epilepsy. *J Neuropsychiatry Clin Neurosci* 2009; **21(4)**:455–462.

145 Cascella NG, Schretlen DJ, Sawa A: Schizophrenia and epilepsy: is there a shared susceptibility? *Neurosci Res* 2009; **63(4)**:227–235.

146 Johnson MR, Shorvon SD: Heredity in epilepsy: neurodevelopment, comorbidity, and the neurological trait. *Epilepsy Behav* 2011; **22(3)**:421–427.

147 Friedman JI, Vrijenhoek T, Markx S et al.: CNTNAP2 gene dosage variation is associated with schizophrenia and epilepsy. *Mol Psychiatry* 2008; **13(3)**:261–266.

148 Schmitz B: Psychiatric side effects of antiepileptic drugs. In: Engel J, Pedley T (eds): *Epilepsy: A Comprehensive Textbook*, 2 edn. Lippincott Williams & Wilkins, Philadelphia, PA, 2008.

149 Sander L, Jacoby A, Leach J: Can a patient-centred approach to epilepsy improve outcomes? *Prog Neurol Psychiatr* 2010; **14(2)**:27–32.

150 Ramaratnam S, Baker GA, Goldstein LH: Psychological treatments for epilepsy. *Cochrane Database Syst Rev* 2008(**3**):CD002029.

151 Diiorio C, Bamps Y, Walker ER, Escoffery C: Results of a research study evaluating WebEase, an online epilepsy self-management program. *Epilepsy Behav* 2011; **22(3)**:469–474.

152 Arida RM, Scorza FA, Cavalheiro EA: Favorable effects of physical activity for recovery in temporal lobe epilepsy. *Epilepsia* 2010; **51(Suppl. 3)**:76–79.

CHAPTER 14

The contribution of sleep and anxiety disorders to quality of life in people with epilepsy

Dee Snape,[1] Ann Jacoby,[1] and Gus Baker[2]

[1] *Department of Public Health and Policy, Institute of Psychology, Health and Society, University of Liverpool, UK*
[2] *Walton Centre for Neurology & Neurosurgery, University of Liverpool, UK*

Introduction

Historically, the most common approach to examining the quality of life (QOL) of people with epilepsy has been to interrogate the effects of different clinical variables, most commonly seizure frequency. It has been reported that the vast majority of individuals who enjoy seizure freedom do not have lower QOL scores than the general population [1,2]. For those continuing to experience seizures, there is evidence that both frequency of seizures and mixed seizure types can adversely affect QOL [3]. While reduction of seizure frequency has been of paramount importance in the clinical management of epilepsy and in assessing the effectiveness of different antiepileptic drugs (AEDs) in clinical trials [4], it has also been important in the context of improving QOL outcomes of epilepsy, and the wide literature focusing on its importance has, understandably, led to calls for further research [2].

In addition to seizures affecting the more tangible aspects of QOL, such as driving or employment, the importance of seizure frequency is also reflected in reported scores of anxiety and depression. Jacoby et al. [5] used the Hospital Anxiety and Depression Scale (HADS) to determine levels of anxiety and depression in a large community population of people with epilepsy and found that both anxiety and depression levels differed markedly according to seizure frequency: only 13% of patients were classified as anxious and 4% classified as depressed in the seizure-free group, compared to 44 and 21%, respectively, in the group experiencing one or more seizures a month. Anxiety and depression

levels also correlated strongly with other self-reported QOL measures, such as perceived impact of epilepsy and stigma. Paradoxically, Goldstein et al. [6] reported that those with very frequent seizures actually scored lower on anxiety measures. Goldstein and Harden [7] subsequently suggested that for these people, seizures become integrated as part of everyday routine, with less time available to feel anxious in anticipation of a seizure. Seizure frequency alone has not been able to adequately predict increased levels of anxiety and depression and Smith et al. [8] suggest that perceived severity of seizures is another important predictor of QOL domain scores, including psychological well-being. The type of epilepsy may also be a factor: Piazzini et al. [9] reported higher levels of depression and anxiety in those with partial epilepsy compared to the idiopathic generalized epilepsy group.

In this chapter, we explore the published literature relating to anxiety in people with epilepsy. We also examine the issue of sleep disorder in the context of epilepsy and how these two indicators of psychological ill-health are related in people with epilepsy.

Anxiety and epilepsy

Definition of anxiety

Anxiety related to epilepsy has only recently been studied in detail, but where anxiety has been investigated it has traditionally been subsumed into the study of psychiatric morbidity and epilepsy collectively [10]. Anxiety and depression are the most commonly

Epilepsy and the Interictal State: Co-Morbidities and Quality of Life, First Edition.
Edited by Erik K. St. Louis, David M. Ficker, and Terence J. O'Brien.
© 2015 John Wiley & Sons, Ltd. Published 2015 by John Wiley & Sons, Ltd.

reported psychological problems among individuals with epilepsy [11–13]. These two disorders therefore warrant further investigation, in order to untangle their biological and psychosocial aspects in relation to epilepsy. Much less attention has been given in the literature on epilepsy and QOL to the prevalence and impact of anxiety disorders than to depression. The term "anxiety" encompasses a wide spectrum of different disorders according to the DSM-IV and ICD-10 classifications [14]. Alongside diagnoses of generalized anxiety disorder (GAD), panic disorders, post-traumatic stress disorder (PTSD), and phobias, the DSM-IV lists a diagnosis of anxiety disorder related to an existing medical condition. Goldstein and Harden [7] point out that individuals with epilepsy could fall under any of these different categories of anxiety, or several of them. Beyenberg et al. [15] point out that the types of anxiety disorders outlined in the DSM-IV may not be applicable to an epilepsy population and that it may be more useful to attempt to identify specific features of anxiety that are associated with the disorder.

Manifestation of anxiety

Anxiety may exist in its own right (biological pathogenesis) or may be related to the chronic features of epilepsy (psychosocial pathogenesis). It may be experienced at different time periods relating to seizures: ictally (during a seizure), postictally (immediately following a seizure), or interictally (in the periods between seizures) [16]. Thus, anxiety can be experienced only as part of a seizure or can be a more long-standing problem, highlighting the difficulty in establishing causes and determining appropriate treatment [17]. "Free-floating" anxiety may be ever present in an individual's life at varying levels [18]. Patients can have symptoms that would fall under the category of generalized anxiety: problems controlling their anxiety and persistent worrying about relatively minor matters [17]. Some phobias present in individuals with epilepsy can be directly traced back to the nature of epilepsy; for example, agoraphobia can manifest as a result of fear of having seizures in public places [18]. Newsom-Davis et al. [19] reported the case of a 26-year-old woman with seizure phobia and concluded that, while true seizure phobia may be rare, psychosocial and emotional factors heavily contributed to the development of the underlying anxiety and necessitated intervention.

Baker et al. [11] reported that of 696 adults with epilepsy in a community-based study, 24% could be classified using HADS as clinically anxious and a further 15% as borderline clinically anxious. Although seizure frequency and drug adverse effects were implicated, the more powerful predictors of anxiety were other psychosocial measures, particularly depression and perceived impact of epilepsy scores. De Souza and Salgado [20] found that 33% of epilepsy patients were experiencing anxiety, with epilepsy patients at much greater risk than nonepileptic controls. Levels of anxiety were unrelated to epilepsy disease variables such as age of onset, duration of epilepsy, or medication type; nor were they related to sociodemographic characteristics such as gender. These authors concluded that perception of seizure control is strongly related to both anxiety and depression, the important factor being how the person concerned *subjectively interprets* frequency of seizures. It has been argued that in some instances, those experiencing more severe forms of epilepsy may adjust to the effects on their lifestyle more positively than those with infrequent seizures [21]. Hermann et al. [21] demonstrated that internal factors such as attributional style (how an individual perceives adverse events and their causes) could be directly related to psychological comorbidities among people with epilepsy, including anxiety. Finally, there is evidence that external factors such as an increased level of social support when a person is faced with a chronic illness may be protective of its negative effects, including for psychological well-being [22].

The role of AEDs in anxiety

The costs to QOL of having seizures must be balanced against any negative effects of treating them. The vast majority of epilepsy patients are prescribed AEDs to control their seizures. The model epilepsy treatment from a patient perspective is seizure control, few side effects, and convenient drug regimes [23], and therefore is not at odds with the clinician perspective [24]. Unfortunately, drug-related side effects of varying severity do continue to affect individuals with epilepsy. In a survey of over 5000 patients across Europe, only 12% considered themselves to be free of any adverse effects of their treatment [3]. In the same study, significant levels of anxiety were reported in half of the patients surveyed, highlighting the importance of tackling anxiety management alongside control of seizures.

Establishing the effects of AEDs on psychiatric problems has proved problematic because of a shortage of studies relating to older drugs and variance in methods of reporting psychiatric problems when testing newer ones [25]. The available evidence is mixed. Fiordelli et al. [12] noted that their patients with multiple drug regimes appeared also to have more psychiatric problems; however, as these individuals were likely also to be those having multiple seizure types, a clear causative link could not be assumed. As in the general population, individuals with epilepsy may have varying susceptibility to developing psychiatric disorders, and personal or familial history of previous problems may predispose certain people to experience disorders [25]. Current thinking is that AEDs generally lean towards anxiolytic (anxiety-reducing) rather than anxiogenic (anxiety-increasing) effects [15]. AEDs have been viewed as beneficial in treating some anxiety disorders [26] and withdrawal from some AEDs has been shown to increase anxiety levels, with levels only decreasing on their reintroduction [27]. Ketter et al. [27] hypothesize that better QOL outcomes could be achieved by treating patients with baseline "activated" profiles (i.e., insomnia, anxiety, agitation) using AEDs with known sedating effects.

Epilepsy and sleep disorder

Manifestation of sleep disorder

Sleep complaints are a frequent concomitant of anxiety disorder [28] and compromised sleep is common among people with epilepsy [24,29]. The influence of the sleep–wake cycle on the manifestation of seizures has been documented in the literature for over a century [29]. Interactions between sleep and epilepsy have been found to take a number of different forms (delay in sleep onset, difficulty staying asleep, waking too early [29]) and have been associated with a number of potential causes, including insufficient sleep syndrome, sleep hygiene, coexisting sleep disorders, the effects of seizures themselves, and the effects of AEDS [30].

A large study conducted by De Haas et al. [31] showed that, over a 6-month period, people with epilepsy had twice the prevalence of subjective sleep disturbance as controls (39 versus 18%) and that the presence of sleep disturbance was associated with a significant reduction in QOL beyond that which was attributable to just

having epilepsy (which was significantly worse than that of matched controls). In addition, sleep disturbance has been highlighted as being particularly problematic among younger people [32]. Hermann [33] included sleep in his list of key domains of QOL for people with epilepsy and highlighted the dearth of research into this domain. Limited attention has been paid by researchers to this aspect of living with epilepsy, so that the literature remains sparse and contradictory. In a cross-sectional survey conducted in Mexico to assess the QOL of 401 people with epilepsy, Alanis-Guevara et al. [34] found the variable most strongly associated with a lower QOL was the presence of sleep disorder. However, as the researchers themselves point out, one major methodological flaw of this study is biased sampling: people with epilepsy were recruited consecutively from a neurology and neurosurgery referral centre and the results cannot be applied generally to people with epilepsy. A number of studies [31,35,36] highlight sleep disruptions as particularly common in patients experiencing partial seizures and find they may be inherent to the condition itself. For example, in one study sleep disturbance was found to be more than twice as prevalent in persons with partial epilepsy as in controls, with most domains of sleep significantly disturbed [35]. Xu et al. [36] concluded that diagnosed and self-reported sleep disturbances in patients with partial-onset epilepsy were frequently overlooked but were negatively associated with everyday functioning and well-being, and as such contributed significantly to the burden of epilepsy. Malow et al. [37] demonstrated that people with epilepsy had increased daytime drowsiness compared with neurology patients without epilepsy (controls). However, epilepsy was not a predictor of more daytime sleepiness when a sleep apnea scale was included. The researchers suggested that the potentially treatable condition of sleep apnea might be responsible for much of the problem in people with epilepsy.

While a more recent study [38] found excessive daytime sleepiness (EDS) and obstructive sleep apnea (OSA) to be more frequent in people with epilepsy than in the general population, the authors found no correlation between EDS and demographic or clinical variables. Furthermore, OSA was shown not to predict EDS. A recent cross-sectional study conducted with a Chinese cohort of 247 adult patients with epilepsy [39] reported findings similar to previous studies:

subjective symptoms of anxiety, depression, and sleep disturbance were independently predictive of lower QOL scores. However, in addition to examining these effects independently, this study sought to quantify the interrelationships between these symptoms and clinical variables, constructing a model to predict QOL scores. The researchers noted that the occurrence of a seizure in the previous 4 weeks and the number of AEDs contributed to the level of depression, whereas symptoms of anxiety and sleep disturbance were mutually dependent. In addition, the degree of anxiety experienced was further influenced by the number of AEDs. The authors argued that the presence of such dynamic interrelationships indicated that these factors should be assessed simultaneously and not in isolation when evaluating the effects of treatment on QOL.

The role of sleep disorder for impaired QOL in people with epilepsy is highlighted by patients themselves, as are their concerns over the possibility that AED treatment may create or exacerbate problems with sleep [40]. Such concerns appear justified by a small but convincing literature identifying the quite different effects AEDs can have on sleep quality [29,30].

In summary, the impact of epilepsy on everyday life cannot solely be explained by clinical factors (Figure 14.1) and particularly not by seizure frequency [11]. Studies of the psychosocial effects of epilepsy highlight how anxiety and sleep disorders are prevalent in individuals with epilepsy, even though their relationship with epilepsy is not yet fully understood. It would appear that levels of psychological comorbidity may need to be considered when establishing epilepsy treatment regimes [41] and that subjective symptoms of anxiety and sleep disorder, as well as epilepsy variables, require simultaneous consideration when evaluating effects of treatment on QOL [39].

Investigating the prevalence and nature of psychological distress in people with epilepsy

In order to address some of the issues highlighted so far in this chapter, we conducted an international comparative study to investigate the nature and extent of anxiety and sleep disorder in people with epilepsy. Data were collected from cohorts of people with epilepsy from four European countries, with eligible participants identified through epilepsy support groups in the United Kingdom (Epilepsy Action), Germany (Deutsche Epilepsievereinigung), the Netherlands (Deutsche Epilepsie Vereimigung eV), and France (d'Epilepsie-France). We aimed to sample 1000 participants per country (4000 in total). In the United Kingdom only, we also asked each person with epilepsy to identify a person without epilepsy to complete a control questionnaire.

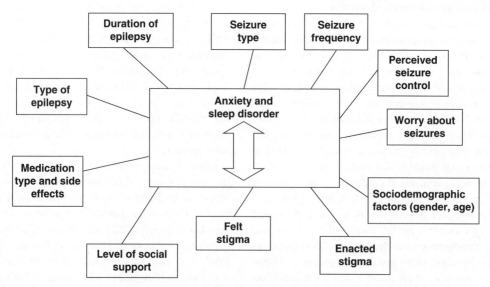

Figure 14.1 Range of potential factors influencing anxiety and sleep disorders.

Data collection was facilitated by the use of two postal self-completion questionnaire booklets (one for people with epilepsy and one for people without) using previously validated scales (see Table 14.1), which included instructions for completion. The figure of 1000 people with epilepsy approached per site assumed a nonresponse rate of 40–50%, based on our previous experience of conducting similar studies using support groups as the sampling frame.

Responders to the study completed the State-Trait Anxiety Inventory (STAI) [42], the Pittsburgh Sleep Quality Index (PSQI) [28], and the Epworth Sleepiness Scale (ESS) [43]. They also completed measures of perceived AED side effects, impact of epilepsy, stigma, social support, and seizure-specific worry (Table 14.1).

The total sample comprised 1645 people with epilepsy and 258 controls. The numbers of people with epilepsy who returned questionnaires per country were: United Kingdom, 751; Germany, 268; Netherlands, 431; France, 195. All questionnaires were reviewed to ensure that inclusion criteria were met and to check for completeness. They were then cleaned and coded prior to analysis.

Participant characteristics

We compared clinical and sociodemographic characteristics across our four samples (Table 14.2). Comparing the four groups for sociodemographic characteristics, the French cohort had slightly younger participants, with a median age of 34 years. A higher proportion of the sample across all four groups was female. Median age at time of first seizure was lowest in the French sample (10.5 years). Participants in the Netherlands were most likely to report being seizure-free: over 50% of this group reported having no seizures during the previous month and over 40% reported seizure freedom during the previous 12 months. Over 90% of all participants were currently taking one or more AED for seizure control. Over half of the participants in the UK (65.1%), German (68.9%), and Dutch (51.5%) samples reported other long-term health problems, compared to only one-third of participants in the French group (Table 14.2).

Prevalence of anxiety and sleep disorder

There were statistically significant differences between the cohorts in median scores for both "state" and "trait" anxiety (Table 14.3). Prevalence of both state

and trait anxiety was higher in the United Kingdom and the Netherlands than in Germany and France. Median scores for night-time sleep quality (PSQI) were highest for the German sample (p < 0.001). Prevalence of night-time sleep problems was 79% for the UK sample and 97, 99, and 95% for the German, Dutch, and French samples, respectively. Prevalence of daytime sleep problems was 40.9% for the UK sample, 25.9% for the German sample, 23.5% for the Dutch sample, and 68.2% for the French sample. The percentage of people reporting their general health as "excellent" or "very good" was 24% of UK respondents, 13.8% of French respondents, 13.3% of German respondents, and 25.2% of Dutch respondents; and 28.5, 26.7, 25.7, and 17.0%, respectively, considered their health now to be worse than it was a year ago. Median AEP scores were lowest for the German sample, although the between-country differences were small. Overall QOL was rated highest by people living in the Netherlands, with 73.9% describing themselves as happy with their QOL (Table 14.3).

Factors contributing to anxiety and sleep disorder

The European data set presents a somewhat complicated picture. People with epilepsy living in the Netherlands appeared at greatest risk of state anxiety, people in France at least risk; in contrast, trait anxiety (median) scores were highest for people in the United Kingdom and lowest for those in Germany. Risk of night-time sleep problems appeared little different across the four countries but daytime sleepiness was a more common problem in France than elsewhere.

When factors contributing to scores for anxiety and sleep disorder were examined in univariate analyses, some patterning in the data emerged. For state anxiety, factors consistently (in at least three of the four countries) significantly associated across the countries were: having fair or poor general health, having worse health compared to a year ago, having other long-term health problems, and having higher total scores for the AEP. For trait anxiety, consistently important factors were: current general health, health compared to a year ago, experiencing four or more seizures in the previous year, worry about past and possible future seizures, AEP total score, levels of social support and felt stigma, marital and employment status, and night- and daytime sleep problems. For problems with daytime

Table 14.1 Previously validated scales included in the People with Epilepsy Questionnaire Booklet.

Variable	Measure	Description
Anxiety	State-Trait Anxiety Inventory (STAI) [42]	Self-administered 40-item measure (20 items relating to "state" anxiety, 20 relating to "trait" anxiety). Uses a four-point scale ("not at all" to "very much so"; "almost never" to "almost always") to examine intensity of anxiety symptoms. Total scores for both state and trait anxiety range from 20 to 80, with a higher score being indicative of a more severe problem
Sleep	Pittsburgh Sleep Quality Index (PSQI) [28]	A 19-item self-rated questionnaire, assessing sleep quality and disturbances over a 1-month period. Patients' responses generate seven "component" scores for subjective sleep quality, sleep latency, sleep duration, sleep efficiency, sleep disturbances, use of medication, and daytime dysfunction, as well as a global score. Total score ranges from 0 to 21, with a higher score being more indicative of a problem
Sleep	Epworth Sleepiness Scale (ESS) [43]	Self-rated questionnaire measuring excessive daytime sleepiness. Uses a four-point scale (0 = no chance of dozing, 1 = slight chance of dozing, 2 = moderate chance of dozing, 3 = high chance of dozing) to examine the intensity of dozing in eight situations. Subscores are added together to provide a total score ranging from 0 to 24, with a score of 10 or over being an indication that specialist help is required
AED side effects	Liverpool Adverse Events Profile (AEP) [44]	Used to report medication-related side effects. This short, self-completed questionnaire lists 19 symptoms known to be associated with AEDs, along with categories relating to how often these symptoms are experienced. Respondents circle the category they feel to be the most representative of their experience of the listed symptoms in the last month, the options ranging from "never a problem" to "always or often a problem." The profile has been shown to detect significant differences in types of side effect reported, depending on the individual's drug therapy [3]
Perceived impact of epilepsy	Impact of Epilepsy Scale [48]	Used to assess perceived impact of epilepsy. Consists of 12 items covering relationship with spouse/partner, relationship with other close family members, social life/social activities, health, work (two items: whether able to work and, if yes, what kind of work), standard of living, relationship with friends, feelings about self, plans/ambitions, driving, and independence. The range for this instrument is 12–60, with higher scores indicating that epilepsy has had a worsening effect
Perceived stigma of epilepsy	Epilepsy-specific Perceived Impact Scale [49]	For each of the items, persons with epilepsy are asked to answer yes or no; an individual's score is the sum of their positive responses. Informants will also be asked about single items relating to experiences of possible epilepsy-related enacted stigma and discrimination. The total score ranges from 0 to 3 (0 indicating no stigma, 3 severe stigma)
Level of social support	Social Support Measure [50]	Assessed using a 19-item measure exploring perceptions of support across four different domains: emotional/informational, tangible, affectionate, and positive social interaction. Respondents answer on a five-point scale from "none of the time" to "all of the time." Data can be analyzed using domain scores or an overall social support index score
Seizure worry	Seizure Worry Scale [51]	A two-item scale asking about worry about past/possible future seizures
Clinical and sociodemographic characteristics	Single items relating to age, gender, attained educational level, and occupational status	Participants are asked to classify their seizures as only tonic–clonic, only other types, or both tonic–clonic and other types. They are also asked to estimate their monthly seizure frequency and their perceptions of the degree of seizure control and to provide information about epilepsy duration and drug type. Finally, they are asked whether they have any chronic illnesses other than epilepsy, whether they are taking any prescribed medication other than AEDS, and how they would describe their health status overall and compared to a year previously (all single items)

Table 14.2 Sample characteristics.

		United Kingdom (Epilepsy Action, n = 751)	Germany (Deutsche Epilepsie Vereinigung, n = 268)	Netherlands (Epilepsie Vereimigung eV, n = 431)	France (d'Epilepsie-France, n = 195)	P value
Gender	Male	283 (38.1%)	109 (41.3%)	204 (47.2%)	92 (47.4)	0.008[a]
	Female	460 (61.9%)	155 (58.7%)	228 (52.8%)	102 (52.6%)	
Age	Median (IQR)	45 (17–92)	47 (11–80)	51 (11–89)	34 (2–77)	
Marital status	Married/partner	400 (53.6%)	133 (51.2%)	298 (69%)	96 (50%)	<0.001[a]
	Divorced/separated	82 (11.0%)	17 (6.5%)	28 (6.5%)	11 (5.7%)	
	Widowed	29 (3.9%)	7 (2.7%)	12 (2.8%)	1 (0.5%)	
	Single	228 (30.6%)	103 (39.6%)	94 (21.8%)	84 (43.8)	
Employment	Paid work (FT/PT)	270 (36.9%)	98 (37.8%)	186 (45.5%)	88 (47.0%)	<0.001[a]
	Unemployed	60 (8.2%)	12 (4.7%)	16 (3.9%)	26 (13.9%)	
	Other	401 (54.9%)	149 (57.5%)	204 (49.8%)	73 (39.0%)	
Other long-term health problems	Yes	488 (65.1%)	182 (68.9%)	220 (51.5%)	71 (36.6%)	<0.001[a]
	No	256 (34.1%)	82 (31.1%)	207 (48.5%)	123 (63.4%)	
Other prescribed medication	No	260 (35.2%)	104 (39.7%)	218 (51.2%)	108 (55.7%)	<0.001[a]
	Yes (one)	177 (24.0%)	75 (28.6%)	97 (22.8%)	52 (26.8)	
	Yes (two to three)	191 (25.8%)	63 (24.0%)	68 (16.0%)	20 (10.3%)	
	Yes (four or more)	111 (15.0%)	20 (7.6%)	43 (10.1%)	14 (7.2%)	
Seizures in past year	None	191 (26.6%)	76 (28.7%)	178 (41.6%)	41 (21.4)	<0.001[a]
	One to three	102 (14.2%)	54 (20.3%)	73 (17.1%)	46 (23.9%)	
	Four or more	426 (59.2%)	135 (50.9%)	177 (41.4%)	105 (54.7%)	
Age at first seizure	Median (IQR)	19 (1–80)	14 (1–71)	20 (1–80)	10.5 (1–62)	<0.001[b]
Age at most recent seizure	Median (IQR)	44 (6–89)	45 (10–80)	45 (1–84)	32 (13–63)	<0.001[b]
Average number of seizures per month	None	272 (36.2%)	112 (44.4%)	231 (55.1%)	72 (38.3%)	<0.001[a]
	One to three	219 (29.2%)	75 (29.8%)	109 (20.0%)	61 (32.4%)	
	Four to five	79 (10.5%)	23 (9.1%)	33 (7.9%)	19 (10.1%)	
	Six or mroe	145 (19.3%)	42 (16.7%)	46 (11.0%)	36 (19.1%)	
Types of seizure	Major	163 (21.7%)	77 (29.6%)	126 (32.3%)	27 (15.1%)	<0.001[a]
	Both	316 (42.1%)	126 (48.5%)	142 (36.4%)	109 (60.9%)	
	Other	228 (30.4%)	57 (21.0%)	122 (31.3%)	43 (24%)	
Drugs for seizure control	Yes	695 (92.5%)	257 (96.6%)	413 (96.3%)	188 (96.4%)	<0.001[a]
	No	32 (4.3%)	9 (3.4%)	16 (3.7%)	7 (3.6%)	
Number of drugs	One	339 (50.7%)	94 (36.7%)	181 (44.5%)	60 (35.9%)	<0.001[a]
	Two	234 (35.0%)	102 (39.8%)	150 (36.9%)	58 (31.5%)	
	Three	80 (12.0%)	50 (19.5%)	59 (14.5%)	44 (23.9%)	
	Four or five	15 (2.2%)	10 (3.9%)	17 (4.2%)	16 (8.7%)	

(continued overleaf)

Table 14.2 (*continued*)

		United Kingdom (Epilepsy Action, n = 751)	Germany (German Epilepsy Union, n = 268)	Netherlands (Deutsche Epilepsie Vereimigung eV, n = 431)	France (d'Epilepsie-France, n = 195)	P value
Seizure control	Very well	249 (34.7%)	83 (32.2%)	186 (44.1%)	53 (27.5%)	<0.001[a]
	Fairly well	279 (38.9%)	124 (48.1%)	146 (34.6%)	81 (42%)	
	Not very well	125 (17.4%)	36 (14.0%)	56 (13.3%)	48 (24.9%)	
	Not at all well	64 (8.9%)	15 (5.8%)	34 (8.1%)	11 (5.7%)	
Worry about past seizures	Fairly/very	391 (54.2%)	123 (46.9%)	126 (29.3%)	132 (68.1%)	<0.001[a]
	A little/not at all	330 (45.8%)	139 (53%)	303 (70.6%)	62 (31.9%)	
Worry about having another seizure	Fairly/very	393 (54.4%)	134 (43.5%)	117 (27.2%)	120 (62.2%)	<0.001[a]
	A little/not at all	329 (45.6%)	148 (56.5%)	313 (73.1%)	73 (37.9%)	

[a]Chi-squared test; [b]Kruskal–Wallis.

Table 14.3 Median scores for and prevalence of anxiety and sleep disorder.

		United Kingdom (Epilepsy Action, n = 751)	Germany (German Epilepsy Union, n = 268)	Netherlands (Deutsche Epilepsie Vereimigung eV, n = 431)	France (d'Epilepsie-France, n = 195)	P value
State A total	Median (IQR)	46 (20)	39 (14)	48 (3)	36 (17)	0.001[b]
Trait A total	Median (IQR)	50 (19)	37 (20)	48 (3)	47 (17)	<0.001[b]
PSQI total	Median (IQR)	9 (6)	11 (5)	9 (6)	10 (5)	<0.001[b]
Epworth total	Normal	441 (59.1%)	197 (74.1%)	329 (76.5%)	62 (31.8%)	<0.001[a]
	Special advice	305 (40.9%)	69 (25.9%)	101 (23.5%)	123 (68.2%)	
Health	Excellent/very good	183 (24.5%)	35 (13.2%)	108 (25.2%)	27 (13.8%)	<0.001[a]
	Good	273 (36.5%)	118 (44.4%)	185 (43.1%)	106 (54.4%)	
	Fair/poor	291 (39.0%)	113 (42.4%)	136 (31.7%)	62 (31.8%)	
Health compared to 1 year ago	Better	185 (24.8%)	78 (29.5%)	125 (29.2%)	62 (43.8%)	0.002[a]
	Same	349 (46.7%)	119 (44.9%)	230 (53.7%)	81 (41.5%)	
	Worse	213 (28.5%)	68 (25.7%)	73 (17.0%)	52 (26.7%)	
AEP total	Median (IQR)	47.5 (13)	44 (14)	48 (4)	45 (18)	<0.001[b]
Overall QOL	Happy	375 (50.3%)	155 (58.7%)	317 (73.9%)	93 (50.3%)	<0.001[a]
	Neutral	128 (17.2%)	54 (20.4%)	62 (14.5%)	36 (19.5%)	
	Unhappy	242 (32.5%)	55 (20.8%)	50 (11.7%)	56 (30.3%)	

[a]Chi-squared test; [b]Kruskal–Wallis.

sleepiness, important factors were: general health, health compared to a year ago, worry about future seizures, AEP total score, felt stigma, and night-time sleep problems. For problems with night-time sleep quality, important factors were general health, other long-term health problems, perceived seizure control, AEP total score, trait anxiety, and daytime sleepiness. For all four outcomes of interest – state and trait anxiety and day and night sleep problems – and across all four country data sets, clinical factors (seizure frequency and type, age of onset of epilepsy, and duration) were unimportant.

Factors contributing to overall QOL

People living in the Netherlands rated their QOL highest overall, with 73.9% reporting they were happy with their overall QOL. In contrast, only around 50% of people with epilepsy in France, Germany, and the UK rated their QOL thus. We used multivariate analysis to examine the role of anxiety and sleep disorders alongside other potentially important factors for overall QOL (Table 14.4). In the UK sample, predictive factors accounted for 52% of variance in overall QOL scores. Key factors related to anxiety were worry about past seizures and level of general health. AEP score was a key factor for both day and night sleep problems. Both anxiety and sleep were found to contribute to overall QOL. In the German sample, our models accounted for 50% of the variance in overall QOL. The only common factor for predicting state and trait anxiety was AEP score, which also predicted day- and night-time sleep problems. Trait anxiety and general health were found to contribute to overall QOL. In the Dutch sample, we were able to account for 51% of the variance in overall QOL. As in the German sample, AEP score was the only factor common to prediction of state and trait anxiety and was also important for night-time sleep. Clinical-demographic factors – age and seizure frequency – emerged as important for overall QOL in the Dutch sample, as did trait anxiety and level of social support. Finally, in the French sample, we were able to account for 48% of the variance in overall QOL. AEP score was a key factor for both state and trait anxiety and day- and night-time sleep problems. AEP score also contributed to overall QOL, alongside trait anxiety and general health.

Collectively, 10 variables were identified as predictive factors for QOL across the four European samples. For

Table 14.4 Summary comparison between European country samples of most important predictive factors (multivariate analysis) for overall QOL.

Predictive variable	United Kingdom	Germany	Netherlands	France
AEP total score				√
Night-time sleep problems	√			
Level of social support	√		√	
Stigma	√			
Worry about possible future seizures	√			
Number of seizures in past year	√		√	
Trait anxiety score	√	√	√	√
Level of treatment compliance		√		
General health		√		√
Age			√	

UK sample: 6 variables account for 52% of variance in overall QOL; German sample: 3 variables account for 50% of variance in overall QOL; Dutch sample: 4 variables account for 51% of variance in overall QOL; French sample: 3 variables account for 48% of variance in overall QOL.

each of the country samples, these variables accounted for half of the variance in overall QOL. Trait anxiety score was identified as the only common predictive factor across all four countries. No other factor emerged as important in more than two countries and the pattern was not consistent. Surprisingly, in light of previous published research indicating its importance [44], France was the only country where AEP score emerged as important for predicting QOL overall.

What does this study add to the current picture?

The data presented here add to our understanding of the nature of anxiety in people with epilepsy and the factors predictive of its two separate dimensions. Speilberger [42] defines trait anxiety as referring to "relatively stable individual differences in anxiety-proneness" and "the tendency to perceive stressful situations as dangerous or threatening." Trait anxiety may also reflect individual differences in the frequency with which anxiety states have been manifested in the past and may be manifested in the future. The stronger the anxiety trait, the more probable that an individual will experience more intense elevations of state anxiety in the face of a threatening situation, such as that presented to a person with epilepsy when experiencing a seizure. High trait anxiety scores are associated with a larger number of self-reported problems in almost every area of life adjustment, with those who are anxiety-prone reporting problems in many areas of daily function, including health, social and intimate relationships, educational and work adjustment, and future planning [42] – a finding with important practical implications in relation to clinical management of people with epilepsy.

Betts [18] notes that experiencing high levels of anxiety for prolonged periods of time can inadvertently make an individual more vulnerable to having a seizure, which may result in a self-perpetuating process of increasing anxiety and higher frequency of seizures. While stress and its association to seizures requires further investigation [45], tackling anxiety about seizures is still important in bolstering the well-being of a person with epilepsy.

Our study confirms an increased prevalence of anxiety in people with epilepsy compared to matched controls. The research demonstrates both trait and state anxiety to be more prevalent in people with epilepsy and identifies contributory factors which include, for state anxiety, worse general health, worse health now than previously, and worry about past seizures; and for trait anxiety, age, seizure worry, and AED side effects. Our study compares and contrasts the prevalence of anxiety across four countries and finds anxiety to be more commonly reported in the United Kingdom and the Netherlands than in Germany and France.

Sleep disturbance creates huge demand for health care services and huge use of over-the-counter medication [46]. Importantly, sleep disorders may also be indicators of major anxiety and depression [47]. Our study indicates that night-time sleep problems are very common even in normal populations but are further elevated in populations with epilepsy. Four-fifths of people with epilepsy report night-time sleep difficulties, and two-fifths report daytime sleepiness. This compares

to only a fifth of the nonepileptic population. Bazil [30] argues that the identified sleep disorders that are common in people with epilepsy are frequently missed by clinicians.

Treatment "success" in epilepsy must include successful management, from the patient's perspective, of comorbidities including anxiety and sleep disorders [24]. The need for increased awareness and screening for such comorbidities by clinicians is essential and questions regarding anxiety management and sleep hygiene should be routinely addressed during clinic consultations. Our study indicates that AEP score is an important contributory factor for sleep problems. The AEP offers an easily administered instrument with the potential to serve as a valuable assessment tool for the presence of sleep disorder in people with epilepsy, enabling AED effects to be systematically addressed and sleep problems appropriately medicated.

Not only do people with epilepsy experience increased rates of anxiety and sleep disorder but they are also more likely to report poor general health and worse health than a year ago than are controls without epilepsy. It is therefore unsurprising that people with epilepsy report poorer QOL overall. Only one-half of people with epilepsy in the UK describe themselves as happy with their QOL, compared to three-quarters of controls. There are also significant between-country differences for QOL. Our finding that people with epilepsy in the Netherlands are the most likely to describe themselves as happy with their QOL supports our previous research in Europe [3]: in that earlier work, people with epilepsy in the Netherlands also reported highest QOL. Trait, but not state, anxiety emerged as a significant contributor to overall QOL of people with epilepsy: sleep quality, though significantly related to anxiety disorder, was not consistently independently associated or predictive of overall QOL.

Conclusion

The study described here goes some way toward identifying the nature and prevalence of anxiety and sleep disorders. Both have clinical management implications, of which clinicians may not always be cognizant. Clinicians treating people with epilepsy need to be vigilant of these two important comorbidities, which clearly influence the day-to-day lives of those concerned.

Acknowledgements

We wish to acknowledge our gratitude to the people with epilepsy and their acquaintances who took the time to participate in this study and to share their experiences with us.

We also wish to thank the epilepsy support organizations located in each of our four European research sites – Epilepsy Action (United Kingdom), Deutsche Epilepsievereinigung (Germany), Epilepsie Vereniging Nederland (the Netherlands), and d'Epilepsie-France (France) – for facilitating participant recruitment and data collection. Without their enthusiasm and dedication to working on behalf of people with epilepsy and their families, this study would not have been possible. Thanks are also due to Barbara Eaton, who cleaned and coded the data, and to Steven Lane, who analyzed it.

Our thanks are also extended to Pfizer Global Pharmaceutical Company for their commitment to user-oriented research and for funding this study.

References

1 Jacoby A: Epilepsy and the quality of everyday life, findings from a study of people with well controlled epilepsy. *Soc Sci Med* 1992; **34**:657–666.
2 Leidy NK, Elixhauser A, Vickrey E et al.: Seizure frequency and the health related quality of life of adults with epilepsy. *Neurology* 1999; **53**:162–166.
3 Baker GA, Jacoby A, Buck D et al.: Quality of life of people with epilepsy: a European study. *Epilepsia* 1997; **38**:353–362.
4 Baker GA, Camfield C, Camfield P et al.: Commission on outcome measurement in epilepsy, 1994–1997; final report. *Epilepsia* 1998; **39**:213–231.
5 Jacoby A, Baker GA, Steen N et al.: The clinical course of epilepsy and its psychosocial correlates: findings from a UK community study. *Epilepsia* 1996; **37**:148–161.
6 Goldstein MA, Harden CL, Ravdin LD et al.: Does anxiety in epilepsy patients decrease with increasing seizure frequency? *Epilepsia* 1999; **40(S7)**:S60–S61.
7 Goldstein MA, Harden CL: Epilepsy and anxiety (review). *Epilepsy Behav* 2000; **1**:228–234.
8 Smith DF, Baker GA, Dewey M: Seizure frequency, patient perceived seizure severity and the psychosocial consequences of intractable epilepsy. *Epilepsy Res* 1991; **9**:231–241.
9 Piazzini A, Canevini MP, Maggiori G: Depression and anxiety in patients with epilepsy. *Epilepsy Behav* 2001; **2**:481–489.

10 Cramer JA, Brandenburg N, Xu X: Differentiating anxiety and depression symptoms in patients with partial epilepsy. *Epilepsy Behav* 2005; **6**:563–569.
11 Baker GA, Jacoby A, Chadwick DW: The associations of psychopathology in epilepsy: a community study. *Epilepsy Res* 1996; **25**:29–39.
12 Fiordelli E, Beghi E, Bogliun G: Epilepsy and psychiatric disturbance, a cross-sectional study. *Br J Psychiatry* 1993; **163**:446–450.
13 Gaitatzis A, Carroll K, Majeed A: The epidemiology of the comorbidity of epilepsy in the general population. *Epilepsia* 2004; **45**:1613–1622.
14 Janca A, Ustun TB, Early TS, Sartorius N: The ICD-10 Symptom Checklist: a companion to the ICD-10 Classification of Mental and Behavioural Disorders. *Social Psychiatry Psychiatr Epidemiol* 1993; **28**:239–242.
15 Beyenberg S, Mitchell AJ, Schmidt D et al.: Anxiety in patients with epilepsy: systematic review and suggestions for clinical management. *Epilepsy Behav* 2005; **7**:161–171.
16 Torta R, Keller R: Behavioural, psychotic, and anxiety disorders in epilepsy: etiology, clinical features and therapeutic implications. *Epilepsia* 1999; **40(Suppl. 10)**:S2–S20.
17 Marsh L, Rao V: Psychiatric complications in patients with epilepsy: a review. *Epilepsy Res* 2002; **49**:11–33.
18 Betts TA: Neuropsychiatry. In: Laidlaw J, Richens A, Chadwick D (eds): *A Textbook of Epilepsy*, 4 edn. Churchill Livingstone, Edinburgh, 1993, pp. 397–457.
19 Newsom-Davis I, Goldstein LH, Fitzpatrick D: Fear of seizures: an investigation and treatment. *Seizure* 1998; **7**:101–106.
20 De Souza EAP, Salgado PCB. A psychosocial view of anxiety and depression in epilepsy. *Epilepsy Behav* 2006; **8**:232–238.
21 Hermann BP, Trenerry MR, Colligan RC et al.: Learned helplessness, attributional style, and depression in epilepsy. *Epilepsia* 1996; **37**:680–686.
22 Amir M, Roziner I, Knoll A et al.: Self-efficacy and social support as mediators in the relation between disease severity and quality of life in patients with epilepsy. *Epilepsia* 1999; **40**:216–224.
23 Fisher RS, Vickrey BG, Gibson P et al.: The impact of epilepsy from the patient's perspective. II: Views about therapy and health care. *Epilepsy Research* 2000; **41**:53–61.
24 Sander JW: Ultimate success in epilepsy – the patient's perspective. *Eur J Neurol* 2005; **12(Suppl. 4)**:3–11.
25 Schmitz B: Effects of antiepileptic drugs on mood and behavior. *Epilepsia* 2006; **47(Suppl. 2)**:S28–S33.
26 Boylan LS, Devinsky O, Barry JJ, Ketter TA: Psychiatric uses of antiepileptic treatments. *Epilepsy Behav* 2002; **3(Suppl. 5)**:54–59.
27 Ketter TA, Post RM, Theodore WH. Positive and negative psychiatric effects of antiepileptic drugs in patients with seizure disorders. *Neurology* 1999; **53(5 Suppl. 2)**:S53–S67.
28 Buysse DJ, Reynolds CF, Monk TH et al.: The Pittsburgh Sleep Quality Index: a new instrument for psychiatric practice and research. *Psychiatry Res* 1989; **28**:193–213.

29 Méndez M, Radtke RA: Interactions between sleep and epilepsy. *J Clin Neurophysiol* 2001; **18**:106–127.

30 Bazil CW: Epilepsy and sleep disturbance. *Epilepsy Behav* 2003; **4(Suppl. 2)**:S39–S45.

31 De Haas S, de Weerd A, Otte A: Epidemiology of sleep disturbance in patients with partial seizures. Paper presented at: 5th European Congress on Epileptology (ECE), October 6–10, 2002, Madrid, Spain.

32 Moran NF, Poole K, Bell G et al.: Epilepsy in the UK: seizure frequency and severity, antiepileptic drug utilisation and impact on life in 1652 people with epilepsy. *Seizure* 2004; **13**:425–433.

33 Hermann BP: Quality of life in epilepsy. *J Epilepsy* 1992; **5**:153–165.

34 Alanis-Guevara I, Pena E, Corona T et al.: Sleep disturbances, socioeconomic status, and seizure control as main predictors of quality of life in epilepsy. *Epilepsy Behav* 2005; **7**:481–485.

35 De Weerd A, de Haas S, Otte A et al.: Subjective sleep disturbance in patients with partial epilepsy: a questionnaire-based study on prevalence and impact on quality of life. *Epilepsia* 2004; **45**:1397–2004.

36 Xu X, Brandenburg NA, McDermott AM, Bazil CW: Sleep disturbances reported by refractory partial-onset epilepsy patients receiving polytherapy. *Epilepsia* 2006; **47**: 1176–1183.

37 Malow BA, Bowes RJ, Lin X: Predictors of sleepiness in epilepsy patients. *Sleep* 1997; **20**:1105–1110.

38 Piperidou C, Karlovasitou A, Triantafyllou N: Influence of sleep disturbance on quality of life of patients with epilepsy. *Seizure* 2008; **17**:588–594.

39 Kwan P, Yu E, Leung H: Association of subjective anxiety, depression, and sleep disturbance with quality of life rating in adults with epilepsy. *Epilepsia* 2008; **50**:1059–1066.

40 Fisher RS, Vickrey BG, Gibson P: The impact of epilepsy from the patient's perspective. I: Descriptions and subjective perceptions. *Epilepsy Res* 2000; **41**:39–51.

41 Johnson EK, Jones JE, Seidenberg M et al.: The relative impact of anxiety, depression and clinical seizure features on health related quality of life in epilepsy. *Epilepsia* 2004; **45**:544–550.

42 Speilberger CD, Gorsuch RL, Luschene RE et al.: *Manual for the State-Trait Anxiety Inventory*. Consulting Psychologists Press, Palo Alto, CA, 1983.

43 Johns MW: A new method for measuring daytime sleepiness: the Epworth Sleepiness Scale. *Sleep* 1991; **14**:540–545.

44 Gilliam F, Fessler AJ, Baker G et al.: Systematic screening allows reduction of adverse antiepileptic drug effects: a randomized study. *Neurology* 2004; **62**:6–7.

45 Betts TA. Epilepsy and stress: time for proper studies of the association. *BMJ* 1992; **305**:378–379.

46 Jenkins CD, Stanton BA, Niemcryk SJ et al.: A scale for measuring effects of treatment on sleep problems. *J Clin Epidemiol* 1988; **41**:313–321.

47 Hermann BP, Seidenberg M, Bell B: Psychiatric comorbidity in chronic epilepsy: identification, consequences and treatment of major depression. *Epilepsia* 2000; **41(Suppl. 2)**: S31–S41.

48 Jacoby A, Baker GA, Smith D et al.: Measuring the impact of epilepsy: the development of a novel scale. *Epilepsy Res* 1993; **16**:83–88.

49 Jacoby A: Felt versus enacted stigma: a concept revisited. Evidence from a study of people with epilepsy in remission. *Soc Sci Med* 1994; **38(2)**:269–274.

50 Sherbourne CD, Stewart AL: The MOS Social Support Survey. *Soc Sci Med* 1991; **32(6)**:705–714.

51 Abetz L, Jacoby A, Baker GA et al.: Patient-based assessment of quality of life in newly diagnosed epilepsy patients: validation of the NEWQOL. *Epilepsia* 2000; **41**:1119–1128.

CHAPTER 15

Epilepsy and personality

Christopher Turnbull, Simon Jones, Sophia J. Adams, and Dennis Velakoulis

Melbourne Neuropsychiatry Centre, University of Melbourne and Neuropsychiatry Unit, Royal Melbourne Hospital, Australia

Introduction

The question of whether people with epilepsy have a different "character" or personality to people without epilepsy has a long history. The concept had its foundations in the ancient belief that people with epilepsy had been possessed by a god or spirit. Associations between epilepsy and religion persisted through the Middle Ages and into the 19th century [1,2]. Psychiatrists working in 19th-century institutional settings observed that patients with epilepsy had chronic changes in the form of personality differences and mental retardation [3]. An environment of stigma and ignorance around the many possible causes of behavioral changes contributed to an attitude that people with epilepsy were somehow different or "inferior" [4].

By the early 20th century, more sophisticated views had emerged. In 1907, Turner wrote, "In earlier days the convulsion or fit was regarded as the sole element of importance in the clinical study of epilepsy, but in more recent years the psychical factor has come to be looked upon as of almost equal importance" [5]. In the 1940s, Lennox considered the potential effects of medications, psychological stress, and social attitudes on people with epilepsy [6]. The idea that people with epilepsy differed because of intellectual impairment or "defective functioning" was replaced by greater consideration of the direct impact of seizures and of broader psychosocial factors [7].

Although much was written about people with epilepsy being different, the concept of "difference" was poorly defined. It was not clear whether it related to fundamental personality difference (traits versus disorder), associated psychopathology, brain injury, or intellectual impairment. Furthermore, most observations were based on institutionalized epilepsy patients and there was limited consideration of different epilepsy types [2]. The discovery in the 1940s that some epilepsy had a temporal focus and that this limbic brain region was important in emotional regulation heralded a new era of research [1].

Early studies into associations between temporal-lobe epilepsy (TLE) and personality change relied on case reports, case series, diagnoses by clinical interview, unstructured questionnaires, and projective tests such as the Rorschach test. Such studies reported personality differences in approximately half of patients with TLE. By modern standards, these early, descriptive studies were limited in several ways. There was considerable variation in the nature of personality disturbance described, little consistency in methodology, and limited consideration of psychopathology. TLE was poorly defined (often without EEG) or considered to be synonymous to epilepsy with "psychomotor seizures," a group now known to include extratemporal seizures [8]. Finally, these studies did not include control groups [9,10]. These and other biases of early studies have been outlined in detail elsewhere [11].

The last 5 decades have seen a steady improvement in the understanding of and ability to characterize epilepsy syndromes. Personality research has developed in parallel to this and the idea of epilepsy-specific personality patterns has received increasing attention. One avenue of research has focused on dimensional personality trait assessment using self-report measures, in an attempt to identify a particular combination of personality features associated with a specific epilepsy syndrome. The two most common approaches have

Epilepsy and the Interictal State: Co-Morbidities and Quality of Life, First Edition.
Edited by Erik K. St. Louis, David M. Ficker, and Terence J. O'Brien.
© 2015 John Wiley & Sons, Ltd. Published 2015 by John Wiley & Sons, Ltd.

been the Minnesota Multiphasic Personality Inventory (MMPI) [12] and Five Factor model instruments, including the Neuroticism-Extroversion-Openness Five Factor Inventory (NEO-FFI) or Personality Inventory (NEO-PI), which measure the five personality traits of neuroticism, extroversion, openness, agreeableness, and conscientiousness [13]. Another avenue of research has investigated associations between epilepsy syndromes and personality disorders, as defined by categorical DSM or ICD frameworks. Finally, a growing body of research has assessed the relationship between epilepsy and personality-associated measures such as attributional style, generally identifying that an optimistic attributional style [14] or problem-solving coping style [15,16] has a lower level of distress, although this is not a consistent finding [17]. This is an evolving area of research that will be addressed with reference to quality of life (QOL), but the remainder of this chapter will focus on the first two, more traditional aspects of personality assessment.

Personality assessment in epilepsy

Epilepsy is a disorder characterized by unpredictable symptoms, variable degrees of comorbid neurological dysfunction, significant stigma [18], and lifelong and at times complicated medication regimes. In assessing personality in epilepsy, it is important to bear in mind that people with epilepsy also have higher rates of depression and other psychiatric disorders [19–21]. Assessment of personality in this context is complex, as personality disorder and personality trait assessment have been shown in some [22–25] (but not all [26,27]) studies to be affected by the presence of depression and to be modified by treatment of depression. In particular, the Five Factor trait neuroticism is associated with depression both in the general population [28] and in the epilepsy population [29]. These studies highlight that in the absence of psychiatric assessment, the interpretation of cross-sectional personality ratings may be problematic.

Further complicating the assessment of personality is the nature of the epilepsy study population. A large number of studies have assessed patients admitted to epilepsy units for assessment of intractable seizures or for epilepsy surgery, biasing samples toward patients with treatment-resistant epilepsy, and with TLE in

particular [1]. The few outpatient studies have often been limited by low response rates [30,31]. The select nature of these populations is a limitation of much epilepsy research, not just research of personality. Compared to research into primary psychiatric diagnoses in epilepsy, there have been relatively few recent studies into personality in epilepsy that have addressed the methodological weaknesses of earlier research [1]. We have summarized the confounders of personality assessment in the epilepsy population in Table 15.1. With these limitations in mind, we aim to provide a review of available studies on personality in epilepsy, with a focus on more recently published studies, and to draw some limited conclusions about the idea of an "epileptic personality" and the impact of personality on QOL in people with epilepsy.

The following two sections discuss two personality syndromes presumed to be related to focal pathology of the temporal lobes (the Geschwind syndrome of TLE) and the frontal lobes (the Janz syndrome of juvenile myoclonic epilepsy, JME). This is followed by a discussion of less specific personality syndromes in epilepsy, the relationship between personality and epilepsy surgery, and finally the relationship between QOL in epilepsy and personality.

TLE and Geschwind syndrome

Geschwind syndrome (also known as Gastaut–Geschwind syndrome) has been highly influential in describing a personality type associated with TLE, but more recent studies have largely failed to validate this concept. Gastaut and colleagues found that a high proportion of TLE patients assessed in an outpatient setting in the 1950s exhibited mental slowness (which they described as "viscosity"), hyposexuality, and episodic irritability. They suggested that such characteristics developed about 2 years after the onset of seizures, with the implication that personality change resulted from changes in the limbic system secondary to seizures [3,32]. Their thinking was influenced by the observation that these characteristics of TLE patients were the opposite of Kluver–Bucy syndrome, a pattern of inattentiveness, placidity, and hypersexuality that follows bilateral temporal-lobe damage [3].

Waxman and Geschwind further expanded on this concept as an "interictal behavior syndrome" of TLE.

Table 15.1 Some frequent limitations of studies investigating interictal personality.

Problems with characterization of epilepsy	Inaccurate localization (limited use of MRI and video EEG monitoring)
	Possible inclusion of patients with psychogenic seizures in epilepsy samples
	Failure to consider potential extratemporal involvement in TLE patients (e.g., frontal lobe)
	Failure to properly differentiate ictal versus periictal phenomena
	Failure to consider seizure variables as potential confounders (e.g., age of onset, duration of epilepsy, seizure frequency and severity)
Problems with characterization of personality	Lack of specificity of personality traits to epilepsy (e.g., differences could reflect psychiatric illness rather than epilepsy)
	Cross-sectional personality assessment rather than longitudinal perspective
	Differences in measurement (e.g., use of self-report versus proxy raters, dimensional versus categorical, personality traits versus personality disorders)
Problems with characterization of psychopathology	Axis I disorders often not considered
	Failure to differentiate between axis I and axis II disorders
	Variable assessment methods: subjective self-reports, clinical assessment, structured diagnostic interviews
	Failure to consider potential effect of intellectual impairment
Problems with characterization of other potential confounders (examples)	Antiepileptic medications
	Level of education
	Socioeconomic status and employment status
	Sense of stigma
	Premorbid personality
Other methodological issues	Small sample sizes and insufficient power of some studies to detect differences
	No control group
	No blinding of raters
	Lack of consecutive sampling, leading to potential selection bias
	Diversity of samples (cases and controls) across studies
	Sampling strategies limiting generalizability of results (e.g., hospitalized patients with chronic epilepsy)

Their 1975 paper outlined three case studies and a number of other case reports in the literature to characterize a "syndrome" that included "alterations in sexual behavior, religiosity, and a tendency toward extensive, and in some cases compulsive, writing and drawing" [33]. Many of the traits of the "syndrome" were similar

to those outlined by Gastaut, and they also attributed it to limbic changes: "interictal spike activity in temporal structures."

The Bear–Fedio Inventory (BFI) was developed to further characterize the interictal personality of TLE, rating 18 behavioral traits [34]. It was designed as an alternative to the MMPI, which in a number of studies had failed to demonstrate consistent differences between epilepsy patients and controls [35,36]. In their original paper, Bear and Fedio demonstrated that all 18 traits were found more frequently in TLE patients than in healthy controls or a neurological comparison group. This study also suggested that the BFI differentiated between right and left TLE [34]. In a subsequent study using the BFI, which included a comparison with psychiatric disorders the authors rejected the concept of a specific behavioral syndrome associated with TLE and proposed that the increased prevalence of the BFI personality traits reflected nonspecific psychopathology [36].

The BFI (or modified versions) and MMPI were used in numerous further studies as a means of allowing more structured evaluation of personality in epilepsy, particularly TLE. Neither instrument was able to reliably identify a Geschwind-like personality as specific to TLE compared to controls. They were also not able to consistently differentiate personality between people with TLE and those without TLE, or between right and left TLE [2,4].

While the Geschwind personality type of TLE could not be consistently identified, other authors have more recently attempted to identify whether there was any specific personality type associated with TLE. However, authors using systematic approaches in the last 5 years have had predominantly negative findings.

Swinkels et al. [8] used two personality inventories (Questionnaire on Personality Traits and the NEO-FFI) in a mixed inpatient and outpatient population to compare personality traits in people with TLE and extra-TLE (E-TLE). They found no differences on any personality subscales between left and right TLE or between TLE and E-TLE. Pung and Schmitz [37] found that TLE patients did not differ from patients with juvenile myoclonic epilepsy (JME) on the NEO-FFI or BFI, although they noted more significant circadian disruption in the JME group. Locke et al. [38] used the NEO-PI-Revised in epilepsy patients admitted for diagnostic assessment and found no differences in any domains or facet trait scales between people with TLE and E-TLE or between right and left TLE. Witt et al. [39] found that, in patients awaiting epilepsy surgery, patients with TLE had lower extroversion scores than patients with E-TLE using a German personality inventory, the *Fragebogen zur Persönlichkeitbei zerebralen Erkrankungen* (FPZ), but no other significant personality differences.

Pizzi et al. used the Personality Assessment Inventory (PAI) to compare personality traits of patients with TLE and frontal-lobe epilepsy (FLE). There was some evidence (p values 0.05–0.10) that patients with FLE had increases on scales that measure emotional lability and relationship difficulties (i.e., mania, borderline features, antisocial, stress, and nonsupport). The authors questioned the clinical significance of the findings, although they proposed that frontal-lobe dysfunction in the FLE patients might contribute to personality or behavior change [40].

Wilson et al. [39] did not find a difference in neuroticism or extroversion scores between patients with mesial TLE and other forms of focal epilepsy, although they did identify an intriguing association between seizure onset in adolescence and elevated neuroticism scores; this association between age of epilepsy onset and personality development has been proposed previously [41] and warrants further investigation.

In summary, the literature fails to define a specific personality type associated with TLE. The ongoing search for such a personality type is often justified on the basis that there are inherent limitations with instruments such as the BFI and MMPI, the diversity of studies, the numerous potential biases, and other methodological weaknesses. These limitations have been outlined in detail by a number of authors [2,4,8,42–44] and are summarized in Table 15.1. Similar methodological limitations exist in some studies that have used other instruments (e.g., Clinical Interview Schedule, Structured Clinical Interview for DSM-III-R, Standard Assessment of Personality) to detect personality disorders [1,8]. However, the more recent studies of personality traits in TLE (post-2005) have addressed many of these methodological weaknesses and have still had predominantly negative results. It remains possible, of course, that such a personality type does not exist.

JME and Janz syndrome

The syndrome of JME, originally described by Janz, has attracted a smaller body of research than the TLE literature, but still a significant one. In Janz's original clinical observations, published mainly in the German literature in the 1950s and 1960s, he described JME patients as having rapid mood swings, lack of discipline, hedonism, and indifference toward the disease [45].

Despite these early descriptions, psychopathology in JME received little attention in English-speaking literature until recent years.

In 2001, Gelisse published a large case series in the French literature [46], which showed a high rate of borderline personality disorder (BPD) in JME, possibly consistent with the personality observations by Janz. This study was limited by its retrospective chart review methodology. In a more methodologically robust study, 100 patients with JME were compared to 100 matched controls using the Structured Clinical Interview for DSM-IV; JME patients had higher rates of personality disorder (20%) – predominantly cluster B (histrionic or borderline, 17%) – compared to controls (4%) [30]. The same researchers showed that the presence of cluster B personality in a JME group was associated with decreased corpus callosum volume [47], reduced thalamic, frontobasal, and mesiofrontal volume [48], and frontal-lobe abnormalities on MRS [49] and that the presence of a cluster B personality disorder reduced the likelihood of seizure remission [50]. These authors have proposed that the cluster B personality matches the personality originally described by Janz [49] and is related to frontal-lobe dysfunction.

A similar proposal of frontal-lobe dysfunction was made by Devinsky et al. [51] and supported by Piazzini et al. [52], who showed that JME patients had dysexecutive findings greater than TLE patients and comparable with FLE patients. Further supporting this, Plattner [53] used a different instrument, the Weinberger Adjustment Inventory, in a teenage population and found a trend toward lower self-restraint (higher impulsiveness) in a JME population compared to controls.

Not all studies have replicated these findings, however. Trinka et al. [31], while replicating the finding of a high rate (23%) of personality disorders using the Structured Clinical Interview for DSM-IV in an Austrian JME population, identified similar levels of cluster A, B, and C personality disorders among these patients. Karachristianou et al. [54] showed no difference between JME patients and a volunteer control group on MMPI scores. As mentioned earlier, Pung and Schmitz [37] found no significant difference between JME and TLE patients on the NEO-FFI or BFI.

On balance, the literature would suggest that JME is associated with a higher prevalence of personality disorder than is found in a control population and that this may reflect frontal brain changes in this disorder.

Studies of personality disorder in patients with mixed epilepsy

The preceding research has attempted to characterize the personality styles of specific epilepsy syndromes, based particularly on the limbic-hyperactivity hypothesis of TLE [3] and the frontal-dysfunction hypothesis of JME [45]. Others have looked at personality traits in general or mixed-epilepsy populations. In these studies, DSM-based categorical approaches have predominated.

In the last 2 decades, several studies have used the Structured Clinical Interview for DSM-IV to assess personality and many have identified similar rates of personality disorder. Lopez-Rodriguez et al. [55] identified a personality disorder (predominantly cluster C) in 21% of patients in a surgical-assessment telemetry population. Victoroff [56] identified a personality disorder (predominantly personality disorder not otherwise specified) in 18% of patients. Arnold and Privitera [57] found a prevalence of 18%, most commonly avoidant personality disorder, in an inpatient monitoring setting using an epilepsy-specific version of the Structured Clinical Interview for DSM-IV. Machanda [58] again found a prevalence of 18% in inpatient epilepsy surgical candidates, again mainly cluster C personality disorders.

Koch-Stoecker [59] systematically examined 100 patients prior to temporal lobectomy using a Structured Clinical Interview for DSM-IV-based clinical interview and found a very high rate of personality disorder of 60%, although half of the personality-disordered patients had comorbid axis I pathology and "organic" personality disorders were most common. Cluster C personalities were most common, followed by cluster B. More recently, in 2009 Harden et al. [60] found similarly high rates of personality disorder in a telemetry population of 60%, albeit in a relatively small sample of 16. Again, cluster C personalities predominated.

In contrast, several studies have failed to show a preponderance of cluster C personality type in patients with epilepsy. Sperli et al. [61] found personality disorders in only 8% of a large presurgical case series, mainly cluster B, using clinical interview. Significantly, in this study an axis II disorder was not noted if an axis I disorder was present. Using a clinical interview, Guanieri et al. [62] identified a 12% prevalence of personality disorders, mainly cluster B. It is noteworthy that both of these studies did not make use of a structured clinical interview and both reported lower rates of personality disorder and a greater preponderance of the more "dramatic" cluster B personalities than did studies using structured interviews.

All of these studies were undertaken in refractory epilepsy populations, admitted for either telemetry or presurgical assessment. One of the few studies of epilepsy and personality conducted outside the refractory epilepsy population, by Matsuura et al. in 2003 [63], found a personality disorder rate of 18% in a large population of first referrals to an epilepsy clinic – a rate consistent with other studies – and differentiated them using the ICD-10 research criteria as "pseudopsychopathic" (50%), "limbic-epileptic" (24%), "apathetic" (14%), or "other" (10%).

In summary, studies in patients with unselected epilepsy subtypes identify a prevalence of personality disorder on the order of 20% (range 8–60%). The type of personality disorder most commonly identified is in the cluster C personality type (i.e., dependant, anxious, avoidant, obsessive–compulsive). While there is not strong evidence for this personality type being associated with a specific epilepsy syndrome, Swinkels et al. [1] noted in their 2005 review that many features of the BFI overlap with cluster C personality disorders and suggest that this might explain earlier findings. The relationship between this personality type and epilepsy may reflect the combined biological and environmental effects of long-standing medically refractory epilepsy, together with the psychosocial consequences of living with the possibility of unpredictable seizures.

Effect of epilepsy surgery

A number of studies have looked at patients undergoing epilepsy surgery from the perspective of cognitive outcomes, seizure burden, and QOL. The smaller number of studies that have looked at personality in this context fall into two areas: 1) those that investigated the effects of surgery on personality traits and 2) those that assessed the effects of personality traits on postoperative adjustment or functioning.

Effects of surgery on personality

Studies assessing the effect of surgery on personality are few and have not shown substantial and consistent changes between the pre- and postoperative state. In 1968, an early study described an improvement in social function, reduction in irritability and improved sexual function in a large proportion of a case series of 27 patients over several years [64]. A larger series in 1973 showed similar findings with regard to social function and epilepsy [65]. However, both studies were limited by the absence of a standard diagnostic system or rating scale.

More recent systematic studies in the last 2 decades have used the MMPI, administered pre- and postoperatively. Trenerry et al. [66] showed a high correlation between pre- and postoperative personality traits using the MMPI, noting "clinically modest" reductions in depression and hypochondriasis (preoccupation with bodily symptoms) scores postoperatively and in psychesthesia (excessive anxiety, doubts, and compulsions) and schizophrenia (a measure of odd thinking and social isolation) in those rendered seizure-free compared to those who were not. Wachi et al. [67] also found some reduction in hypochondriasis, psychesthenia, and schizophrenia scores. Derry et al. [68] showed decline in the MMPI hypochondriasis scale in patients assessed prior to surgery and then 2 years after surgery. The authors attributed this change over time to questions that related specifically to seizure symptoms rather than personality and reported that there was "no meaningful difference" in MMPI profile between pre- and postoperative measurements regardless of seizure outcome. Meldolesi et al. [69] suggested that the MMPI profile was "relatively stable" up to 2 years after surgery but noted a decrease in "paranoid" and "social introversion" scales and an increase in "lie" and "defensiveness" scales, which the authors interpreted as reduced interpersonal withdrawal and sensitivity and increased social desirability and self-control. While showing small QOL improvements associated with decreased depression scores postoperatively, this study made no comment about association of any personality traits with QOL changes [69].

In summary, the available longitudinal data suggest that personality measures do not change substantially in patients following surgery; the most consistent finding is a modest reduction in anxiety and obsessive symptoms, odd thought patterns, and bodily preoccupation and concern with physical health. However, the relatively short (up to 2 years) follow-up of the more recent studies may be insufficient to detect gradual changes in personality and self-identity.

Effects of personality on postoperative outcomes

A larger body of work has assessed the effect of personality on postsurgical outcome. Seminal work by Taylor and Falconer [70] in 1968 showed that, while seizure freedom was important, good "premorbid adjustment" resulted in improved postoperative outcome. More recent studies have examined this relationship by looking at personality scales (e.g., MMPI) or by assessing the effects of personality disorders.

MMPI studies

In one of the first studies, Rausch et al. [71] assessed 10 patients pre- and postoperatively and found that of 7 patients with "poor" premorbid function, those with "disorganized" styles managed better than those with "rigid" or obsessional traits. Hermann et al. [72] combined the MMPI, the Washington Psychosocial Seizure Inventory (WPSI), and the General Health Questionnaire into one psychosocial measure and concluded that preoperative psychosocial adjustment and seizure-free outcome best predicted postoperative psychosocial outcomes. Rose et al. [73] showed that high preoperative neuroticism correlated with poor outcomes on psychosocial adjustment and QOL postoperatively, although they did not assess comorbid depression. Wheelock et al. [74] showed that MMPI scores for depression and psychesthenia reduced following surgery but that high levels of both correlated with low satisfaction with surgical outcome. The elimination of seizures postoperatively was identified as leading to significant improvements in psychological and psychosocial functioning [74].

Studies using other personality rating scales

A number of studies have examined other aspects of personality in terms of postoperative outcomes using a variety of measures.

Chovaz et al. [75] showed that resourcefulness and depression, interpreted as measures of learned helplessness, were predictors of psychosocial function postoperatively, whereas locus of control was not. Seizure control was also a very important predictor of postoperative psychosocial function [75]. Canizares et al. [76] showed that neuroticism, measured using a Spanish version of the Eysenck Personality Questionnaire, predicted cognitive complaints postoperatively, whereas objective cognitive function did not. In 2010,

Wilson et al. [77] showed that patients with higher neuroticism and lower extroversion had higher rates of depression at 3 months after surgery and that high-neuroticism patients had more family disruption and more difficulty in adjusting to the "burden of normality" after surgery. These authors also found that patients with adolescent- or preadolescent-onset epilepsy had the greatest perception of self-change and improvement in QOL after epilepsy surgery [77].

Studies in patients with personality disorders

In one of the few studies to examine the effect of personality disorders on postsurgical outcome, Koch-Stoecker [59] showed in 2002 that the presence of personality disorder increased the risk of postoperative psychiatric hospitalization regardless of the presence of an axis I disorder. More recently, Guarnieri et al. [62] found in 2009 that the presence of psychiatrist-diagnosed personality disorders preoperatively increased the risk of persistent auras postoperatively.

In summary, premorbid personality, in particular neuroticism and the presence of diagnosed personality disorder, is correlated with poorer psychological and psychosocial outcome postoperatively. It is important to note that many studies show that the strongest predictor of postoperative psychosocial outcome is seizure elimination or a significant reduction in seizure frequency. Personality factors such as neuroticism should be considered in the work-up of patients destined for surgery as a marker of poorer postoperative psychosocial adjustment, especially in the presence of ongoing seizures.

Relationship between personality and QOL

Epilepsy is a chronic disorder, even when well managed, and as a result QOL has become an important way of measuring health outcomes [78,79]. It is well recognized that QOL issues represent a significant burden for people with epilepsy [80–82]. QOL in people with personality disorders has been reported to be globally poor [83]. The complex interaction between epilepsy and personality makes it important to assess the effect of personality on QOL in epilepsy specifically [84]. The literature that exists in this area can be generally grouped into studies looking at coping mechanisms, studies investigating the relationship between QOL and personality traits or disorders, and studies looking at the impact of personality on QOL after epilepsy surgery.

Coping mechanisms such as resilience, optimism [85], locus of control [86,87], and spirituality [88] have been reported to have an impact on the QOL for people with epilepsy. Optimism, or attributional style, can have an indirect effect on QOL. In the general population, optimistic people report higher QOL [89]. The expectation that good things will happen is a relatively stable personality trait. Optimistic people may be more likely to pursue and persist with treatment options and to cope in times of adversity [89], perhaps through the promotion of a healthy lifestyle, adaptive behaviors and cognitive responses, greater flexibility, or problem-solving capacity [90].

In the epilepsy population, those patients with a perception of poor seizure control report a poorer QOL [91]. In several studies, the negative impacts of epilepsy severity were alleviated by resilience factors. Pais-Ribeiro et al. [85] reported that optimists showed an improved perception of their physical and mental state of health and reported higher QOL compared to pessimists. Amir [92] reported a high sense of mastery and social support contributing to improved QOL. Higher optimistic orientation also correlated with better perception of cognitive functioning, although it did not correlate with seizure perception in the same study [85]. It may be that epilepsy-specific optimism is an important clinical variable, rather than optimism in itself.

It is likely that the majority of people are able to respond to a serious life event in a resilient manner. This accounts for the relatively good QOL within 1–2 years of a first seizure event and return to almost normal functioning. In studies documenting this process, most people were able to restore some sense of control over their lives, regardless of the reported high loss of control at diagnosis [93].

A study comparing epilepsy patients and healthy controls with a range of social questionnaires, including the Eysenck Personality Questionnaire [94], reported that patients with epilepsy were more likely to be introverted, with more changeable emotions than the healthy population. The extent of the correlation between well-being, personality, and emotional variables led the authors to suggest that personality characteristics may be the main influence on well-being for people with epilepsy. There is one other article looking at specific personality traits, but only with regard to sexual QOL, which was shown to be reduced with lower extroversion [95].

Overall, the impact of personality on QOL for people living with epilepsy is assumed to be relevant yet is understudied. At this time, it appears that neuroticism as a personality trait may be a key feature to be identified in people with epilepsy, in that it may negatively influence perceptions of the impact of epilepsy. As neuroticism is a personality trait associated with a range of psychiatric comorbidities [96–98], as well as increased all-cause mortality in the general population [99], proactive identification and treatment designed to enhance resilience may be advisable.

Conclusion

The study of personality in epilepsy has a long history and the literature reports systematic studies for over half a century. Over the same period, there has been a substantial change in the characterization and treatment of epilepsy and personality disorder, as well as in study methodologies. As a consequence, the literature on the topic is difficult to interpret and at times conflicting. Nevertheless, it is possible to conclude from the evidence that personality dysfunction of various forms is more common in patients with intractable epilepsy than in the general population. Given that the majority of studies have focused on hospitalized patients or patients attending specialist referral centers, it is difficult to know whether this finding can be generalized to the wider epilepsy population.

Early investigation and clinical observation suggested that TLE was associated with a particular personality type. More recent studies based on modern rating scales or standardized interviews have generally not supported this. The DSM-IV construct of "cluster C" personality disorders bears some resemblance to early descriptions of the "epileptic personality," and the apparent increase in cluster C personality disorders in epilepsy patients admitted for video-EEG monitoring may provide some indirect support for this concept.

The idea of the impulsive, irresponsible personality style associated with JME has received less attention, but recent reports of increase in cluster B personality disorders and frontal-lobe dysfunction in this population may explain early clinical observations.

Finally, there is consistent evidence that certain personality traits, especially neuroticism, are associated with poorer QOL and poorer adjustment following epilepsy surgery. While this finding is not necessarily specific to epilepsy, and personality assessment is often confounded by comorbid depression, it highlights the importance of understanding personality in epilepsy patients and of being aware of factors that may impact on patients' QOL.

References

1 Swinkels WA, Kuyk J, van Dyck R, Spinhoven P: Psychiatric comorbidity in epilepsy. *Epilepsy Behav* 2005; **7**:37–50.
2 Ritaccio AL, Devinsky O: Personality disorders in epilepsy. In: Ettinger AB, Kanner AM (eds): *Psychiatric Issues in Epilepsy: A Practical Guide to Diagnosis and Treatment.* Lippincott Williams and Wilkins, Philadelphia, PA, 2001.
3 Blumer D: Evidence supporting the temporal lobe epilepsy personality syndrome. *Neurology* 1999; **53**:S9–S12.
4 Devinsky O, Najjar S: Evidence against the existence of a temporal lobe epilepsy personality syndrome. *Neurology* 1999; **53**:S13–S25.
5 Turner WA: *Epilepsy: A Study of the Idiopathic Disease.* Macmillan, London, 1907; quoted in Chua P: Personality aspects of temporal lobe epilepsy. Master of Medicine thesis, University of Melbourne, 1995.
6 Lennox W: Personality in seizure states. In: Hunt J (ed.): *Personality and the Behaviour Disorders.* The Ronald Press, New York, NY, 1944, pp. 952–964.
7 Guerrant JAW, Fischer A, Weinstein MR et al.: *Personality in Epilepsy.* Charles C. Thomas, Springfield, IL, 1962.
8 Swinkels WA, van Emde Boas W, Kuyk J et al.: Interictal depression, anxiety, personality traits, and psychological dissociation in patients with temporal lobe epilepsy (TLE) and extra-TLE. *Epilepsia* 2006; **47**:2092–2103.
9 Gibbs FA: Ictal and non-ictal psychiatric disorders in temporal lobe epilepsy. *J Nerv Ment Dis* 1951; **113**:522–528.
10 Bingley T: Mental symptoms in temporal lobe epilepsy and temporal lobe gliomas with special reference to laterality of lesion and the relationship between handedness and brainedness; a study of 90 cases of temporal lobe epilepsy and 253 cases of temporal lobe glioma. *Acta Psychiatr Neurol Scand Suppl* 1958; **120**:1–151.
11 Tizard B: The personality of epileptics: a discussion of the evidence. *Psychol Bull* 1962; **59**:196–210.
12 Butcher JNE: *MMPI-2: A Practitioner's Guide.* American Psychological Association, Washington, DC, 2005.
13 McCrae RR, John OP: An introduction to the five-factor model and its applications. *J Personality* 1992; **60**:175–215.
14 Hermann BP, Trenerry MR, Colligan RC: Learned helplessness, attributional style, and depression in epilepsy. Bozeman Epilepsy Surgery Consortium. *Epilepsia* 1996; **37**:680–686.
15 Piazzini A, Ramaglia G, Turner K et al.: Coping strategies in epilepsy: 50 drug-resistant and 50 seizure-free patients. *Seizure* 2007; **16(3)**:211–217.
16 Cengel-Kültür SE, Ulay HT, Erdağ G: Ways of coping with epilepsy and related factors in adolescence. *Turk J Pediatr* 2009; **51(3)**:238–247.
17 Donnelly KM, Schefft BK, Howe SR et al.: Moderating effect of optimism on emotional distress and seizure control in adults with temporal lobe epilepsy. *Epilepsy Behav* 2010; **18(4)**:374–380.
18 Jacoby A, Gorry J, Gamble C, Baker GA: Public knowledge, private grief: a study of public attitudes to epilepsy in the United Kingdom and implications for stigma. *Epilepsia* 2004; **45(11)**:1405–1415.
19 Kanner AM: Depression and epilepsy: a review of multiple facets of their close relation. *Neurol Clin* 2009; **27**:865–880.
20 LaFrance WC Jr, Kanner AM, Hermann B: Psychiatric comorbidities in epilepsy. *Int Rev Neurobiol* 2008; **83**:347–383.
21 Adams SJ, O'Brien TJ, Lloyd J et al.: Neuropsychiatric morbidity in focal epilepsy. *Br J Psychiatry* 2008; **192(6)**:464–469.
22 Mulder RT, Joyce PR, Frampton CM: Personality disorders improve in patients treated for major depression. *Acta Psychiatr Scand* 2010; **122(3)**:219–225.
23 Melartin TK, Haukka J, Rytsälä HJ et al.: Categorical and dimensional stability of comorbid personality disorder symptoms in DSM-IV major depressive disorder: a prospective study. *J Clin Psychiatry* 2010; **71**:287–295.
24 Griens AM, Jonker K, Spinhoven P, Blom MB: The influence of depressive state features on trait measurement. *J Affect Disord* 2002; **70(1)**:95–99.
25 Tang TZ, DeRubeis RJ, Hollon SD et al.: Personality change during depression treatment: a placebo-controlled trial. *Arch Gen Psychiatry* 2009; **66(12)**:1322–1330.
26 Morey LC, Shea MT, Markowitz MD et al.: State effects of major depression on the assessment of personality and personality disorder. *Am J Psychiatry* 2010; **167**:528–535.
27 Santor DA, Bagby RM, Joffe RT: Evaluating stability and change in personality and depression. *J Pers Soc Psychol* 1997; **73(6)**:1354–1362.

28 Klein DN, Kotov R, Bufferd SJ: Personality and depression: explanatory models and review of the evidence. *Ann Rev Clin Psychol* 2011; **7**:269–295.

29 Wilson SJ, Wrench JM, McIntosh AM et al.: Personality development in the context of intractable epilepsy. *Arch Neurol* 2009; **66(1)**:68–72.

30 de Araújo Filho GM, Pascalicchio TF, Sousa Pda S et al.: Psychiatric disorders in juvenile myoclonic epilepsy: a controlled study of 100 patients. *Epilepsy Behav* 2007; **10(3)**: 437–441.

31 Trinka E, Kienpointner G, Unterberger I et al.: Psychiatric comorbidity in juvenile myoclonic epilepsy. *Epilepsia* 2006; **47(12)**:2086–2091.

32 Blumer D: Personality in epilepsy. *Semin Neurol* 1991; **11**: 155–166.

33 Waxman SG, Geschwind N: The interictal behavior syndrome of temporal lobe epilepsy. *Arch Gen Psychiatry* 1975; **32**:1580–1586.

34 Bear DM, Fedio P: Quantitative analysis of interictal behavior in temporal lobe epilepsy. *Arch Neurol* 1977; **34**:454–467.

35 Geschwind N: Behavioural change in temporal lobe epilepsy. *Arch Neurol* 1977; **34**:453.

36 Mungas D: Interictal behavior abnormality in temporal lobe epilepsy: a specific syndrome or nonspecific psychopathology? *Arch Gen Psychiatry* 1982; **39**:108–111.

37 Pung T, Schmitz B: Circadian rhythm and personality profile in juvenile myoclonic epilepsy. *Epilepsia* 2006; **47(Suppl. 2)**:111–114.

38 Locke DE, Fakhoury TA, Berry DT et al.: Objective evaluation of personality and psychopathology in temporal lobe versus extratemporal lobe epilepsy. *Epilepsy Behav* 2010; **17**:172–177.

39 Witt JA, Hollmann K, Helmstaedter C: The impact of lesions and epilepsy on personality and mood in patients with symptomatic epilepsy: a pre- to postoperative follow-up study. *Epilepsy Res* 2008; **82**:139–146.

40 Pizzi AM, Chapin JS, Tesar GE, Busch RM: Comparison of personality traits in patients with frontal and temporal lobe epilepsies. *Epilepsy Behav* 2009; **15(2)**:225–229.

41 Viberg M, Blennow G, Polski B: Epilepsy in adolescence: implications for the development of personality. *Epilepsia* 1987; **28**:542–546.

42 Swinkels WA, Duijsens IJ, Spinhoven P: Personality disorder traits in patients with epilepsy. *Seizure* 2003; **12**:587–594.

43 Trimble MR: Personality disturbances in epilepsy. *Neurology* 1983; **33**:1332–1334.

44 Perini GI, Tosin C, Carraro C et al.: Interictal mood and personality disorders in temporal lobe epilepsy and juvenile myoclonic epilepsy. *J Neurol Neurosurg Psychiatry* 1996; **61**:601–605.

45 Janz D: The psychiatry of idiopathic generalized epilepsy. In: Trimble MR, Schmitz B (eds): *The Neuropsychiatry of Epilepsy*, Cambridge University Press, Cambridge, 2002, pp. 41–61.

46 Gélisse P, Genton P, Samuelian JC et al.: [Psychiatric disorders in juvenile myoclonic epilepsy]. *Rev Neurol (Paris)* 2001; **157(3)**:297–302.

47 Filho GM, Jackowski AP, Lin K et al.: The integrity of corpus callosum and cluster B personality disorders: a quantitative MRI study in juvenile myoclonic epilepsy. *Prog Neuropsychopharmacol Biol Psychiatry* 2010; **34(3)**:516–521.

48 de Araújo Filho GM, Jackowski AP, Lin K et al.: Personality traits related to juvenile myoclonic epilepsy: MRI reveals prefrontal abnormalities through a voxel-based morphometry study. *Epilepsy Behav* 2009; **15(2)**:202–207.

49 de Araújo Filho GM, Lin K, Lin J et al.: Are personality traits of juvenile myoclonic epilepsy related to frontal lobe dysfunctions? A proton MRS study. *Epilepsia* 2009; **50(5)**: 1201–1209.

50 Guaranha MS, Filho GM, Lin K et al.: Prognosis of juvenile myoclonic epilepsy is related to endophenotypes. *Seizure* 2011; **20(1)**:42–48.

51 Devinsky O, Gershengorn J, Brown E et al.: Frontal functions in juvenile myoclonic epilepsy. *Neuropsychiatry Neuropsychol Behav Neurol* 1997; **10(4)**:243–246.

52 Piazzini A, Turner K, Vignoli A et al.: Frontal cognitive dysfunction in juvenile myoclonic epilepsy. *Epilepsia* 2008; **49(4)**:657–662.

53 Plattner B, Pahs G, Kindler J et al.: Juvenile myoclonic epilepsy: a benign disorder? Personality traits and psychiatric symptoms. *Epilepsy Behav* 2007; **10**:560–564.

54 Karachristianou S, Katsarou Z, Bostantjopoulou S et al.: Personality profile of patients with juvenile myoclonic epilepsy. *Epilepsy Behav* 2008; **13(4)**:654–657.

55 Lopez-Rodriguez F, Altshuler L, Kay J et al.: Personality disorders among medically refractory epileptic patients. *J Neuropsychiatry Clin Neurosci* 1999; **11**:464–469.

56 Victoroff J: DSM-III-R psychiatric diagnoses in candidates for epilepsy surgery: lifetime prevalence. *Neuropsychiatry Neuropsychol Behav Neurol* 1994; **7**:87–97.

57 Arnold LM, Privitera MD: Psychopathology and trauma in epileptic and psychogenic seizure patients. *Psychosomatics* 1996; **37**:438–443.

58 Manchanda R, Schaefer B, McLachlan RS et al.: Psychiatric disorders in candidates for surgery for epilepsy. *J Neurol Neurosurg Psychiatry* 1996; **61(1)**:82–89.

59 Koch-Stoecker S: Personality disorders as predictors of severe postsurgical psychiatric complications in epilepsy patients undergoing temporal lobe resections. *Epilepsy Behav* 2002; **3(6)**:526–531.

60 Harden CL, Jovine L, Burgut FT et al.: A comparison of personality disorder characteristics of patients with nonepileptic psychogenic pseudoseizures with those of patients with epilepsy. *Epilepsy Behav* 2009; **14(3)**:481–483.

61 Sperli F, Rentsch D, Despland PA et al.: Psychiatric comorbidity in patients evaluated for chronic epilepsy: a differential role of the right hemisphere? *Eur Neurol* 2009; **61(6)**:350–357.

62 Guarnieri R, Walz R, Hallak JE et al.: Do psychiatric comorbidities predict postoperative seizure outcome in temporal lobe epilepsy surgery? *Epilepsy Behav* 2009; **14(3)**:529–534.

63 Matsuura M, Oana Y, Kato M: A multicentre study on the prevalence of psychiatric disorders among new referrals for epilepsy in Japan. *Epilepsia* 2003; **44(1)**:107–114.

64 Hill D, Pond DA, Mitchell W, Falconer MA: Personality changes following temporal lobectomy for epilepsy: 1957. *Epilepsy Behav* 2004; **5**:603–610.

65 Falconer MA: Reversibility by temporal-lobe resection of the behavioral abnormalities of temporal-lobe epilepsy. *New Engl J Med* 1973; **289(9)**:451–455.

66 Trenerry MR, Hermann BP, Barr WB et al.: MMPI scale elevations before and after right and left temporal lobectomy. *Assessment* 1996; **3**:307–315.

67 Wachi M, Tomikawa M, Fukuda M et al.: Neuropsychological changes after surgical treatment for temporal lobe epilepsy. *Epilepsia* 2001; **42(Suppl. 6)**:4–8.

68 Derry PA, Harnadek MC, McLachlan RS et al.: A longitudinal study of the effects of seizure symptoms on the Minnesota Multiphasic Personality Inventory-2 (MMPI-2) clinical interpretation. *J Clin Psychol* 2002; **58(7)**:817–826.

69 Meldolesi GN, Di Gennaro G, Quarato PP et al.: Changes in depression, anxiety, anger, and personality after resective surgery for drug-resistant temporal lobe epilepsy: a 2-year follow-up study. *Epilepsy Res* 2007; **77(1)**:22–30.

70 Taylor DC, Falconer MA: Clinical, socio-economic, and psychological changes after temporal lobectomy for epilepsy. *Br J Psychiatry* 1968; **114(515)**:1247–1261.

71 Rausch R, McCreary C, Crandall PH: Psychosocial functioning following successful surgical relief from seizures: evidence of prediction from preoperative personality characteristics. *J Psychosom Res* 1977; **21(2)**:141–146.

72 Hermann BP, Wyler AR, Somes G: Preoperative psychological adjustment and surgical outcome are determinants of psychosocial status after anterior temporal lobectomy. *J Neurol Neurosurg Psychiatry* 1992; **55(6)**:491–496.

73 Rose KJ, Derry PA, McLachlan RS: Neuroticism in temporal lobe epilepsy: assessment and implications for pre- and postoperative psychosocial adjustment and health-related quality of life. *Epilepsia* 1996; **37**:484–491.

74 Wheelock I, Peterson C, Buchtel HA: Presurgery expectations, postsurgery satisfaction, and psychosocial adjustment after epilepsy surgery. *Epilepsia* 1998; **39**:487–494.

75 Chovaz CJ, McLachlan RS, Derry PA, Cummings AL: Psychosocial function following temporal lobectomy: influence of seizure control and learned helplessness. *Seizure* 1994; **3(3)**:171–176.

76 Cañizares S, Torres X, Boget T et al.: Does neuroticism influence cognitive self-assessment after epilepsy surgery? *Epilepsia* 2000; **41(10)**:1303–1309.

77 Wilson SJ, Wrench JM, McIntosh AM et al.: Profiles of psychosocial outcome after epilepsy surgery: the role of personality. *Epilepsia* 2010; **51(7)**:1133–1138.

78 Jacoby A: Stigma, epilepsy, and quality of life. *Epilepsy Behav* 2002; **3**:10–20.

79 Jacoby A: Epilepsy and the quality of everyday life: findings from a study of people with well-controlled epilepsy. *Soc Sci Med* 1992; **34(6)**:657–666.

80 Cramer JA: Quality of life for people with epilepsy. *Neurol Clin* 1994; **12(1)**:1–13.

81 Devinsky O, Vickrey BG, Cramer J et al.: Development of the quality of life in epilepsy inventory. *Epilepsia* 1995; **36(11)**:1089–1104.

82 Jacoby A, Snape D, Baker GA: Determinants of quality of life in people with epilepsy. *Neurol Clin* 2009; **27**:843–863.

83 Narud K, Mykletun A, Dahl AA: Quality of life in patients with personality disorders seen at an ordinary psychiatric outpatient clinic. *BMC Psychiatry* 2005; **5**:10.

84 Wilson S, Bladin P, Saling M: The "burden of normality": concepts of adjustment after surgery for seizures. *J Neurol Neurosurg Psychiatry* 2001; **70(5)**:649–656.

85 Pais-Ribeiro J, da Silva AM, Meneses RF, Falco C: Relationship between optimism, disease variables, and health perception and quality of life in individuals with epilepsy. *Epilepsy Behav* 2007; **11(1)**:33–38.

86 Hermann B, Jacoby A: The psychosocial impact of epilepsy in adults. *Epilepsy Behav* 2009; **15(Suppl. 1)**:S11–S16.

87 Gramstad A, Iversen E, Engelsen BA: The impact of affectivity dispositions, self-efficacy and locus of control on psychosocial adjustment in patients with epilepsy. *Epilepsy Res* 2001; **46(1)**:53–61.

88 Giovagnoli AR, Meneses RF, da Silva AM: The contribution of spirituality to quality of life in focal epilepsy. *Epilepsy Behav* 2006; **9(1)**:133–139.

89 Scheier MF, Carver CS: Effects of optimism on psychological and physical well-being: theoretical overview and empirical update. *Cog Ther Res* 1992; **16(2)**:201–228.

90 Conversano C, Rotondo A, Lensi E et al.: Optimism and its impact on mental and physical well-being. *Clin Pract Epidemiol Ment Health* 2010; **6**:25–29.

91 Smith D, Baker GA, Jacoby A, Chadwick DW: The contribution of the measurement of seizure severity to quality of life research. *Qual Life Res* 1995; **4(2)**:143–158.

92 Amir M, Roziner I, Knoll A, Neufeld MY: Self-efficacy and social support as mediators in the relation between disease severity and quality of life in patients with epilepsy. *Epilepsia* 1999; **40(2)**:216–224.

93 Velissaris SL, Wilson SJ, Saling MM et al.: The psychological impact of a newly diagnosed seizure: losing and restoring perceived control. *Epilepsy Behav* 2007; **10(2)**:223–233.

94 Zhu DT, Jin LJ, Xie GJ, Xiao B: Quality of life and personality in adults with epilepsy. *Epilepsia* 1998; **39(11)**:1208–1212.

95 Mölleken D, Richter-Appelt H, Stodieck S, Bengner T: Influence of personality on sexual quality of life in epilepsy. *Epileptic Disord* 2010; **12(2)**:125–132.

96 Spinhoven P, de Rooij M, Heiser W et al.: The role of personality in comorbidity among anxiety and depressive disorders

in primary care and specialty care: a cross-sectional analysis. *Gen Hosp Psychiatry* 2009; **31(5)**:470–477.

97 Lahey BB: Public health significance of neuroticism. *Am Psychol* 2009; **64(4)**:241–256.

98 Rhebergen D, Batelaan NM, de Graaf R et al.: The 7-year course of depression and anxiety in the general population. *Acta Psychiatr Scand* 2011; **123(4)**:297–306.

99 Grossardt BR, Bower JH, Geda YE et al.: Pessimistic, anxious, and depressive personality traits predict all-cause mortality: the Mayo Clinic cohort study of personality and aging. *Psychosom Med* 2009; **71(5)**:491–500.

CHAPTER 16

Psychogenic attacks and epilepsy

Bláthnaid McCoy[1] and Selim R. Benbadis[2]

[1] Department of Pediatric Neurologist and Epileptologist, The Hospital for Sick Children Assistant Professor of Pediatrics, University of Toronto

[2] Department of Neurology & Neurosurgery, University of South Florida and Tampa General Hospital, USA

Introduction

Over the years, the landscape of epilepsy care has evolved and expanded. Seizure freedom remains a major goal of treatment but is not the only goal. We strive to minimize morbidity and maximize our patients' QOL. We want patients to actively participate in life and reach their potentials. Unfortunately, when it comes to managing psychogenic symptoms, they are often underrecognized and mismanaged among patients both with and without epilepsy. The strikingly negative impact of psychogenic nonepileptic seizures or psychogenic attacks is well known. Clinicians need to have a clear approach to psychogenic attacks in order to recognize and manage them appropriately in a timely manner to maximize outcomes.

Historically, psychogenic attacks were recognized as a form of hysteria. In the late 1800s, Charcot described them as "hysteroepilepsy" [1]. More recently, the terms "hysterical" and "pseudoseizure" have been replaced by less pejorative terms such as "psychogenic nonepileptic seizures" [2]. However, use of the term "seizure" in reference to psychogenic attacks is confusing to patients and families and may impact initial impression of the diagnosis, which may in turn negatively impact their receptiveness and response to treatment [3]. Preferable terminology might be "psychogenic nonepileptic attacks" or "psychogenic spells," although this debate remains unresolved [3].

A psychogenic attack is defined as an episode of disturbance of motor, sensory, autonomic, cognitive, and/or emotional functions that resembles an epileptic seizure but is associated with psychopathology and not with ictal electrical discharges in the brain [4–7]. Psychogenic attacks are considered a physical manifestation of a psychological distress in which symptoms of a psychiatric nature are expressed in a neurological fashion [8]. Psychogenic attacks are listed as "psychogenic nonepileptic seizures" under the heading of "dissociative disorders" in the ICD-10 and under "somatoform or conversion disorders" in the DSM-IV [9,10]. Psychogenic attacks do not include nonepileptic events with a physiological basis such as syncope, childhood breath-holding spells, or movement disorders. Rather, the term "psychogenic attacks" is reserved for events that arise through unconscious psychological mechanisms and should be distinguished from willful factitious seizures.

Beyond semantics and terminology, the impact of psychogenic attacks on patients, their families, and health services is sizeable and demands our attention. There are significant risks associated with incorrect or delayed diagnosis, such as inappropriate treatment with antiepileptic drugs (AEDs) leading to toxicity, poor prognosis, and impaired quality of life (QOL). Furthermore, there are significant health costs associated with psychogenic attacks, both direct costs of health utilization and indirect costs of absenteeism and reliance on social welfare payments [11]. The misdiagnosis of psychogenic attacks as epileptic seizures has an estimated annual cost of USS650–4000 million [12]. Health care utilization costs are significantly reduced in the 6 months following accurate diagnosis of psychogenic attacks with video-EEG [13].

The key to successful management of psychogenic attacks is to reach a correct and timely diagnosis, to formulate an appropriate treatment plan, and to clearly

Epilepsy and the Interictal State: Co-Morbidities and Quality of Life, First Edition.
Edited by Erik K. St. Louis, David M. Ficker, and Terence J. O'Brien.
© 2015 John Wiley & Sons, Ltd. Published 2015 by John Wiley & Sons, Ltd.

communicate both the diagnosis and the treatment plan to the patient and their family.

Epidemiology

The incidence of psychogenic attacks is reported by two epidemiological studies as 1.4–3.0 per 100 000 persons annually [14,15]. The prevalence has been estimated as 2–33 cases per 100 000 persons in the general population, paralleling that of multiple sclerosis and of trigeminal neuralgia [16]. Prevalence is increased among those with learning disabilities or neuropsychological deficits [17]. Women make up 75–85% of those with psychogenic attacks [18]. Psychogenic attacks are also seen in children, with most patients showing an initial onset of their symptoms between the ages of 10 and 19 years [19], but many remaining undiagnosed until adulthood. The mean latency between onset of events and diagnosis is 7–16 years [20]. During this time, over three-quarters of patients receive inappropriate antiepileptic medication, often with multiple medications trialed [21].

Psychogenic attacks represent 20–40% of patients referred to epilepsy centers [22–24]. While estimates of comorbid epilepsy diagnosis range from 5 to over 60% [2], only 5–10% meet strict diagnostic criteria for coexistent epilepsy [24]. Of five patients treated for refractory epilepsy, one likely does not have epilepsy at all [25].

Pathophysiology

In order to appropriately counsel patients with psychogenic attacks, an understanding of the often complex, intertwined psychological or biological pathophysiology is necessary. In psychological terms, the disorders are classified according to the international classifications of the DSM-IV and ICD-10 as somatoform, conversion, or dissociative disorders. Somatoform disorders are characterized by physical complaints that are unaccompanied by identifiable medical explanations and have a psychological origin. This group includes conversion disorder [26]. It is generally accepted that psychogenic attacks represent conversion disorders and are unintentionally created as a result of a stressor [27]. These are to be distinguished from rare psychogenic attacks as part of a factitious disorder [28]. In essence,

psychogenic attacks represent a maladaptive coping strategy [29]. A psychological conflict is translated into a physical symptom: the seizure. This provides a means of expressing distress in a way that is dissociated from the conscious experience of the causative trauma [30]. The differing terminology between the ICD-10 and DSM-IV classifications has been questioned and uniform classification of psychogenic attacks as dissociative disorders in both classifications has been proposed [31]. Concurrent psychiatric disorders in occur in 43–100% of psychogenic attacks [32]. When compared with an age- and education-matched group of women with left temporal-lobe epilepsy (TLE), women with psychogenic attacks did not display any severe neurocognitive impairments, supporting a psychologically versus neurologically derived pathology of psychogenic attacks [33].

Several biological pathways have been proposed to explain the pathogenesis of psychogenic attacks, based on chemical imbalances. Modern functional imaging techniques have been employed to study potential biological mechanisms. With regard to "stress," cortisol and norepinephrine have been studied. The hypothalamic–pituitary–adrenal (HPA) axis has been examined to analyze cortisol flux among patients with psychogenic attacks. A significant increase in salivary cortisol has been detected among patients with psychogenic attacks, which is unexplained by depression, medication, or other external factors [34]. Similar changes in norepinephrine levels as part of a "stress" response have been reported in patients with psychogenic attacks [35]. Functional imaging has enabled some interesting observations of patients with psychogenic disorders. Positron emission tomography (PET) scanning has shown glucose hypometabolism in the frontal lobes of patients with depression and anxiety [36] and fMRI can detect distinctive patterns of activation among patients with conversion disorders [37].

Etiology

A trauma, triggering event, or "unspeakable dilemma" can be identified in as many as 84% of patients [30,38,39] and approximately one-third of patients have experienced sexual abuse [42]. The particular event is thought to play an important role in the development of psychogenic attacks by traumatizing a patient with underlying vulnerabilities and triggering a response mechanism of psychogenic symptoms. Five self-reported, trauma-related psychometric scales have been shown to discriminate between patients with psychogenic attacks and epileptic seizures [40]. Another study among patients with psychogenic attacks found that verbal memory deficits paralleled those of adult survivors of childhood abuse [41].

Many patients have coexisting psychiatric diagnoses, especially mood disorders and anxiety [32]. Particular groups of patients may experience a different etiology and pattern of psychogenic attacks. The presentation of prolonged psychogenic attacks, often termed "pseudostatus," is particularly challenging to identify [43] and is highly concerning because unnecessary and potentially dangerous procedures such as intravenous cannulation and intubation or treatment with emergency AEDs is often administered to these patients, placing them at undue risk. Pseudostatus is reported particularly among those with comorbid psychiatric disorders and learning disabilities [44,45].

Patients with intellectual learning difficulties have different clinical features than psychogenic attack patients as a whole because they are more frequently male and have immediate, situational, or emotional triggers for attacks and a less frequent antecedent sexual abuse history [44].

Among the most challenging psychogenic attack cases are patients with coexisting epilepsy. The prevalence is similar among children (11%) and adults (16%) [46]. In a study of 219 children and adults, coexistent epilepsy was the most frequent etiology of psychogenic attacks and conversion disorder was seen in only one-quarter of AED-resistant patients, suggesting that psychogenic attacks are more likely secondary to epilepsy than conversion disorder [46]. Since epilepsy often precedes the onset of psychogenic attacks, it may be the reason for psychogenic attacks in some patients [47].

New-onset psychogenic attacks following epilepsy surgery occurs in 2–9% of cases [48,49], usually beginning within the first postoperative year and often within 3 months [48]. Low IQ, preoperative psychopathology (including psychosis), and major surgical complications are identified as risk factors [48]. When patients with seizures are confronted with new stress or increased social demands or expectations after surgery, they may express it by reenacting their chronic disease [50].

Diagnosis

Although only 17% of physicians express doubt about the underlying diagnosis of children referred to an epilepsy center, 39% do not to have epilepsy [51]. Similar issues of diagnostic inaccuracy arise with first admissions to a hospital, with incorrect epilepsy diagnosis occurring in 13.9% of patients admitted to a neurological intensive care unit and failure to diagnose epilepsy in 15.6% of emergency department cases [52]. Box 16.1 outlines the most common clinical historical and ictal semiologic spell features enabling accurate diagnosis of psychogenic attacks.

Box 16.1 Clinical features suggestive of psychogenic attacks.

Historical features

- Event occurrence solely during wakefulness (especially only when available witnesses are present).
- Unusually frequent events.
- Duration longer than usual epileptic seizures (several minutes or longer).
- Waxing and waning clinical course.
- Ictal eye closure or crying.
- Falling with lack of injury.

Clinical semiologic features

- Ictal eye closure.
- Crying during spell.
- "No-no" type head-shaking.
- Nonanatomical spread of movements.
- Wrongly sequenced movements (i.e., clonic then tonic progression).
- Absence of postictal state.

Note

Particular caution is advised against placing too much weight on history or observation alone, since each of these features may also occur in true epileptic seizures.

Clinical features

The history is the most critical variable in teasing out the description of any paroxysmal spell, whether epileptic or nonepileptic in nature. Features of the event, the patient's premorbid personality, potential triggers, and the wider social surrounds are considered when determining whether an event might be nonepileptic [53,54]. History and eye-witness accounts may accurately diagnose psychogenic attacks in as many as 68% of children [55]. Certain features are highly suggestive of psychogenic attacks, including events occurring solely during wakefulness (especially those occurring only at times when a witness is present), unusually frequent events, a duration longer than usual epileptic seizures, a waxing and waning clinical course, and ictal eye closure or crying [53,54,56]. There are age-dependent features, with prepubertal patients more likely to have events of unresponsiveness and pubertal patients more likely to display motor events [57]. Ictal heart rate can be used to distinguish psychogenic attacks from epileptic seizure, with a reported positive predictive value of 97%, using a cut-off of ≥30% above baseline [58]. However, caution is advised as no single feature has absolute accuracy. One major concern is that some atypical events or motor events, especially at night, may represent frontal-lobe seizures and may be misinterpreted as psychogenic attacks. A commonly held belief is that events arising from true sleep recording are epileptic events, whereas psychogenic attacks arise from wakefulness or pseudosleep (patients look as though they are asleep but if video-EEG monitoring is performed, clear EEG features of wakefulness are recorded). However, caution is still advised in this setting because psychogenic attacks may infrequently arise from sleep or within a few seconds of arousal [59].

In distinguishing psychogenic attacks from epileptic seizures, a sensitive screening test is needed. A self-administered psychogenic attack screening test using demographic, clinical, seizure-related, and psychosocial information has a sensitivity of 94% and a specificity of 83% and may be useful in the initial assessment of patients at epilepsy centers [60].

Diagnostic investigations

Increased serum prolactin levels were initially reported to differentiate generalized tonic–clonic seizures from psychogenic attacks over 30 years ago [61]. Prolactin increase may be mediated by ventral thalamic activation by generalized motor seizure activity [62]. Elevated serum prolactin, when measured 10–20 minutes after a suspected event, is a useful adjunct in differentiating a seizure from psychogenic attacks in adults and children [63]. Sensitivity and specificity are uncertain, with

reports of elevation after syncope [64]. Creatine phosphokinase levels are elevated for up to 15 hours after an epileptic event, widening the spectrum for clinical use in comparison to prolactin, with a reported sensitivity of 75% and specificity of 86% for the diagnosis of generalized tonic–clonic seizures [65].

Many clinicians perform routine EEGs as part of their initial assessment of a patient with paroxysmal events. However, the yield of EEG applied in a nonspecific manner is low. Nonspecific abnormalities in addition to overzealous EEG reporting can lead to erroneous diagnoses [66]. One reason is the common misconception that phase reversals indicate abnormality [66]; in addition, epileptiform abnormalities may be found in a small percentage of the population who have not had a seizure and their significance is unclear.

In a similar fashion, performing neuroimaging to aid decision-making as to whether or not an event is epileptic is unlikely to yield useful information. Moreover, detection of nonspecific or nondiagnostic abnormalities can add to patient distress and confusion with the diagnosis of psychogenic attacks.

Certain patterns of neuropsychological dysfunction are reported commonly among patients with psychogenic attacks, similar to those described among patients with post-traumatic stress disorder (PTSD).

The "gold standard" for diagnosis of psychogenic attacks is video-EEG telemetry [67]. When compared to EEG alone, video increases the diagnostic yield [68], although psychogenic attacks are more likely to occur off-camera than epileptic seizures [69]. The duration of monitoring required to record events and diagnose psychogenic attacks is usually 3–7 days, but can occasionally be longer [70]. Provocation of psychogenic attacks may shorten the required duration of video-EEG monitoring, including simple suggestion, activation techniques of photic stimulation and hyperventilation, and the use of an injected placebo. Habitual nonepileptic events by simple activation and suggestion techniques during short-term outpatient video-EEG monitoring (ranging from 40 minutes to 2 hours) are reported in 50–76% of patients [71–73]. Distinguishing an event as habitual by eyewitness account is essential to avoiding misdiagnosis. The advantages of using provocation include obviating the need for an inpatient admission and achieving a specificity for diagnosing psychogenic attacks approaching 100% [74]. Disadvantages include the potential to miss a coexisting epilepsy and limited interictal EEG recording [75]. The ethics of provocation are controversial [74–76]. Nondisclosure of provocation is a potential "abuse" of a vulnerable person. However, neither placebo saline injection nor nondisclosure is necessary when attempting provocation of psychogenic attacks. Among epileptologists surveyed, 40% use provocation techniques, the majority using hyperventilation with suggestion. However, half report using saline [68] and 23% acknowledge some ethical conflict [68]. Our feeling is that when spell provocation, with or without preceding disclosure, is motivated from the perspective of physician beneficence (acting in the patient's best interest – a valid ethical perspective competing with patient autonomy), the accurate diagnosis that enables effective treatment of psychogenic attacks argues instead in favor of provocation.

Analysis of EEG is often difficult in patients with psychogenic attack and inter-rater reliability is lower than for epileptic seizures [77]. The EEG recording may be obscured by rhythmic movement artifact during "convulsive" psychogenic or epileptic events. However, in psychogenic attacks, EEG frequency remains stable, whereas in epileptic seizures, frequency evolves during the event [78]. In order to minimize error, more than one habitual event should be recorded, to ensure lack of event stereotypy and to provide diagnostic confidence that events are not true epileptic seizures; when doubt remains, repeating inpatient video- EEG monitoring is always appropriate.

Treatment

Another challenge of psychogenic attacks is to effectively communicate the diagnosis to the patient and their family. When the initial communication goes well, symptoms settle in most patients [79]. The approach to treatment is outlined in Box 16.2. A team approach to sharing the diagnosis is important and should include the physician, psychology, social work support, psychiatry, and additional members as appropriate (such as a child protection agency, counselor, family physician, or nursing support). However, there are often fundamental differences in how individual team members think; for example, psychiatrists may view video-EEG as inaccurate, while neurologists may think that the predominant factor contributing to a patient's outcome is their own psychopathology rather than the doctors'

impact in promptly and effectively communicating the accurate diagnosis [80]. The team should meet first and clarify the diagnosis, clearly plan the therapeutic interventions, and discuss close follow-up plans. An honest and clear approach discussing reasons for concluding the patient does not have epilepsy, clearly describing the diagnosis of psychogenic attacks (emphasizing that they are not suspected of "faking" the attacks), reassuring the patient and their family of a lack of clearly associated psychopathology (when appropriate), and discussing triggering factors and etiological factors that may be involved should follow [81,82]. Close multidisciplinary follow-up is important. A suggested model for approaching treatment includes creating a list of predisposing, precipitant, and perpetuating factors with the patient once the diagnosis is disclosed [28]. Appropriate psychotherapy or pharmacologic therapy can then be offered. In 2005, an international interdisciplinary group gathered to discuss developments in the treatment of patients with psychogenic attacks. The group highlighted the need for further research to evaluate existing therapeutic interventions and to identify new ones [83]. Since then, a small number of studies have been published for both drug therapy and cognitive behavioral therapy (CBT).

Box 16.2 Approach to relaying diagnosis and treating patients with psychogenic attack.

- Honestly and clearly discuss reasons for concluding the spells are not epileptic in nature.
- Clearly describe the diagnosis of psychogenic attacks.
- Emphasize that the patient is not suspected of "faking" attacks.
- Reassure the patient and their family concerning the lack of clearly associated psychopathology, when appropriate.
- Invite the patient to privately discuss any triggering and underlying causative psychological or stress-related factors that might be involved.
- Establish prompt and close multidisciplinary follow-up.
- Provide psychological care with cognitive behavioral therapy.
- Consider psychotherapy.
- Consider pharmacological treatment with an antidepressant medication.

Pharmacologic agents may be helpful in treating some patients with psychogenic attacks. A small double-blind, randomized, placebo-controlled study evaluating sertraline, a selective serotonin reuptake inhibitor (SSRI), found that psychogenic attacks were reduced in patients treated with sertraline, while they were slightly increased in those treated with placebo [84]. A larger-scale study is necessary to corroborate this class II evidence. In another study, seizure event frequency was reduced, as were depressive or anxiety symptoms [85].

Most neurologists endorse psychotherapy for patients with psychogenic attacks but data on its effectiveness are limited. Class III evidence suggests that CBT in addition to standard medical care significantly reduces attack frequency [86]. Health care utilization also declines significantly following psychotherapy [87].

In most cases, the essential role of patient support is provided by psychology and social work teams, but they should not work in isolation. Recent evidence of antidepressant agent efficacy in treating psychogenic attacks may encourage more active participation from the psychiatric community, which unfortunately thus far has devoted little attention to somatoform disorders, including psychogenic attacks [88,89].

Prognosis

Children with psychogenic attacks have a better outcome than their adult counterparts, with up to 66% becoming "seizure-free" [90]. Causes of psychogenic attacks among children are more likely to be external, more easily identified, and more amenable to prompt intervention. Outcome figures for adults show significantly lower rates of "seizure freedom," varying from 33 to 40% [79,91,92]. Significant morbidity of psychogenic attacks is also reported, with over half of patients dependent on social security [91] and 44% having a poor outcome (continued spells and significantly impaired function, including unemployment), figures even worse than those for newly diagnosed epilepsy [91]. A good outcome is associated with shorter history of psychogenic attacks, less acute psychiatric dysfunction, a history of acute emotional trauma preceding event onset, lack of coexisting epilepsy, and living an independent lifestyle [93,94].

Follow-up

Close multidisciplinary follow-up is crucial. Patients are often confused and uncertain about their diagnosis and treatment. Often their neurologist has been managing their care since the onset of their events and sudden transition to a psychiatrist or other health care provider is unhelpful. Rather, neurology, psychiatry, and psychology teams should work together. The best scenario is an initial joint clinic visit, enabling a clear consensus on the plan for the patient.

The grey zone: driving and psychogenic attacks

There is no clear guideline or consensus on managing antiepileptic medication and driving permission among patients with psychogenic attacks [95–97]. A US physician survey reported that almost 50% of respondents would apply the same restrictions for patients with psychogenic attacks as for epilepsy, 32% would place no restrictions on driving, and 19% would decide on a case-by-case basis. [95] In German and British surveys, most respondents reported imposing driving restrictions on patients with psychogenic attacks [96,97].

Certainly, all approaches must consider safety as paramount. Decisions need to be tailored to the individual patient, but in most cases we suggest gradually tapering and withdrawing antiepileptic medications. If a new type of event occurs or events escalate during medication withdrawal, admission for repeat video-EEG to categorize them is suggested. If continued clinical events lead to loss of control, driving is unsafe regardless of an epileptic or nonepileptic cause. If the patient is stable and events have resolved, resumption of driving may be considered. Our usual approach is to wean antiepileptic medication and ensure the patient is stable prior to restoring driving privileges. The risk of motor vehicle accidents in patients with psychogenic attacks requires further study; it is essential to establish a consensus and provide sufficient evidence-based guidance for patients and their clinicians [97].

Conclusion

When it comes to managing comorbidities of epilepsy, positive therapeutic leaps comparable to those achieved in surgical epilepsy practice have yet to be achieved. For patients with psychogenic attacks, we must maintain a high index of suspicion, promptly employ diagnostic video-EEG monitoring to allow an accurate and certain diagnosis, clearly and compassionately communicate the diagnosis to the patient and their family, and deploy a team-based therapeutic and follow-up approach to maximize patient outcomes. Certainly, the general lack of interest shown by the professional mental health organizations, at least in the United States [98], is a contributor to poor outcome and to patients feeling abandoned.

References

1 Goetz CG: *Charcot, The Clinician: The Tuesday Lessons*. Raven Press, New York, NY, 1987, pp. 102–122.

2 Gates JR: Epidemiology and classification of non-epileptic events. In: Gates JR, Rowan AJ (eds): *Nonepileptic Seizures*, 2 edn. Butterworth-Heinemann, Boston, MA, 2000, pp. 3–14.

3 Benbadis SR: Psychogenic nonepileptic "seizure" or "attacks"? It's not just semantics: attacks. *Neurology* 2010; **75(1)**: 84–86.

4 Ozkara C, Dreifuss FE: Differential diagnosis in pseudoepileptic seizures. *Epilepsia* 1993; **34(2)**:294–298.

5 DeToledo JC, Lowe MR, Puig A: Nonepileptic seizures in pregnancy. *Neurology* 2000; **55(1)**:120–121.

6 Reuber M, Mitchell AJ, Howlett S, Elger CE: Measuring outcome in psychogenic nonepileptic seizures: how relevant is seizure remission? *Epilepsia* 2005; **46(11)**:1788–1795.

7 Siket MS, Merchant RC: Psychogenic seizures: a review and description of pitfalls in the acute diagnosis and management in the emergency department. *Emerg Med Clin North Am* 2011; **29(1)**:73–81.

8 Bourgeois JA, Chang CH, Hilty DM et al.: Clinical manifestations and management of conversion disorders. *Curr Treat Options Neurol* 2002; **4**:487–497.

9 World Health Organization: *The ICD-10 Classification of Mental and Behavioural Disorders: Clinical Descriptions and Diagnostic Guidelines*. WHO, Geneva, 1992.

10 American Psychiatric Association: *Diagnostic and Statistical Manual of Mental Disorders*, 4 edn. American Psychiatric Association, Washington, DC, 1994.

11 Whitaker JN: The confluence of quality of care, cost-effectiveness, pragmatism, and medical ethics in the diagnosis of nonepileptic seizures. *Arch Neurol* 2001; **56**: 2066–2067.

12 Nowack WJ: Epilepsy: a costly misdiagnosis. *Clin Electroencephalogr* 1997; **28**:225–228.

13 Martin RC, Gilliam FG, Kilgore M et al.: Improved healthcare resource utilization following video-EEG-confirmed diagnosis of nonepileptic seizures. *Seizure* 1998; **7**:185–190.

14 Sigurdardottir KR, Olafsson E: Incidence of psychogenic seizures in adults: a population-based study in Iceland. *Epilepsia* 1998; **39**:749–752.

15 Szaflarski JP, Ficker DM, Cahill WT, Privitera MD: Four-year incidence of psychogenic nonepileptic seizures in adults in Hamilton County, OH. *Neurology* 2000; **55**:1561–1563.

16 Benbadis SR, Hauser WA: An estimate of the prevalence of psychogenic non-epileptic seizures. *Seizure* 2000; **9**: 280–281.

17 Reuber M, Elger CE: Psychogenic nonepileptic seizures: review and update. *Epilepsy Behav* 2003; **4(3)**:205–216.

18 Lesser RP: Psychogenic seizures. *Neurology* 1996; **46**: 1499–1507.

19 Reuber M, Mitchell AJ, Howlett JS et al.: Functional symptoms in neurology: questions and answers. *J Neurol Neurosurg Psychiatry* 2005; **76**:307–314.

20 de Timary P, Fouchet P, Sylin M et al.: Non-epileptic seizures: delayed diagnosis in patients presenting with electroencephalographic (EEG) or clinical signs of epileptic seizures. *Seizure* 2002; **11(3)**:193–197.

21 Benbadis SR: How many patients with pseudoseizures receive antiepileptic drugs prior to diagnosis? *Eur Neurol* 1999; **41(2)**:114–115.

22 Benbadis SR, Hauser WA: An estimate of the prevalence of psychogenic non-epileptic seizures. *Seizure* 2000; **55**: 1904–1905.

23 Lancman ME, Lambrakis CHC, Steinhardt MJ: Psychogenic pseudoseizures: a general overview. In: Ettinger AB, Kanner AM (eds): *Psychiatric Issues in Epilepsy*. Lippincott Williams & Wilkins, Philadelphia, PA, 2001, pp. 341–354.

24 Benbadis SR, Agrawal V, Tatum WO 4th,: How many patients with psychogenic nonepileptic seizures also have epilepsy. *Neurology* 2001; **57(5)**:915–917.

25 Hovorka J, Nezadal T, Herman E et al.: Psychogenic nonepileptic seizures, prospective clinical experience: diagnosis, clinical features, risk factors, psychiatric co-morbidity, treatment outcome. *Epileptic Disord* 2007; **9(Suppl. 1)**: S52–S58.

26 Andreason NC, Black DW: Somatoform and related disorders. In: Andreason NC, Black DW (eds): *Introductory Textbook of Psychiatry*, 3 edn. American Psychiatric Publishing, Washington, DC, 2001.

27 Reilly J, Baker GA, Rhodes J, Salmon P: The association of sexual and physical abuse with somatisation: characteristics of patients presenting with irritable bowel syndrome and non-epileptic attack disorder. *Psychol Med* 1999; **29**:399–406.

28 LaFrance WC, Devinsky O: Treatment of nonepileptic seizures. *Epilepsy Behav* 2002; **3(5 Suppl.)**:19–23.

29 Alper KA, Devinsky O, Perrine K et al.: Nonepileptic seizures and childhood sexual and physical abuse. *Neurology* 1993; **43**:1950–1953.

30 Bowman ES, Markand ON: Psychodynamics and psychiatric diagnoses of pseudoseizure subjects. *Am J Psychiatry* 1996; **153**:57–63.

31 Brown RJ, Cardena E, Nijenhuis E, van der Hart O: Should conversion disorder be reclassified as dissociation disorder in DSM-V. *Psychosomatics* 2007; **48**:369–378.

32 Bowman ES: Psychopathology and outcome in pseudo-seizures. In: Ettinger AB, Kanner AM (eds): *Psychiatric Issues in Epilepsy: A Practical Guide to Diagnosis and Treatment.* Lippincott Williams & Wilkins, Philadelphia, PA, 2001, pp. 355–377.

33 Strutt AM, Hill SW, Scott BM et al.: A comprehensive neuropsychological profile of women with psychogenic nonepileptic seizures. *Epilepsy Behav* 2011; **20(1)**:24–28.

34 Bakvis P, Spinhoven P, Giltay EJ et al.: Basal hypercortisolism and trauma in patients with psychogenic nonepileptic seizures. *Epilepsia* 2010; **51(5)**:752–759.

35 Katz L, Fleisher W, Kjernisted K et al.: A review of the psychobiology and pharmacotherapy of posttraumatic stress disorder. *Can J Psychiatry* 1997; **42**:467–475.

36 Drevets WC: Functional neuroimaging studies of depression: the anatomy of melancholia. *Annu Rev Med* 1998; **49**: 341–361.

37 Stone J, Zeman A, Simonotto E et al.: FMRI in patients with motor conversion symptoms and controls with simulated weakness. *Psychosom Med* 2007; **69(9)**:961–969.

38 Reolofs K, Keijsers GPJ, Hoogduin CAL et al.: Childhood abuse in patients with conversion disorder. *Am J Psychiatry* 2002; **159**:1980–1913.

39 Bowman ES, Markand ON: The contribution of life events to pseudoseizure occurrence in adults. *Bull Menninger Clin* 1999; **63**:70–88.

40 Fleisher W, Staley D, Krawetz P et al.: Comparative study of trauma-related phenomena in subjects with pseudo-seizures and subjects with epilepsy. *Am J Psychiatry* 2002; **159**:660–663.

41 Bremner JD, Randall P, Scott PM et al.: Deficits in short-term memory in adult survivors of childhood abuse. *Psychiatry Res* 1995; **59**:97–107.

42 Wyllie E, Glazer JP, Benbadis SR et al.: Psychiatric features of children and adolescents with pseudoseizures. *Arch Pediatr Adolesc Med* 1999; **153**:244–248.

43 Dworetzky BA, Bubrick EJ, Szaflarski JP, Nonepileptic Seizure Task Force: Nonepileptic psychogenic status: markedly prolonged psychogenic seizures. *Epilepsy Behav* 2010; **19(1)**:65–68.

44 Duncan R, Oto M: Psychogenic nonepileptic seizures in patients with learning disability: comparison with patients with no learning disability. *Epilepsy Behav* 2008; **12(1)**: 183–186.

45 Papavasiliou A, Vassilaki N, Paraskevoulakos et al.: Psychogenic status epilepticus in children. *Epilepsy Behav* 2004; **5(4)**:539–546.

46 Rotge JY, Lambrecq V, Marchal C et al.: Conversion disorder and coexisting nonepileptic seizures in patients with refractory seizures. *Epilepsy Behav* 2009; **16(2)**:350–352.

47 Ramsay RE, Cohen A, Brown MC: Coexisting epilepsy and non-epileptic seizures. In: Gates JR, Rowan AJ (eds): *Non-Epileptic Seizures.* Butterworth-Heinemann, Boston, MA, 1993, pp. 47–54.

48 Ney GC, Barr WB, Napolitano C et al.: New-onset psychogenic seizures after surgery for epilepsy. *Arch Neurol* 1998; **55**:726–730.

49 Glosser G, Robert D, Glosser DS: Nonepileptic seizures after resective epilepsy surgery. *Epilepsia* 1999; **40(12)**: 1750–1754.

50 Krahn LE, Rummans TA, Sharbrough FW et al.: Pseudo-seizures after epilepsy surgery. *Psychosomatics* 1995; **36**: 487–493.

51 Uldall P, Alving J, Hansen LK et al.: The misdiagnosis of epilepsy in children admitted to atertiary epilepsy center with paroxysmal events. *Arch Dis Child* 2006; **91**:219–221.

52 Boesebeck F, Freermann S, Kellinghaus C, Evers S: Misdiagnosis of epileptic and non-epileptic seizures in a neurological intensive care unit. *Acta Neurol Scand* 2010; **122(3)**:189–195.

53 Reuber M: Psychogenic nonepileptic seizures: diagnosis, aetiology, treatment and prognosis. *Arch Neurol Psychiatr* 2005; **156**:47–57.

54 Mellers JDC: The approach to patients with "non-epileptic seizures." *Postgrad Med* 2005; **81**:498–504.

55 Tamer SK: The pediatric non-epileptic seizure. *Indian J Pediatr* 1997; **64(5)**:671–676.

56 Bergen D, Ristanovic R: Weeping as a common element of pseudoseizures. *Arch Neurol* 1993; **50(10)**:1059–1060.

57 Verotti A, Agostinelli S, Mohn A et al.: Clinical features of psychogenic non-epileptic seizures in pre-pubertal and pubertal patients with idiopathic epilepsy. *Neurol Sci* 2009; **30(4)**:319–323.

58 Opherk C, Hirsch LJ: Ictal heart rate differentiates epileptic from non-epileptic seizures. *Neurology* 2002; **58(4)**:636–638.

59 Orbach D, Ritaccio A, Devinsky O: Psychogenic, nonepileptic seizures associated with video-EEG-verified sleep. *Epilepsia* 2003; **44(1)**:64–68.

60 Syed TU, Arozullah AM, Loparo KL et al.: A self-administered screening instrument for psychogenic nonepileptic seizures. *Neurology* 2009; **72(19)**:1646–1652.

61 Trimble MR: Serum prolactin in epilepsy and hysteria. *BMJ* 1978; **2(6153)**:1682.

62 Gallaghjer BB, Flanigan HF, Kind DW, Littleton WH: The effect of electrical stimulation of the medial temporal lobe structures in epileptic patients upon stimulation of ACTH, prolactin and growth hormone. *Neurology* 1987; **37**: 299–303.

63 Chen DK, So YT, Fischer RS: Use of serum prolactin in diagnosing epileptic seizures. Report of the Therapeutics and Technology Assessment Subcommittee of the American Academy of Neurology. *Neurology* 2005; **65**;668–675.

64 Lusic I, Pintaric I, Hozo I et al.: Serum prolactin levels after seizure and syncopal attacks. *Seizure* 1999; **8**:218–222.

65 Petramfar P, Yaghoobi E, Nemati R, Asadi-Pooya AA: Serum creatine phosphokinase is helpful in distinguishing generalized tonic-clonic seizures from psychogenic nonepileptic seizures and vasovagal syncope. *Epilepsy Behav* 2009; **15(3)**:330–332.

66 Benbadis SR: The EEG in nonepileptic seizures. *J Clin Neurophys* 2006; **23(4)**:340–352.

67 Benbadis SR, Lafrance WC, Korabathina K, Lin K, Papandonatos GD, Kraemer H: Interrater reliability of EEG-video monitoring. *Neurology* 2009; **73**:843–846.

68 Schachter SC, Fraser B, Rowan AJ: Provocation testing for non-epileptic seizures: attitudes and practices in the United States among American Epilepsy Society members. *J Epilepsy* 1996; **9**:249–252.

69 Watemberg N, Tziperman B, Dabby R et al.: Adding video recording increases the diagnostic yield of routine Electroencephalograms in children with frequent paroxysmal events. *Epilepsia* 2005; **46(5)**:716–719.

70 Friedman DE, Hirsch LJ: How long does it take to make an accurate diagnosis in an epilepsy monitoring unit. *J Clin Neurophysiol* 2009; **26(4)**:213–217.

71 McGonigal A, Russell AJC, Mallik AK et al.: Use of short term video EEG in the diagnosis of attack disorders. *J Neurol Neurosurg Psychiatry* 2004; **75**:771–772.

72 McGonigal A, Oto M, Russell AJC et al.: Outpatient video EEG reocirding in the diagnosis of non-epileptic seizures: a randomized controlled trial of simple suggestion techniques. *J Neurol Neurosurg Psychiatry* 2002; **75**:549–551.

73 Varela HL, Taylor DS, Benbadis SR: Short-term outpatient EEG-video monitoring with inducation in a veterans administration population. *J Clin Neurophysiol* 2007; **24(5)**: 390–391.

74 Benbadis SR: Provocation techniques should be used for the diagnosis of psychogenic seizures. *Arch Neurol* 2001: **58**: 2063–2065.

75 Gates JR: Provocation techniques should not be used for nonepileptic seizures. *Arch Neurol* 2001; **58**:2065–2066.

76 Benbadis SR: Provocative techniques should be used for the diagnosis of psychogenic nonepileptic seizures. *Epilepsy Behav* 2009; **15(2)**:106–109.

77 Benbadis SR, LaFrance WC, Papandonatos GD et al.: Interrater reliability of EEG-video monitoring. *Neurology* 2009; **73**:843–846.

78 Vinton A, Carino J, Vogrin S et al.: "Convulsive" nonepileptic seizures have a characteristic pattern of rhythmic artifact distinguishing them from convulsive epileptic seizures. *Epilepsia* 2004; **45(11)**:1344–1350.

79 Carton S, Thompson PJ, Duncan JS: Non-epileptic seizures: patients' understanding and reaction to the diagnosis and impact on outcome. *Seizure* 2003; **12**:287–294.

80 Harden CL, Burgut FT, Kanner AM: The diagnostic significance of video-EEG monitoring findings on pseudoseizure patients differs between neurologists and psychiatrists. *Epilepsia* 2003; **44(3)**:453–456.

81 Friedman JH, LaFrance C: Psychogenic disorders the need to speak plainly. *Arch Neurol* 2010; **67**:753–755.

82 Mellers JDC: The approach to patients with "non-epileptic seizures." *Postgrad Med J* 2005; **81**:498–504.

83 LaFrance WC Jr, Alper K, Babock D et al.: Nonepileptic seizures treatment workshop summary. *Epilepsy Behav* 2006; **8(3)**:451–461.

84 LaFrance WC Jr, Keitner GI, Papandonatos GD et al.: Pilot pharmacologic randomized controlled trial for psychogenic non-epileptic seizures. *Neurology* 2010; **75(13)**:1166–1173.

85 Pintor L, Bailles E, Matrai S et al.: Efficiency of Venlafaxine in patients with psychogenic nonepileptic seizures and anxiety and/or depressive disorders. *J Neuropsych Clin Neurosci* 2010; **22**:401–408.

86 Goldstein LH, Chalder T, Chigwere C et al.: Cognitive–behavioral therapy for psychogenic nonepileptic seizures: a pilot RCT. *Neurology* 2010; **74**:1986–1994.

87 Mayor R, Howlett S, Grunewald R, Reuber M: Long-term outcome of brief augmented psychodynamic interpersonal therapy for psychogenic nonepileptic seizures:seizure control and health care utilization. *Epilepsia* 2010; **51**: 1169–1176.

88 Benbadis SR: The problem of psychogenic symptoms: Is the psychiatric community in denial? *Epilepsy Behav* 2005; **6**:9–14.

89 Benbadis SR: Mental health organizations and the ostrich policy. *Neuropsychiatry* 2013; **1**:5–7.

90 Irwin K, Edwards M, Robinson R: Psychogenic non-epileptic seizures: management and prognosis. *Arch Dis Child* 2000; **82**:474–478.

91 Reuber M, Pukrop R, Bauer J et al.: Outcome in psychogenic nonepileptic seizures: 1 to 10 year follow-up in 164 patients. *Ann Neurol* 2003; **53(3)**:305–311.

92 Bowman ES: Nonepileptic seizures: psychiatric framework, treatment and outcome. *Neurology* 1999; **53(5 Suppl. 2)**: S84–S88.

93 Guberman A: Psychogenic pseudo-seizures in non-epileptic patients. *Can J Psych* 1982; **27**:401–404.

94 Meierkord H, Will B, Fish D, Shorvon S: The clinical features and prognosis of pseudoseizures diagnosed using video-telemetry. *Neurology* 1991; **41**:1643–1646.

95 Benbadis SR, Blustein JN, Sunstadt L: Should patients with pseudoseizures be allowed to drive? *Epilepsia* 2000; **41**:895–897.

96 Spect U, Thorbecke R: Should patients with psychogenic nonepileptic seizures be allowed to drive? Recommendations of German experts. *Epilepsy Behav* 2009; **16(3)**: 547–550.

97 Morrison I, Razvi SSM: Driving regulations and psychogenic non-epileptic seizures: perspectives from the United Kingdom. *Seizure* 2011; **20(2)**:177–180.

98 Benbadis SR: Mental health organizations and the ostrich policy. *Neuropsychiatry* 2013; **1**:5–7.

General health and epilepsy

CHAPTER 17

Obesity and epilepsy

Sandra J. Petty[1] and Alison M. Pack[2]

[1] The Florey Institute of Neuroscience and Mental Health, Ormond College, and, Department of Medicine, Royal Melbourne Hospital, University of Melbourne, Australia

[2] Neurological Institute, Columbia University, USA

Introduction

The obesity epidemic is well recognized in Western society [1] and is increasing globally [2]. The prevalence of obesity has sometimes been found to be higher among patients with epilepsy, but the problem is less studied in this patient group than in the general population [3]. Prevalence rates of obesity in epilepsy vary across available studies and are likely to be interrelated with activity levels and other health factors. The potential for cardiovascular risk [4] and metabolic syndrome [4,5], reduced antiepileptic drug (AED) treatment adherence [6], and psychosocial effects of weight gain and obesity [7] all require attention and the mechanisms of weight gain and strategies for prevention of obesity require further study [8]. The problem of obesity in epilepsy requires longitudinal research into risk factors, treatment strategies, weight loss effectiveness, and secondary prevention of complications.

Weight gain is common in association with treatment with some AEDs. It has been long recognized that patients taking sodium valproate may experience weight gain, and more recently the metabolic syndrome has been detected [9]. There can be a rapid weight increase early in therapy and close weight monitoring is recommended [8]. In addition, longer-term monitoring of weight is recommended for patients taking valproate [10]. Weight gain can also be associated with use of carbamazepine, gabapentin, pregabalin, and vigabatrin [6,11].

Interestingly, the problem of obesity in patients with epilepsy has also been found in AED treatment-naive children, and thus the occurrence of obesity in epilepsy does not rest solely upon a medication side effect [12]. Prevalence is likely to depend on additional factors, including physical activity levels, dietary intake, and the association of obesity with more refractory seizures and AED polytherapy [13].

Whether there are direct neural or hormonal factors [14] linking epilepsy and obesity requires further research [15]. In a retrospective cohort study, after adjustment for age, gender, and smoking status, the incidence rate of seizures was found to be increased in extremely obese patients (BMI $\geq$40) when compared to those of normal weight [16], with an incidence rate ratio of 1.7 (95% CI 0.7, 3.9), but the difference was not statistically significant. Factors related to obesity in the general population – broadly, the positive imbalance between caloric intake and energy expenditure, the presence of other medical conditions or medications causing weight gain (e.g., thyroid disease, depression, use of glucocorticoid, some antipsychotics), and diet and lifestyle factors – also need to be considered.

The health consequences of obesity are important to assess in patients with epilepsy. For example, extreme obesity and associated cardiovascular disease may raise valid operative risk concerns in patients being assessed for epilepsy surgery. However, a retrospective study of body mass index (BMI) as a predictor did not show an increased perioperative risk or differing seizure outcomes in patients undergoing anterior temporal lobectomy with amygdalohippocampectomy [17]. There was a statistically significant increase in later mortality in the extremely obese group, although data on cause of death were limited [17]. The authors discussed a potential limitation whereby medical prescreening

Epilepsy and the Interictal State: Co-Morbidities and Quality of Life, First Edition.
Edited by Erik K. St. Louis, David M. Ficker, and Terence J. O'Brien.
© 2015 John Wiley & Sons, Ltd. Published 2015 by John Wiley & Sons, Ltd.

might have prevented surgical management of some patients with extreme obesity and significant cardiovascular comorbidity, meaning this group may have been underrepresented [17]. In addition, the risk of acute myocardial infarction and a subsequent poor outcome may be increased in patients with epilepsy [18]. In some cases, accessibility of MRI or other scanning techniques is limited if the scanner manufacturer's weight safety limits or the machine's physical dimensions are exceeded.

Weight management, and carefully supervised weight reduction (where indicated) after assessment of cardiovascular and exercise injury risks, may improve fitness and well-being and reduce the risk of adverse health consequences of obesity. Weight gain and obesity are important issues for consideration in some patients with epilepsy and should ideally form part of care for epilepsy patients, in both primary care and specialist centers.

Epidemiology

The incidence and prevalence of obesity among patients with epilepsy has received limited study. Reported studies suggest that adults and children with epilepsy have higher rates of obesity. In a population-based sample of over 8000 persons, patients with epilepsy were more likely to be obese (34.1 versus 23.7% rate of obesity in adults with and without epilepsy, respectively) [19]. Likewise, children with newly diagnosed untreated epilepsy had higher BMI Z scores compared to standard Centers for Disease Control and Prevention (CDC) growth charts (p < 0.0001) and a healthy control cohort (p < 0.0002) [12]. Among the epilepsy cohort, 38.6% were overweight or obese. Factors contributing to obesity among patients with epilepsy include physical inactivity, secondary effects on hormones, AED treatment, and comorbid depression.

Pathophysiology

Although obesity is reported commonly in persons with epilepsy, the mechanisms explaining this association are not well defined. The impact of hormonal changes, the effect of AEDs, limited physical activity, and comorbid mood changes may all contribute to the risk of obesity in patients with epilepsy.

Epilepsy and hormonal changes

Alterations in hormonal profiles have been described in patients with epilepsy. Hormonal changes can result in multiple clinical sequelae, including obesity. Abnormalities in sex steroid hormones, thyroid hormones, leptin, and ghrelin are all associated with obesity. These hormones can be affected in patients with epilepsy treated with AEDs.

Reproductive hormones may be altered in men and women with epilepsy. These alterations are likely secondary to a complex relationship between the sex steroid hormone axis, the epilepsy itself, and AED therapy [20,21]. The concentration and metabolism of estrogen, testosterone, and dehydroepiandrosterone may be modified in persons with epilepsy. These endocrinologic changes can be secondary to epilepsy itself. In those with temporal-lobe epilepsy (TLE), extensive connections between limbic structures and the hypothalamus and pituitary may cause changes in sex steroid hormones. Interestingly, in a cohort of women with partial epilepsy, free estradiol and progesterone were more significantly affected in those with more frequent seizures, supporting the notion that epilepsy itself affects reproductive hormones and function [22]. AED therapy can also affect sex hormones and their binding proteins, resulting in reproductive abnormalities [23]. Polycystic ovarian syndrome (PCOS) is a common hormonal or endocrine disorder associated with obesity. It occurs in 10–25% of women with epilepsy, independent of AED treatment [21]. In the general population, reported percentages are between 5 and 6%. Some studies suggest that sodium valproate therapy may increase the risk of PCOS [21]. This is not a consistent finding in all studies, however. Given the higher prevalence of PCOS among women with epilepsy, PCOS should be considered in obese women with epilepsy.

Abnormalities in thyroid function, specifically hypothyroidism, can result in increased weight and obesity. Thyroid function is not affected by epilepsy itself [20]. Although alterations have been described in association with some AEDs (carbamazepine, phenytoin), these patients are typically euthyroid [20]. As such, clinically relevant thyroid disorders are not commonly described specifically in association with epilepsy and AED treatment. Thyroid dysfunction related to epilepsy and AEDs is therefore not a significant factor contributing to obesity in patients with epilepsy.

Leptin is an adipokine expressed primarily in adipocytes. Although leptin has a number of actions, its most important role is in regulation of body weight. Leptin concentration in adipocytes is directly related to obesity severity and positively correlates with BMI and insulin concentrations. No reported studies suggest an independent effect of epilepsy itself on leptin concentrations. Increased concentrations of leptin in association with sodium valproate therapy are found [8]. This increase may be secondary to obesity itself, however. In one study, after a year of treatment, increased leptin concentrations were seen only in obese subjects and not in those who were nonobese [24]. Abnormalities in leptin have not been described in association with other AEDs, including carbamazepine and oxcarbazepine [25–27].

Ghrelin is an adipokine produced in the stomach that is a potent appetite-stimulating hormone [28]. Plasma ghrelin levels increase before meals and decrease postprandially. In the literature, there are no clear associations between changes in gherlin and obesity. Patients treated with sodium valproate who are obese have reduced gherlin levels [8,29,30]. Carbamazepine therapy also appears to reduce gherlin levels [30]. The clinical consequences of these reductions remain unclear.

Antiepileptic drugs

Numerous AEDs are commonly associated with weight gain (sodium valproate, gabapentin, pregabalin, carbamazepine). Sodium valproate treatment can result in weight gain and subsequent obesity. The reported frequency of weight gain in the literature is variable, ranging from 10 to 70% [8]. Studies suggest that weight gain is more common in women than in men [27,31,32]. While as a group both men and women experienced significant weight gain in one study of 106 subjects (55 women and 51 men), the women gained weight more frequently (43.6 versus 23.5% of women and men, respectively) and in larger amounts [31]. Weight gain has been reported to occur within the first 3 months of treatment, with a peak at the sixth month [8,33]. The exact mechanism to explain the association between sodium valproate, weight gain, and obesity is unclear and requires further study. Postulated mechanisms include dysregulation of the hypothalamus (as evidenced by reported increased appetite and thirst), effects on adipokine levels, hyperinsulinemia, and insulin resistance [8]. Gabapentin is also associated with weight gain. In an open-label study of patients treated

with high-dose gabapentin therapy and followed for over 12 months, 57% gained more than 5% of their baseline body weight, with 10 patients gaining more than 10% of their original body weight [34]. Similarly, pregabalin therapy can result in weight gain. In double-blind, placebo-controlled studies for epilepsy, 12–14% of patients in the highest treatment group of 600 mg/day gained weight, compared to about 6% in the placebo group and 10% in the 150 mg/day group [35,36]. Although not as well studied, carbamazepine is associated with weight gain [6].

Exercise

Patients with epilepsy are less likely to exercise and participate in activities that promote a healthy lifestyle. In a Canadian national population-based survey of the health status and health behaviors of Canadian adolescents and adults, 60% of patients with epilepsy were physically inactive, compared to 50% of the general population [3]. After adjusting for age, gender, education, and income, those with epilepsy were 1.4 times more likely to be inactive than the general population (odds ratio (OR) 1.4, 95% CI 1.1–1.7). Another Canadian study in children and adolescents found that those with epilepsy participated in fewer sport activities and were more likely to be overweight [3]. The only epilepsy-specific factor correlating to activity level was seizure frequency. Among 178 Korean subjects with epilepsy, 58% were described as being inactive and 40% did not participate in any leisure-time physical activity. Inactive persons were more likely to be on AED polytherapy, have anxiety, or have had previous seizure experiences during activities [37]. The reported lack of exercise in patients with epilepsy can result in weight gain and obesity.

Psychiatric comorbidities

Psychiatric comorbidities, including depression and anxiety, are common among patients with epilepsy [38]. Prospective studies find that depression and obesity are associated [39,40]. A longitudinal cohort of over 4000 black and white young adults found that respondents who started out with higher levels of depressive symptoms experienced a faster rate of increase in BMI (white youths only) and waist circumference (black and white youths) over time [41]. The study did not evaluate the effect of potential mediators, including antidepressant medication. Although not studied in patients with epilepsy, these results would suggest that those who have comorbid depression may be at increased risk for weight gain and obesity. Further study should evaluate the effect of mood on weight among patients with epilepsy.

Evaluation

There are no specific formal guidelines for how clinicians should assist patients with epilepsy in weight assessment and management. A useful approach for the physician and patient in clinic would include awareness and education, dietician referral, weight monitoring, and assessment and treatment for obesity causes, related conditions, and complications. Patient-based epilepsy support groups may be a good resource and can provide practical information to patients.

Weight record

At the time of diagnosis of epilepsy (or at commencement of AED therapy), it is useful to record the patient's baseline weight and height for current health assessment and as a future reference point. If a weight-management problem is identified, strategies for weight reduction (if indicated) and prevention of weight gain should be discussed. A dietician and primary care physician can assist with further assessment and management.

Anthropometry
Adults

BMI is an index calculated as weight (kg)/height squared (m^2). This can stratify weight into classifications including underweight, normal weight, overweight, and obese (see Table 17.1). Further BMI subclassifications can be found at http://apps.who.int/bmi/index.jsp?introPage=intro_3.html (last accessed July 15, 2014). It should be noted that some variations in the BMI classification criteria apply in different ethnic populations [42] and that there are some limitations on the use of BMI, such as where patients have a muscular build.

In clinic, the use of a waist circumference (>94 cm in men and >80 cm in women), and in particular a waist/hip ratio (>0.95 in men and >0.8 in women), indicates increased cardiovascular risk [43]. The waist/hip ratio in older people is utilized as a measure to detect relative abdominal obesity and may be a useful indicator of a higher risk of circulatory mortality [44].

Table 17.1 Body mass index (BMI) criteria.

Classification	BMI (kg/m^2)
Underweight	<18.5
Normal weight	18.5–24.99
Overweight	≥25
Obese	≥30

However, it should be noted that these simple clinical measures and cut-offs have some variability with age, gender, and ethnicity [45].

Skinfold fat testing can be arranged but it is time-consuming and is probably not practical in the epilepsy clinic setting, although it may be available through an obesity or metabolic clinic.

Children

In the United States, childhood obesity is currently classified as ≥95th percentile for BMI for age, and overweight as >85th and <95th percentile for BMI for age [46].

Assessment of factors contributing to weight gain and obesity

Assessment of other factors contributing to weight gain and obesity should be performed [47]. This would include a detailed medical history, medication review, and diet and physical activity history. Comorbidities that might affect the safety of an exercise program should be assessed for, and referrals made where appropriate. Potential referrals may include: cardiologist for cardiovascular conditions, hypertension, dyslipidaemia, and risk-factor modification; endocrinology for assessment of endocrine obesity causes and associations, such as hyperinsulinemia, polycystic ovarian syndrome [48], type 2 diabetes mellitus, and potentially vitamin D deficiency [49]; respiratory physician assessment if complications such as obstructive sleep apnea or type 2 respiratory failure are suspected; physiotherapy for balance assessment; and rheumatologist for bone, muscle, and joint symptoms. A specific metabolic or weight-management clinical service may also be recommended for assistance with management of obesity. Psychological factors that can be associated with epilepsy [38] and which might contribute to unhealthy eating and lifestyle habits (e.g., anxiety, stress response, depression) should be considered and managed.

Cardiovascular risk-factor assessment

Cardiovascular risk assessment also forms an important part of the evaluation of patients with epilepsy, given their known increase in cardiovascular risk factors [50] and cardiovascular mortality [51].

Laboratory markers and investigations

These may be tailored to the needs of the individual patient but can include tests such as:

- Fasting blood sugar level and HbA1C ± insulin level.
- Fasting cholesterol, high- or low-density lipoproteins (HDL or LDL), and triglycerides.
- Homocysteine level.
- Serum vitamin D level (25 hydroxyvitamin D).
- Liver function tests (LFTs) and liver ultrasound (fatty liver, gallstones).
- Thyroid-stimulating hormone (TSH).
- Hormonal profile.
- ECG and referral for further assessment (if arrhythmia or other cardiac disease is suspected).
- 24-hour urinary cortisol (if Cushing syndrome is clinically suspected).

Treatment

There are no published randomized controlled trials of treatment strategies for obesity in patients with epilepsy.

Clinician–patient discussion to promote awareness of issues of weight gain and obesity in epilepsy and associated secondary effects, as well as weight-management strategies, are likely to be of benefit.

Education and health promotion

Promotion of healthy lifestyle and eating habits should be aimed for, in order to instigate lifestyle changes that promote sustained and achievable weight loss, working within any limitations of the underlying epilepsy and any other comorbidities. *Screening tests, as well as cardiologist, respiratory physician, and other specialist referrals, may be required prior to embarking upon an exercise program.*

Where prescribed medications are known to be associated with weight gain in some patients, this should be included in a discussion of the benefits and risks of treatment, and strategies for limiting such weight gain should be provided. The patient can be encouraged to self-monitor for weight gain, work with the treatment team to limit the extent or impact of weight gain, and identify other contributing factors to weight gain, such as high caloric intake, medical symptoms, or mood problems.

The risk following sudden and/or unsupervised cessation of AED treatment should be discussed (including exacerbation of seizures, risk of mortality, and exclusion from driving). The patient should be encouraged to involve their treatment team in weight-management strategies and decisions on any therapeutic changes.

Lifestyle and risk-factor modification

Lifestyle changes, including changes in diet and physical activity, are important factors in the prevention and management of obesity. They can improve health and cardiometabolic risk markers in patients with obesity [52], although they have not been specifically studied in patients with epilepsy.

Behavior modification is required, including instigation of a diet and exercise program that is sustainable for the patient. Participation in organized sports and exercise should be encouraged in children and adults (within any limitations of their epilepsy). Exercise-induced seizures do occasionally occur, but many sports are considered safe for patients with epilepsy, with appropriate medical assessment, monitoring, and preparation, and may produce positive health benefits [53]. Studies suggest that limitation of physical activity and reduced physical fitness are more prevalent among patients with epilepsy [54,55]. Many sports, including some contact sports such as football and soccer, have not been shown to induce seizures [7]. When choosing a sport, sensible exclusions should be considered, including those that involve heights or situations where timely rescue may be limited or unavailable (e.g., hang-gliding, free-climbing, and scuba diving) and those with a high risk of physical or head injury or of loss of awareness or consciousness (e.g., boxing and martial arts) [7].

Cardiovascular risk factors should be monitored for and, where possible, modified. Patients should not smoke. Blood pressure should be monitored and well managed. Any identified causes or associations of obesity should be monitored and managed on an individualized basis.

Weight monitoring and dietician advice

The patient should monitor their weight regularly at home, where possible. It may be useful to record this as part of their seizure diary. This should also assist in assessment of any weight changes following a change in AED therapy, which can be reviewed in clinic.

Similarly, a complete dietary record (usually as a short-term exercise, e.g., 1 week) can be useful in highlighting overall food intake and any dietary indiscretions. This can be reviewed by a dietician to enable education and personalized dietary improvement strategies.

For adults, a tailored dietary plan, targeting a sustainable weight loss of approximately 1.0–1.5 kg/week, can be supervised by a dietician or primary care provider. When a target healthy weight is achieved, a maintenance diet and exercise plan can be implemented.

For management of obesity in children, education of parents would generally be recommended. Specialist input may be required, as growth and BMI need to be factored into the overall strategy.

Cultural variations in perception of obesity and dietary habits should also be taken into consideration when preparing a diet and exercise plan.

Alcohol intake should be discouraged (noting interactions of alcohol with seizures, lifestyle, and AEDs, as well as weight gain and cardiovascular risk). Intake of foods high in saturated fats and sugar should be avoided; input from a dietician or primary care provider into a suitable diet plan can be sought.

Medications

Consider changing AED therapy if weight gain on one agent is problematic, balancing this against the desire to use the best agent for control of the type of epilepsy and the risks of changing therapy. The AEDs topiramate and zonisamide may have the side effect of weight loss in some patients, although their primary indication is for treatment of epilepsy and they are not registered or approved as "diet pills."

Caution should be advised regarding the use of over-the-counter (or Internet-promoted) weight-loss preparations, which may contain stimulants or agents that can interact with epilepsy medications and management. In some countries, these products are not subject to the level of analysis required for licensing of prescription medications and data on their safety, efficacy (if any), impact on seizure control, and interaction with prescribed medications may not be available.

Treatment of any underlying causes or complications of obesity should be managed on an individual basis, with appropriate specialist consultation.

Management of any identified psychological or psychiatric factors affecting weight control, where relevant to the individual patient, should be initiated with referral to appropriate psychologists or psychiatrists. In some cases, this may require a combined approach to treatment of obesity and psychiatric comorbidities, including cognitive–behavioral therapy (CBT) and specific counseling and medications for anxiety and/or depression [56]. There are no specific studies on this approach in epilepsy and further research into management of obesity in epilepsy is urgently required.

Prognosis

The consequences of obesity for the patient and the community are well acknowledged, including increased rates of morbidity from cardiovascular disease, stroke, and diabetes, as well as arthritis and possible associations of increased waist circumference with some malignancies. The increased mortality seen in patients with extreme obesity in long-term follow-up after epilepsy surgery, although not thought to be a result of the surgery itself, provides vital insight into the chronic problems induced by obesity in the epileptic population [17]. In a retrospective analysis of 244 adult patients who underwent epilepsy surgery, while BMI was not predictive for duration of ICU or hospital stay, perioperative morbidity and long-term seizure-control mortality during follow-up were increased for patients with extreme obesity ($p < 0.007$) [17]. Studies of effective weight-loss strategies in epilepsy and any subsequent gains in health outcomes of such an intervention are required.

References

1 Azagury DE, Lautz DB: Obesity overview: epidemiology, health and financial impact, and guidelines for qualification for surgical therapy. *Gastrointest Endosc Clin N Am* 2011; **21(2)**:189–201.

2 James WP: WHO recognition of the global obesity epidemic. *Int J Obes (Lond)* 2008; **32(Suppl. 7)**:S120–S126.

3 Hinnell C, Williams J, Metcalfe A et al.: Health status and health-related behaviors in epilepsy compared to other chronic conditions: a national population-based study. *Epilepsia* 2010; **51(5)**:853–861.

4 Verrotti A, Manco R, Agostinelli S et al.: The metabolic syndrome in overweight epileptic patients treated with valproic acid. *Epilepsia* 2010; **51(2)**:268–273.

5 Verrotti A, Agostinelli S, Parisi P et al.: Nonalcoholic fatty liver disease in adolescents receiving valproic acid. *Epilepsy Behav* 2011; **20(2)**:382–385.

6 Ben-Menachem E: Weight issues for people with epilepsy: a review. *Epilepsia* 2007; **48(Suppl. 9)**:42–45.

7 Howard GM, Radloff M, Sevier TL: Epilepsy and sports participation. *Curr Sports Med Rep* 2004; **3(1)**:15–19.

8 Verrotti A, D'Egidio C, Mohn A et al.: Weight gain following treatment with valproic acid: pathogenetic mechanisms and clinical implications. *Obes Rev* 2011; **12(5)**:e32–e43.

9 Kim JY, Lee HW: Metabolic and hormonal disturbances in women with epilepsy on antiepileptic drug monotherapy. *Epilepsia* 2007; **48(7)**:1366–1370.

10 Petty SJ, Kantor S, Lawrence KM et al.: Weight and fat distribution in patients taking valproate: a valproate-discordant gender-matched twin and sibling pair study. *Epilepsia* 2014 (In Press).

11 Jallon P, Picard F: Bodyweight gain and anticonvulsants: a comparative review. *Drug Saf* 2001; **24(13)**:969–978.

12 Daniels ZS, Nick TG, Liu C et al.: Obesity is a common comorbidity for pediatric patients with untreated, newly diagnosed epilepsy. *Neurology* 2009; **73(9)**:658–664.

13 Janousek J, Barber A, Goldman L, Klein P: Obesity in adults with epilepsy. *Epilepsy Behav* 2013; **28(3)**:391–394.

14 Obici S: Molecular targets for obesity therapy in the brain. *Endocrinology* 2009; **150(6)**:2512–2517.

15 Trevathan E, Dietz WH: Obesity in neurology practice: a call to action. *Neurology* 2009; **73(9)**:654–655.

16 Gao S, Juhaeri J, Dai WS: The incidence rate of seizures in relation to BMI in UK adults. *Obesity (Silver Spring)* 2008; **16(9)**:2126–2132.

17 Kang C, Cascino GD: The effect of preoperative body mass index on outcome after temporal lobe epilepsy surgery. *Epilepsy Res* 2009; **87(2–3)**:272–276.

18 Janszky I, Hallqvist J, Tomson T et al.: Increased risk and worse prognosis of myocardial infarction in patients with prior hospitalization for epilepsy: the Stockholm Heart Epidemiology Program. *Brain* 2009; **132(10)**:2798–2804.

19 Kobau R, DiIorio CA, Price PH et al.: Prevalence of epilepsy and health status of adults with epilepsy in Georgia and Tennessee: Behavioral Risk Factor Surveillance System, 2002. *Epilepsy Behav* 2004; **5(3)**:358–366.

20 Pennell PB: Hormonal aspects of epilepsy. *Neurol Clin* 2009; **27(4)**:941–965.

21 Verrotti A, D'Egidio C, Mohn A et al.: Antiepileptic drugs, sex hormones, and PCOS. *Epilepsia* 2011; **52(2)**:199–211.

22 Murialdo G, Magri F, Tamagno G et al.: Seizure frequency and sex steroids in women with partial epilepsy on antiepileptic therapy. *Epilepsia* 2009; **50(8)**:1920–1926.

23 Morrell MJ, Flynn KL, Seale CG et al.: Reproductive dysfunction in women with epilepsy: antiepileptic drug effects on sex-steroid hormones. *CNS Spectr* 2001; **6(9)**: 771–772,783–786.

24 Verrotti A, Basciani F, Morresi S et al.: Serum leptin changes in epileptic patients who gain weight after therapy with valproic acid. *Neurology* 1999; **53(1)**:230–232.

25 Uludag IF, Kulu U, Sener U et al.: The effect of carbamazepine treatment on serum leptin levels. *Epilepsy Res* 2009; **86(1)**:48–53.

26 Cansu A, Serdaroglu A, Cinaz P: Serum insulin, cortisol, leptin, neuropeptide Y, galanin and ghrelin levels in epileptic children receiving oxcarbazepine. *Eur J Paediatr Neurol* 2011; **15(6)**:527–531.

27 Hamed SA, Fida NM, Hamed EA: States of serum leptin and insulin in children with epilepsy: risk predictors of weight gain. *Eur J Paediatr Neurol* 2009; **13(3)**:261–268.

28 Hillman JB, Tong J, Tschop M: Ghrelin biology and its role in weight-related disorders. *Discov Med* 2011; **11(61)**: 521–528.

29 Greco R, Latini G, Chiarelli F et al.: Leptin, ghrelin, and adiponectin in epileptic patients treated with valproic acid. *Neurology* 2005; **65(11)**:1808–1809.

30 Prodam F, Bellone S, Casara G et al.: Ghrelin levels are reduced in prepubertal epileptic children under treatment with carbamazepine or valproic acid. *Epilepsia* 2010; **51(2)**: 312–315.

31 El-Khatib F, Rauchenzauner M, Lechleitner M et al.: Valproate, weight gain and carbohydrate craving: a gender study. *Seizure* 2007; **16(3)**:226–232.

32 Stephen LJ, Kwan P, Shapiro D et al.: Hormone profiles in young adults with epilepsy treated with sodium valproate or lamotrigine monotherapy. *Epilepsia* 2001; **42(8)**: 1002–1006.

33 Abaci A, Saygi M, Yis U et al.: Metabolic alterations during valproic acid treatment: a prospective study. *Pediatr Neurol* 2009; **41(6)**:435–439.

34 DeToledo JC, Toledo C, DeCerce J, Ramsay RE: Changes in body weight with chronic, high-dose gabapentin therapy. *Ther Drug Monit* 1997; **19(4)**:394–396.

35 Arroyo S, Anhut H, Kugler AR et al.: Pregabalin add-on treatment: a randomized, double-blind, placebo-controlled, dose-response study in adults with partial seizures. *Epilepsia* 2004; **45(1)**:20–27.

36 Beydoun A, Uthman BM, Kugler AR et al.: Safety and efficacy of two pregabalin regimens for add-on treatment of partial epilepsy. *Neurology* 2005; **64(3)**:475–480.

37 Han K, Choi-Kwon S, Lee SK: Leisure time physical activity in patients with epilepsy in Seoul, South Korea. *Epilepsy Behav* 2011; **20(2)**:321–325.

38 Gilliam FG, Mendiratta A, Pack AM, Bazil CW: Epilepsy and common comorbidities: improving the outpatient epilepsy encounter. *Epileptic Disord* 2005; **7(Suppl. 1)**:S27–S33.

39 Stunkard AJ, Faith MS, Allison KC: Depression and obesity. *Biol Psychiatry* 2003; **54(3)**:330–337.

40 Faith MS, Matz PE, Jorge MA: Obesity-depression associations in the population. *J Psychosom Res* 2002; **53(4)**: 935–942.

41 Needham BL, Epel ES, Adler NE, Kiefe C: Trajectories of change in obesity and symptoms of depression: the CARDIA study. *Am J Public Health* 2010; **100(6)**:1040–1046.

42 World Health Organization: Appropriate body-mass index for Asian populations and its implications for policy and intervention strategies. *Lancet* 2004; **363(9403)**:157–163.

43 Han TS, van Leer EM, Seidell JC, Lean ME: Waist circumference action levels in the identification of cardiovascular risk factors: prevalence study in a random sample. *BMJ* 1995; **311(7017)**:1401–1405.

44 Price GM, Uauy R, Breeze E et al.: Weight, shape, and mortality risk in older persons: elevated waist-hip ratio, not high body mass index, is associated with a greater risk of death. *Am J Clin Nutr* 2006; **84(2)**:449–460.

45 Canoy D: Coronary heart disease and body fat distribution. *Curr Atheroscler Rep* 2010; **12(2)**:125–133.

46 Ogden CL, Carroll MD, Curtin LR et al.: Prevalence of overweight and obesity in the United States, 1999–2004. *JAMA* 2006; **295(13)**:1549–1555.

47 Aronne LJ: Classification of obesity and assessment of obesity-related health risks. *Obes Res* 2002; **10(Suppl. 2)**: S105–S115.

48 Luef G, Abraham I, Haslinger M et al.: Polycystic ovaries, obesity and insulin resistance in women with epilepsy: a comparative study of carbamazepine and valproic acid in 105 women. *J Neurol* 2002; **249(7)**:835–841.

49 McGill AT, Stewart JM, Lithander FE et al.: Relationships of low serum vitamin D3 with anthropometry and markers of the metabolic syndrome and diabetes in overweight and obesity. *Nutr J* 2008; **7**:4.

50 Elliott JO, Jacobson MP, Haneef Z: Cardiovascular risk factors and homocysteine in epilepsy. *Epilepsy Res* 2007; **76(2–3)**:113–123.

51 Annegers JF, Hauser WA, Shirts SB: Heart disease mortality and morbidity in patients with epilepsy. *Epilepsia* 1984; **25(6)**:699–704.

52 Goodpaster BH, Delany JP, Otto AD et al.: Effects of diet and physical activity interventions on weight loss and cardiometabolic risk factors in severely obese adults: a randomized trial. *JAMA* 2010; **304(16)**:1795–1802.

53 Arida RM, de Almeida AC, Cavalheiro EA, Scorza FA: Experimental and clinical findings from physical exercise as complementary therapy for epilepsy. *Epilepsy Behav* 2013; **26(3)**:273–278.

54 Wong J, Wirrell E: Physical activity in children/teens with epilepsy compared with that in their siblings without epilepsy. *Epilepsia* 2006; **47(3)**:631–639.

55 Steinhoff BJ, Neususs K, Thegeder H, Reimers CD: Leisure time activity and physical fitness in patients with epilepsy. *Epilepsia* 1996; **37(12)**:1221–1227.

56 Donini LM, Savina C, Castellaneta E et al.: Multidisciplinary approach to obesity. *Eat Weight Disord* 2009; **14(1)**:23–32.

CHAPTER 18

Epilepsy in the elderly: vascular disease, the aging brain, and selection of appropriate therapies

Katherine H. Noe and Joseph I. Sirven

Department of Neurology, Mayo Clinic, USA

Introduction

Epilepsy affects between 1.5 and 3 million people in the United States annually. It is often mistakenly perceived as a childhood disorder but in fact the most common time to develop seizures is after age 60. The prevalence of epilepsy in persons aged 65 or older is twice that in young adults, and it continues to increase with age (Figure 18.1) [1–3]. Failure to recognize the importance of epilepsy in the older adult may contribute to misdiagnoses. Epilepsy in the elderly is distinct in its etiologies and presentation, which along with increased medical comorbidity adds to the difficulty of appropriate diagnosis and evaluation of seizures in the older adult compared to younger patients. Once recognized, the goals of seizure treatment in the elderly are the same as those for younger adults, namely to prevent future seizures and related injury and to maintain quality of life (QOL). In practice, however, epilepsy treatment in the elderly presents unique challenges. A higher incidence of drug side effects, medication interactions, and altered pharmacokinetics are of particular concern. Unfortunately, there is a dearth of evidence-based data regarding use of antiepileptic drugs (AEDs) in this population. Management of the older epilepsy patient is often based on information extrapolated from younger patients, without consideration for the unique problems and issues associated with a geriatric population. This review will discuss issues of diagnosis and treatment of epilepsy unique to the older age group.

Epidemiology/etiologies/pathophysiology

Seizures occur more frequently in the elderly, in part because they are often secondary to conditions more common in patients over age 60, including ischemic stroke, cerebral hemorrhage, tumor, and neurodegenerative diseases such as Alzheimer dementia. Therefore, to gain a clear understanding of the incidence of seizure disorders in this age group, distinctions must be made between acute symptomatic seizures and epilepsy. Acute symptomatic seizures are those directly attributable to or provoked by an acute insult to the central nervous system (CNS) or by a systemic metabolic derangement. In contrast, epilepsy is a condition of repeated unprovoked seizures and is diagnosed only when two or more such seizures have occurred. Epilepsy can occur without a clear underlying etiology (idiopathic epilepsy) or on the basis of a chronic CNS lesion such as encephalomalacia from old stroke (remote symptomatic epilepsy). The evaluation and management of each of these seizure presentations will be discussed.

Acute seizures

Acute symptomatic seizures are not uncommon in the elderly. In a population-based study, the incidence was 82 per 100 000 person years between ages 66 and 74, rising to 123 per 100 000 in those aged 75 or more [4]. In elderly patients, about half of all acute symptomatic seizures are attributed to cerebrovascular

Epilepsy and the Interictal State: Co-Morbidities and Quality of Life, First Edition.
Edited by Erik K. St. Louis, David M. Ficker, and Terence J. O'Brien.
© 2015 John Wiley & Sons, Ltd. Published 2015 by John Wiley & Sons, Ltd.

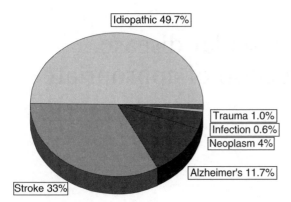

Figure 18.1 Etiology of epilepsy in the elderly.

disease (seizures occurring within 1 week of an ischemic or hemorrhagic stroke) [4–6]. Other frequently cited etiologies included toxic/metabolic derangements, trauma, neoplastic disease, and medication or alcohol withdrawal [3,4,7,8]. Hypoglycemia associated with insulin use and nonketotic hyperglycemia are often causes of seizures in diabetics [9,10]. Hyponatremia, uremia, and hypocalcemia are frequent seizure triggers [11]. Abrupt discontinuation of sedative and anxiolytic drugs such as barbiturates and benzodiazepines may cause withdrawal seizures in this age group [12–14]. Many commonly prescribed medications can also lower seizure threshold, including antipsychotics, antidepressants, theophylline, antibiotics such as quinolones, and certain pain medications, especially meperidine [12,13]. The herbal supplement ginko biloba may also have this effect [15,16]. CNS infection is a relatively uncommon cause of acute seizures in the elderly in the United States but should be suspected in the setting of fever, meningeal signs, or immunosuppression. Acute symptomatic seizures are associated with increased 30-day mortality, with a case fatality in patients aged 65 or older of 30–40% [17], but it is unknown whether mortality reflects the severity of the underlying brain insult or an independent effect of seizure activity.

Chronic seizures: epilepsy

The number of epilepsy cases also rises steadily after age 60. The annual incidence of epilepsy in the United States and Europe is 134 per 100 000 in those aged 65 years or older [1,2,11,18,19]. The prevalence of chronic seizures may be even higher in the institutionalized elderly, as up to 10% of nursing home residents have documented

seizure activity and/or receive AED therapy [20,21]. Epilepsy in this age group is commonly related to remote CNS insults or to chronic progressive neurologic disease, including cerebrovascular disease in 33%, dementia in 11.7%, neoplasm in 4%, infection in 0.6%, and trauma in 1% [3] (Figure 18.1); in the remaining half of patients, no definitive cause can be identified [3]. Another study of newly diagnosed epilepsy in patients aged 60 and above found that the most common etiology was stroke (43%), followed by arteriosclerosis (16%), unknown etiology (24%), and head trauma (7%) [22]. The majority of older adults experience partial seizures consistent with the presence of underlying acquired etiologies. In persons with epilepsy aged 65 and over, 13% have simple partial seizures, 49% complex partial, and 29% generalized or myoclonic seizures [1], in contrast with children, in whom the most prevalent seizure types are generalized (50%), with 11% having simple partial and 23% complex partial events.

Status epilepticus

Status epilepticus, defined as more than 30 minutes of continuous seizure activity or of intermittent seizures without return to consciousness, is also more common in older adults. The incidence of status epilepticus in the elderly is two to five times higher than in young adults [23,24]. Status epilepticus does not occur only in the setting of a known seizure disorder but can also be the first presentation of epilepsy or occur as a result of acute symptomatic derangements. Of all acute symptomatic seizures in older people, 30% present as status epilepticus [25]. The elderly are both more likely to develop status epilepticus and more likely to die as a result of it. In a database of status epilepticus cases, mortality rate for all adults was 26%, rising to 38% after age 60 and 50% after age 80 [23,26]. In the elderly, 40% of status epilepticus cases are attributable to acute or chronic stroke [27]. Although acute stroke is likely to contribute significantly to overall morbidity and mortality, the mortality of stroke with status epilepticus is three times greater than that for stroke alone [28]. Status epilepticus following anoxic brain injuries, such as postcardiopulmonary arrest, has a mortality rate close to 100% [28].

Diagnostic evaluation

Misdiagnosis is a significant obstacle in the treatment of epilepsy in older adults. In one study of new-onset epilepsy in elderly patients, a seizure disorder was not seriously considered at first evaluation in 25% of cases [29]. Common misdiagnoses were syncope/blackout (46%), altered mental status (42%), and dementia (7%). Diagnosis of ongoing seizures was delayed by almost 5 days in confused elderly patients in a recent analysis at our center [30]. While it is relatively easy to recognize a classic generalized tonic–clonic seizure, older adults are more likely to experience partial seizures with clinical manifestations unique compared to those often seen in younger patients, perhaps due to epileptic foci in older adults involving the frontal and parietal lobes rather than the temporal lobe [31]. Thus, elderly patients are less likely to experience auras such as déjà vu and other symptoms classically associated with temporal-lobe epilepsy (TLE). Rather, older adult patients with partial seizures may complain of dizziness, posturing, paresthesias, and other symptoms related to frontal- and parietal-lobe function. Further diagnostic confusion may arise from multiple comorbidities, polypharmacy, and difficulty obtaining an accurate history due to underlying cognitive impairment in some patients and collateral history providers. Postictal periods may last for days in older adults, mimicking delirium or dementia, further confounding diagnosis.

Diagnosis requires a detailed and accurate history. Patients are often unaware of their own seizure symptoms and behavior, so obtaining collateral history from an eyewitness is invaluable. Syncope, transient ischemic attacks, transient global amnesia, and vertigo are common conditions in elderly patients that present similarly to seizures [32]. Table 18.1 lists common discriminators of nonepileptic events and seizures. Although historical variables may be helpful, they remain nonspecific. Carefully detailed questions about the episodes and about epilepsy risk factors, including minor or major head trauma and concomitant medications, must be asked.

Further diagnostic testing is often needed to confirm or clarify the etiology of a seizure-like spell. Depending on the history, evaluation for metabolic derangements, cardiac disease, cerebrovascular disorders, or vestibular dysfunction may be considered, as appropriate. For epilepsy evaluation, EEG and neuroimaging are standard tests. The values and limitations of these tests are discussed further in this section.

EEG

EEG is a cornerstone of seizure evaluation in all age groups. However, elderly patients are more likely to have nonspecific or non-epilepsy-related EEG changes, which can add to diagnostic errors by unwary interpreters. Findings related to normal aging may include mild slowing or decreased amplitude of background

Table 18.1 Variables that distinguish between common spells in the elderly.

Variable	Seizure	Syncope	TIA	TGA	Vertigo
Warning/aura	Sometimes	Faint feeling	None	None	None
Duration	1–2 minutes	Seconds to minutes	Minutes to hours	4–24 hours	Minutes to days
Effect of posture/positional change	None	None	Frequent	Rare	Frequent
Spell symptoms	Tonic–clonic movements, variable confusion, altered consciousness	Loss of tone/brief clonic jerks	Deficits along a vascular pattern	Confusion/ amnesia	Nausea, ataxia, tinitus
Incontinence	Variable	Variable	None	None	None
Heart rate	Increased	Irregular/decreased	Variable	No effect	Rare?
Post-spell symptoms	Confusion, sleep	Alert	Alert	Alert	Alert
EEG during event	Epileptiform pattern	Diffuse slowing	Focal slowing	Normal, rarely slowing	Normal

TIA, transient ischemic attack; TGA, transient global amnesia.

rhythms and intermittent slowing over temporal head regions [33,34]. EEG in elderly individuals may also show benign patterns that can easily be misinterpreted as epileptogenic by inexperienced readers, such as small sharp spikes, wicket spikes, or subclinical rhythmic electrical discharges of adulthood (SREDA), the latter occurring nearly exclusively in older adults [34–38]. Adding to diagnostic confusion, truly epileptogenic findings such as spikes or sharp waves appear less commonly in the EEGs of elderly individuals with epilepsy than in those of young patients. Only 26–37% of older patients with epilepsy demonstrate epileptiform abnormalities on routine EEG [31,39]. Thus, absence of epileptiform abnormalities on EEG should not exclude the diagnosis of seizures or epilepsy. When epileptogenic discharges are present, they are strongly suggestive of a seizure diagnosis but must be interpreted cautiously, with the clinical history in mind. Epileptiform transients may be seen in patients with diseases other than epilepsy, such as dementia, stroke, neoplasms, and prion diseases [39–41]. The "gold standard" of epilepsy diagnosis is an actual recorded seizure. Therefore, when the diagnosis of seizures or epilepsy remains in question, prolonged inpatient video-EEG or ambulatory EEG monitoring should be strongly considered.

Neuroimaging

Imaging studies (MRI/CT) should be performed as part of the initial evaluation of all older patients with epilepsy to identify and treat etiologies such as CNS hemorrhage, tumor, and abscess. MRI is the procedure of choice, given superiority to CT in detecting all pathologic processes except subarachnoid hemorrhage [42]. CT is helpful in emergent situations or when MRI is contraindicated.

Treatment

When should antiepileptic drugs be initiated?

The main reason for prescribing AED therapy is to prevent further seizures. Related goals are preventing seizure-related morbidity and mortality and maintaining QOL. For many elderly patients, critical issues are the continued ability to drive and to maintain independent living. A single seizure with an obvious precipitating cause does not imply an underlying tendency toward seizure recurrence requiring AED treatment. For example, an individual having seizures caused by a new medication or electrolyte disturbance does not require initiation of AED therapy; rather, the offending medication should be discontinued or the underlying electrolyte imbalance corrected. Patients found to have a history of two or more prior seizures are at high risk for future events and should be treated [43].

After a single idiopathic seizure, the decision to initiate treatment is based on an assessment of recurrence risk. Risk stratification is generally based on studies of younger adults as this issue has not been adequately evaluated in the elderly. Partial seizures, postictal paralysis, family history of epilepsy, epileptiform EEG, and abnormal neurologic examination are all associated with a higher risk of recurrence in studies of younger adults [44–46]. Older age itself also may predict risk, since older patients appear more likely to have seizure recurrence [44], but older patients should not necessarily be placed on an AED after a first seizure. Rather, appropriate investigation is needed to better identify risk factors that are likely to lead to seizure recurrence. In general, individuals with a single seizure and a structural cortical lesion (i.e., tumor, encephalomalacia from a stroke or trauma) identified on neuroimaging have a higher risk of seizure recurrence and benefit from AED treatment. However, primary prophylaxis with AEDs for patients with new stroke or tumor but without clinical seizure occurrence is not routinely recommended [47,48].

Choosing a medication

An ideal AED would be highly effective and avoid adverse side effects, drug interactions, complex dosing regimens, and undue expense. No perfect drug exists, and AED selection must therefore rely on careful consideration of what is best for a given individual. Effectiveness for seizure type, side-effect profile, dosing regimen, medication interaction, and cost are among the important factors to consider. The great majority of elderly patients have partial seizures, for which all currently available AEDs except ethosuximide are potentially efficacious. Lamotrigine and gabapentin are recommended as first-line agents for partial epilepsy in the elderly [22,49] (level A evidence). Similarly, expert consensus favors lamotrigine as a treatment of choice for the older patient, followed by gabapentin or levetiracetam [50] (level C evidence). For the rare older patient who has primary generalized epilepsy, a broad-spectrum AED such as valproate, lamotrigine, topirimate, or levetiracetam would be an appropriate choice [50] (level C evidence) .

In a recent retrospective review, lamotrigine was the most effective AED in older adults, based on 12-month retention and seizure freedom, followed by levetiracetam [51] (level B evidence). Oxcarbazepine was consistently less effective (less tolerable) than most other AEDs [51] (level B evidence). Table 18.2 summarizes all currently approved AEDs, showing their side-effect profiles and relative costs. The older AEDs phenobarbital, phenytoin, valproate, and carbamazepine continue to be highly prescribed. More than 50% of elderly patients on AEDs, both in the community and in nursing home populations, are prescribed phenytoin [20,52]. However, multiple newer AEDs introduced over the last decade are now available. Table 18.3 outlines the potential advantages and disadvantages of the new AEDs compared with standard therapy in the older population.

Side effects

AEDs are one of the most common sources of adverse medication side effects in the elderly [53,54]. In general, older and newer AEDs appear to have similar efficacy for partial seizures, but the newer agents may offer advantages in side-effect profile and tolerability. There are few clinical trials comparing new and old AEDs directly in elderly patients. A randomized controlled trial of carbamazepine, lamotrigine, and gabapentin for treatment of new-onset partial seizures in patients

Table 18.2 Antiepileptic drugs (AEDs) currently used in elderly patients.

Antiepileptic drug	Drug interactions	Common adverse effects	Cost
Carbamazepine	++	Diplopia, dizziness, idiosyncratic aplastic anemia, rash, hyponatremia, osteoporosis	$$
Felbamate	+++	Dizziness, headache, idiosyncratic hepatic failure or aplastic anemia, insomnia, weight loss	$$$
Gabapentin	0	Fatigue, transient gastrointestinal distress	$$$
Lacosamide	0	Headache, dizziness	$$$$
Lamotrigine	+	Dizziness, headache	$$$
Levetiracetam	0	Somnolence, coordination difficulties	$$$
Oxcarbazepine	+	Dizziness, diplopia, ataxia, hyponatremia	$$$
Phenobarbital	++	Cognitive effects, respiratory depression, sedation	$
Phenytoin	++	Ataxia, gingival hyperplasia, hirsutism, lymphadenopathy, nystagmus, osteoporosis	$
Pregabalin	0	Weight gain, sedation	$$$$
Primidone	++	Sedation, depression, dizziness	$
Rufinamide	++	Sedation, cardiac disturbances	$$$$
Tiagabine	+	Gastrointestinal distress, cognitive effects	$$$
Topiramate	++	Impaired memory, weight loss, word-finding difficulty	$$$
Valproate	+	Weight gain	$$
Vigabatrin	+	Weight loss, peripheral visual loss	$$$$$
Zonisamide	+	Somnolence, dizziness, agitation, difficulty concentrating, weight loss	$$$

+/++/+++, least to most drug interactions; $/$$/$$$/$$$$/$$$$$, least to most expensive in US dollars/month.

Table 18.3 Advantages and disadvantages of antiepileptic drugs (AEDs) for elderly patients.

Antiepileptic drug	Advantages	Disadvantages
Carbamazepine	Inexpensive	Rash
	Efficacy for partial seizures	Bone disease
		Hyponatremia
		Drug interactions
Felbamate	Broad spectrum of coverage	Serious idiosyncratic side effects
	Efficacy for refractory seizures	Expensive
		Complex drug interactions
Gabapentin	No drug interactions	Multiple daily doses
	Renal excretion	Expensive
Lacosamide	No drug interactions	Dizziness commonly reported
	Intravenous formulation	Expensive
Lamotrigine	Broad spectrum of coverage	Slow to initiate
	Well tolerated	Rash
	Once- or twice-daily dosing	Expensive
Levetiracetam	Easy to initiate	Behavioral/mood problems
	No drug interactions	Expensive
	Renal excretion	
	Intravenous formulation	
Oxcarbazepine	Well tolerated	Hyponatremia
		Expensive
Phenobarbital	Inexpensive	Sedation
	Once-daily dosing	Cognitive adverse effects
		Behavioral/mood problems
		Bone disease
Phenytoin	Inexpensive	Sedation
	Once-daily dosing	Narrow therapeutic window
		Imbalance
		Bone disease
		Idiosyncratic cerebellar ataxia and neuropathy
		Cosmetic issues (gingival hyperplasia, hirsuitism)
		Drug interactions
Pregabalin	No drug interactions	Weight gain
		Expensive
Rufinamide	Some drug interactions	Not well studied in older adults (unclear effectiveness for partial seizures)

Table 18.3 (*continued*)

Antiepileptic drug	Advantages	Disadvantages
Topiramate	Broad spectrum of coverage	Cognitive adverse effects
	Weight loss	Expensive
		Drug interactions (inducer at high doses; i.e., >200 mg/day)
Tiagabine	Limited drug interactions	Multiple daily doses
		Cognitive adverse effects
		Expensive
Valproate	Broad spectrum of coverage	Weight gain
		Tremor
		Bone disease
Vigabatrin	Effective	Peripheral visual field loss
		Extremely expensive in United States
Zonisamide	Well tolerated	Sedation
	Once-daily dosing	Expensive

aged 60 and over [22] (level A evidence) found similar efficacy for all three drugs, but carbamazepine users were significantly more likely to experience adverse medication side effects, resulting in early discontinuation. Another randomized prospective study comparing lamotrigine with carbamazepine for newly diagnosed seizures in patients 65 and older also found carbamazepine users to be more than twice as likely to experience adverse side effect-related medication discontinuation [55] (level A evidence). A pooled data analysis confirmed the superior tolerability of lamotrigine versus carbamazepine and phenytoin in elderly patients [56] (level B evidence). An open-label study of levetiracetam as add-on therapy in patients over age 65 also found this to be a well-tolerated medication [57] (level B evidence). Common side effects of individual AEDs are summarized in Table 18.2.

Drug interactions

Drug interaction is one of the more important considerations regarding choice of AED therapy. For community-dwelling elderly people in the United States, the average number of annual filled prescriptions is 30, rising to 40 or more in persons with at least three chronic medical conditions [20]. Interactions

resulting from multiple drug therapies can lead to significant adverse effects and to concerns about compliance and expense.

There are two broad types of drug interaction: pharmacokinetic and pharmacodynamic. Pharmacokinetic drug interactions are defined as resulting from altered absorption, distribution, metabolism, or elimination. The most common pharmacokinetic drug interaction is altered hepatic metabolism. Drugs that induce or inhibit hepatic metabolism of other drugs may either increase toxicity or reduce the effectiveness of other medications. Among the AEDs, phenobarbital, primidone, phenytoin, and carbamazepine are inducers of cytochrome P450 enzymes, while valproate is an inhibitor [58]. Therefore, these agents may be problematic for the older patient taking multiple drugs. Medications taken for comorbid medical or psychiatric conditions may cause similar adverse alterations in AED metabolism. For example, macrolide antibiotics such as erythromycin inhibit hepatic enzyme induction, so concomitant erythromycin and carbamazepine use can easily result in carbamazepine toxicity. For older patients on warfarin, combined use with hepatic enzyme-inducing AEDs may result in decreased anticoagulant effect, with potentially serious outcomes [58]. Pharmacodynamic drug interactions are defined as occurring when medications have mechanisms of action that are either synergistic or antagonistic. For example, both benzodiazepines and barbiturates have an additive effect when combined because both affect the $GABA_A$ binding site. Therefore, choosing an AED with a unique mechanism of action and limited hepatic metabolism may be most beneficial in older patients. Most of the newer AEDs may be better choices for older adults with seizures. A detailed discussion of AED drug interactions is provided by two excellent references: [58] and [59].

Initiating and monitoring drug therapy

When starting AEDs in elderly patients, it is wise to "start low and go slow." Complex pharmacokinetic changes with aging, such as altered gastrointestinal absorption, changes in serum protein binding, decreased hepatic metabolism, and renal clearance, can all affect AED serum levels in complex and unpredictable ways. Once AED therapy is established, adjustment of medication is primarily guided by clinical seizure control and side effects. Measuring AED concentrations can be of value in assessing compliance and ascertaining toxicity. It becomes even more important in older patients, who may have problems with memory, making compliance difficult. Pharmacokinetic changes associated with advancing age, such as decreased drug clearance and reduced metabolism, may contribute to toxicity, which can be prevented by monitoring serum concentrations [60].

However, modification of AED dosing according to changes in AED levels alone is not recommended, since the serum concentration of certain AEDs, especially phenytoin, fluctuate unpredictably and substantially even within individual patients. Phenytoin levels varied two- to threefold over time in individual elderly nursing home patients known to be highly compliant with their medications, which were received during scheduled administrations of stable dosages. Intraindividual phenytoin level variability in these patients was thought to result from achloridia and resultant variable absorption through the elderly gastric mucosa, since phenytoin relies on a relatively acidic environment for optimal absorption and bioavailability [61]. Recommended serum level ranges for antiepileptic medications are based on populations of predominantly younger patients and, therefore, blood levels thought to be in a "therapeutic" or "toxic" range for a population of

patients may not be applicable to specific individuals, or to older patients in particular. Older adults may be more sensitive to the sedative and cognitive effects of AEDs and may experience difficulties at lower than expected doses. For drugs such as phenytoin, older people may have a narrow therapeutic window, placing them at greater risk for toxicity. For highly protein-bound drugs, lower protein binding in older patients can result in a higher than expected free level of medication. Serum concentrations of phenytoin, carbamazepine, and valproic acid should be monitored as total and free plasma concentrations. In contrast, the majority of the new AEDs are not highly protein bound and do not yet have well-defined or generally accepted therapeutic serum concentration ranges, so checking serum drug levels for many newer agents is not required and is often not helpful in determining toxicity or therapeutic effect. As in other patient populations, a patient's outcomes on AED therapy, with careful consideration of resultant clinical efficacy and reported adverse effects, should be the chief factor guiding AED dose adjustments, rather than arbitrarily altering AED doses to achieve specific serum concentrations.

Falls and fractures

Seizures may lead to falls and subsequent fractures [62,63], which can have profound consequences in an older individual's life, including loss of mobility, placement in a nursing home, and death. Persons with epilepsy have twice the fracture rate of the general population [64]. Falling and fracture in elderly epilepsy patients is a complex issue, reflecting both seizure-related trauma and the adverse effects of AEDs, which may cause instability and bone density loss. Older AEDs have been associated with imbalance, with the exception of gabapentin and levetiracetam [65]. AEDs that induce hepatic enzyme metabolism can contribute to the development of osteoporosis via inactivation of vitamin D, leading to decreased calcium absorption [66]. Both osteoporosis and osteopenia are significantly increased in patients chronically exposed to these drugs [67,68]. For older patients at risk for development of bone disease or in whom osteoporosis is already present, newer AEDs may again be a better choice. All patients taking AEDs should be placed on prophylactic vitamin D and calcium supplementation and have serial bone density measurements followed.

Nonmedication therapies
Vagus nerve stimulation

Vagus nerve stimulation (VNS) is a reasonable treatment option for medically refractory seizures in patients who are not good candidates for traditional epilepsy surgery. In experienced surgical hands, the VNS implantation procedure has a low complication rate. Although usually done under general anesthesia, use of regional anesthesia is an option. The sole analysis of VNS effectiveness in older adults found an average seizure reduction of 31% at 3 months, with 50–60% of patients achieving at least a 50% reduction by 1 year [69] (level B evidence). No patients were seizure-free. Few adverse effects were found, consisting of hoarseness, coughing, and paresthesias. No clinically significant episodes of bradycardia were reported postoperatively. QOL significantly improved. VNS efficacy compares favorably to medications, but VNS is almost always used as an adjunctive therapy rather than a replacement for AEDs. VNS is a contraindication for subsequent body MRI and may complicate mammography; therefore, its use should be carefully considered in patients with a history of malignancy or another condition in which serial imaging is indicated.

Epilepsy surgery

In about 30–40% of all epilepsy patients, seizures are refractory and incompletely controlled by medical therapy. Epilepsy surgery is considered when disabling seizures continue despite appropriate AED therapy and when control of seizures would significantly improve QOL. Temporal lobectomy, the most common surgical procedure for epilepsy, has proliferated recently as its efficacy and safety are now well documented [70]. In a randomized controlled trial of temporal lobectomy versus medical management for younger adults with refractory seizures, surgery was significantly more effective (58 versus 8% seizure-free at 1 year) and resulted in improved QOL [71]. Elderly patients are often not considered to be appropriate candidates for epilepsy surgery, due to underlying medical comorbidities or to seizure etiology (e.g., a demented nursing home resident). Unfortunately, older patients without contraindications have traditionally not been considered surgical candidates due to concerns about age-related surgical complications and decreased efficacy due to longstanding epilepsy duration. However, several retrospective studies have investigated surgical outcomes in selected patients over the age of 50 and have found the rate of seizure-free outcomes to be similar to that of younger age groups, without significant decline in memory function [72–76]. Although more studies are needed, older adults should not be excluded from surgical consideration based solely on age. Rather, exclusion criteria should be similar to those for younger patients, which would include lack of a definite epileptic focus and a seizure focus in an inoperable location, such as the motor strip or areas of language and/or memory functioning. While surgical complication rates in previous studies were at acceptable levels, the candidates were highly selected. Careful consideration of surgical risk and potential improvement in seizure control and overall QOL must be made on an individual basis.

Which treatment? Medications versus surgery

Figure 18.2 illustrates an algorithm for management of seizures in the older adult. Treatment is initiated after a second seizure. If seizures persist despite a trial of antiepileptic medication with documentation of a therapeutic level or adverse effects then other AEDs are tried. If two or three appropriately selected and administered AEDs have been tried and seizures persist then surgery should be considered. Surgery should only be pursued in individuals where there is likely to be an improvement in patient QOL or in order to prevent injurious seizures. A patient with dementia and seizures would usually not be an appropriate candidate for surgery. In sum, the benefits must outweigh the risks. If the patient is not a candidate for surgery or fails to respond to surgery then VNS may be an appropriate option.

Psychosocial implications of seizures in older people

Seizures can impact the lives of older people in many ways. However, the study of QOL issues in epilepsy remains largely neglected in this age group. In older adults with epilepsy living in the community, medication side effects (64%) and issues related to driving and transportation (64%) are the most commonly noted concerns [77]. In the United States, while specific laws vary from state to state, a recent seizure generally results in suspension of driving privileges for a period

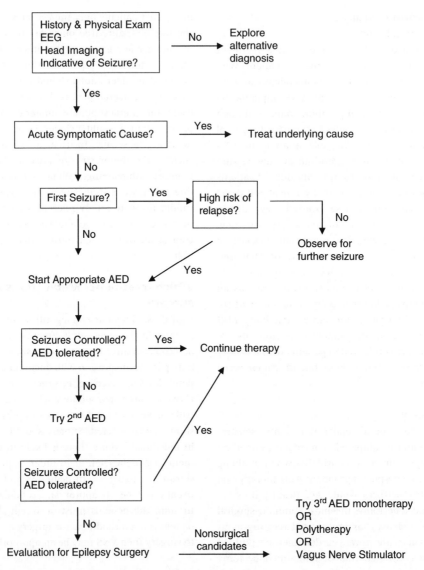

Figure 18.2 Algorithm for the treatment of epilepsy in older adults.

of at least several months. Loss of driving privileges can be even more devastating to older than younger patients and may impact their ability to maintain independent living, especially if there is a lack of adequate public transportation. Among elderly people with epilepsy, 36% report concerns about embarrassment or social restrictions [77]. Social stigma of epilepsy may particularly impact elderly patients, who were often raised during a time when seizures were mistakenly considered a sign of mental illness, moral weakness,

or even a cause for institutionalization. The common misperception that seizures are a condition of the young may contribute to a lack of acceptance of an epilepsy diagnosis. Medical care providers should be aware of the psychosocial implications of a seizure diagnosis for elderly individuals and must recognize that these concerns can add to a patient's reluctance to accept diagnosis and treatment. Adequate counseling and education of patients and family members is a crucial component of care.

Practical advice and pearls

- Epilepsy in older people is a major public health problem with significant pathological, psychosocial, and economical burdens on both individuals and society.
- With aging of the global population, epilepsy is likely to become even more prevalent.
- The impact of epilepsy and newer AED and nonpharmacological treatments have not been investigated as systematically in older patients as in younger ones.
- Seizures in older adults may present in a more subtle manner than in younger patients, delaying diagnosis and therapy.
- There is level A evidence to favor the use of either lamotrigine and gabapentin over carbamazepine as initial therapy for older adults with epilepsy.
- AED therapy should be started at lower doses and at a slower titration rate in the elderly than in younger adults, to improve drug retention and minimize adverse effects.
- Future research into the pathophysiology of the aging brain and epilepsy and into the treatment of epilepsy in older people is fundamental to adequately treating the burgeoning aged population with epilepsy.
- Suggested resources include the Web sites of the American Epilepsy Society (www.aesnet.org) and the Epilepsy Foundation of America/Epilepsy Therapy Project (www.epilepsy.com) (both last accessed July 15, 2014).

References

1 Hauser WA: Seizure disorders: the changes with age. *Epilepsia* 1992; **33(Suppl. 4)**:S6–S14.
2 Hauser WA, Annegers JF, Kurland LT: Incidence of epilepsy and unprovoked seizures in Rochester, Minnesota: 1935–1984. *Epilepsia* 1993; **34**:453–468.
3 Hauser WA: *Epidemiology of Seizures and Epilepsy in the Elderly.* Butterworth-Heinemann, Boston, MA, 1997, pp. 7–18.
4 Annegers JF, Hauser WA, Lee JR et al.: Incidence of acute symptomatic seizures in Rochester, Minnesota 1935–1984. *Epilepsia* 1995; **36**:327–333.
5 So EL, Annegers JF, Hauser WA et al.: Population-based study of seizure disorders after cerebral infarction. *Neurology* 1996; **46**:350–355.
6 Giroud M, Gras P, Fayolle H et al.: Early seizures after acute stroke: a study of 1,640 cases. *Epilepsia* 1994; **35(5)**: 959–964.

7 Sanders JWA, Hart YM, Johnson AL et al.: Natural General Practice Study of Epilepsy: newly diagnosed epileptic seizures in general population. *Lancet* 1990; **336**: 1267–1270.
8 Ettinger AB, Shinnar S: New-onset seizures in an elderly hospitalized population. *Neurology* 1993; **43**:489–492.
9 Malouf R, Brust JCM: Hypoglycemia: causes, neurologic manifestations, and outcomes. *Ann Neurol* 1985; **17**: 421–430.
10 Singh BM, Gupta DR, Strobos RJ: Nonketotic hyperglycemia and epilepsia partialis continua. *Arch Neurol* 1973; **29**:187–190.
11 Loiseau P: Pathologic processes in the elderly and their association with seizures. In: Rowan AJ, Ramsey RE (eds): *Seizures and Epilepsy in the Elderly.* Butterworth-Heinemann, Boston, MA, 1997, pp. 63–68.
12 Messing RO, Closson RG, Simon RP: Drug-induced seizures: a 10-year experience. *Neurology* 1984; **34**:1582–1586.
13 Zaccara G, Muscas GC, Messori A: Clinical features, pathogenesis and management of drug-induced seizures. *Drug Safety* 1990; **5**:109–151.
14 Thomas P, Lebrun C, Chatel M: De novo absence status epilepticus as a benzodiazepine withdrawal syndrome. *Epilepsia* 1993; **34**:355–358.
15 Kupiec T, Raj V: Fatal seizures due to potential herb-drug interactions with Ginko biloba. *J Anal Toxicol* 2005; **29**: 755–758.
16 Granger AS: Ginko biloba precipitating epileptic seizures. *Age Ageing* 2001; **30**:523–525.
17 Hesdorffer DC, D'Amelio M: Mortality in the first 30 days following incident acute symptomatic seizures. *Epilepsia* 2005; **46(Suppl. 11)**:S43–S45.
18 Luhdorf K, Jensen LK, Plesner AM: Epilepsy in the elderly: incidence, social function, and disability. *Epilepsia* 1989; **30**: 389–399.
19 Tallis R, Hall G, Craig I et al.: How common are epileptic seizures in old age? *Age Ageing* 1991; **20**:442–448.
20 Lackner TE, Cloyd JC, Thomas LW, Leppik IE: Antiepileptic drug use in nursing home residents: effect of age, gender, and comedication on patterns of use. *Epilepsia* 1998; **39**: 1083–1087.
21 Garrard J, Cloyd J, Gross C et al.: Factors associated with antiepileptic drug use among elderly nursing home residents. *J Gerontol A Biol Sci Med Sci* 2000; **55**:384–392.
22 Rowan AJ, Ransay RE, Collins JF et al.: New onset geriatric epilepsy: a randomized study of gabapentin, lamotrigine, and carbamazepine. *Neurology* 2005; **64**:1868–1873.
23 DeLorenzo RJ, Hauser WA, Towne AR et al.: A prospective population-based epidemiologic study of status epilepticus in Richmond, Virginia. *Neurology* 1996; **46**: 1029–1035.
24 Vignatelli L, Tonon C, D'Allessandro R et al.: Incidence and short-term prognosis of status epilepticus in adults in Bologna, Italy. *Epilepsia* 2003; **44**:964–968.

25 Cascino GD, Hesdorffer D, Logroscino G, Hauser WA: Morbidity of nonfebrile status epilepticus in Rochester, Minnesota 1965–1984. *Epilepsia* 1998; **39**:829–832.

26 DeLorenzo RJ, Pellock JM, Towne AR et al.: Epidemiology of status epilepticus. *J Clin Neurophys* 1995; **12**:316–325.

27 Waterhouse EJ, Vaughan JK, Barnes TY et al.: Synergistic effect of status epilepticus and ischemic brain injury on mortality. *Epilepsy Res* 1998; **29**:175–183.

28 Waterhouse EJ, DeLorenzo RJ: Status epilepticus in older patients: epidemiology and treatment options. *Drugs Aging* 2001; **18**:133–142.

29 Ramsay RE, Rowan AJ, Pryor FM: Special considerations in treating the elderly patient with epilepsy. *Neurology* 2004; **62(Suppl. 2)**: S24–S29.

30 Sheth RD, Drazkowski J, Sirven J et al.: *Arch Neurol* 2006; **63(4)**:529–532.

31 Ramsey RE, Pryor F: Epilepsy in the elderly. *Neurology* 2000; **55(Suppl. 1)**:S9–S14.

32 Tinuper P: The altered presentation of seizures in the elderly. In: Rowan AJ, Ramsey RE (eds): *Seizures and Epilepsy in the Elderly*. Butterworth-Heinemann, Boston, MA, 1997, pp. 123–130.

33 Otomo E: Electroencephalography in old age: dominant alpha rhythm. *Electrencephalogr Clin Neurophysiol* 1966; **21**: 489–491.

34 Klass DW, Brenner RP: Electroencephalography of the elderly. *J Clin Neurophysiol* 1995; **12**:116–131.

35 Roubicek J: The electroencephalogram in the middle aged and the elderly. *J Am Geriatr Soc* 1977; **25**:145–152.

36 Silverman AJ, Busse EW, Barnes RH: Studies in the process of aging: electroencephalographic findings in 400 elderly subjects. *Electroencephalogr Clin Neurophysiol* 1955; **7**:67–77.

37 Westmoreland BF, Klass DW: A distinctive rhythmic EEG discharge of adults. *Electroencephalogr Clin Neurophysiol* 1981; **51**:186–191.

38 Westmoreland BF: Benign variants and patterns of uncertain clinical significance. In: Daly DD, Pedley TA (eds): *Current Practice of Clinical Electroencephalography*, 2 edn. Raven Press, New York, NY, 1990, pp. 243–252.

39 Drury I, Beydoun A: Interictal epileptiform activity in elderly patients with epilepsy. *Electroencephalogr Clin Neurophysiol* 1998; **106**:369–373.

40 Muller HF, Kral VA: The EEG in advanced senile dementia. *J Am Geriatr Soc* 1967; **15**:415–426.

41 Chatrian GE, Shaw CM, Leffman H: The significance of periodic lateralized epileptiform discharges in EEG: an electrographic, clinical, and pathological study. *Electroencephalogr Clin Neurophysiol* 1964; **17**:177–193.

42 Zimmerman R: Diagnostic methods. II: Imaging studies. In: Rowan AJ, Ramsay RE (eds): *Seizures and Epilepsy in the Elderly*. Butterworth-Heinemann, Boston, MA, 1997, pp. 159–177.

43 Hauser WA, Rich SS, Lee JR et al.: Risk of recurrent seizures after two unprovoked seizures. *N Engl J Med* 1998; **338**:429–434.

44 Hopkins A, Garman A, Clarke C: The first seizure in adult life: value of clinical features, electroencephalography and computerized tomographic scanning in prediction of seizure recurrence. *Lancet* 1988; **1**:721–726.

45 Berg AT, Shinnar S: The risk of seizure recurrence following a first unprovoked seizure: a quantitative review. *Neurology* 1991; **41**:965–972.

46 Annegers JF, Shirts SB, Hauser WA et al.: Risk of seizure recurrence after an initial unprovoked seizure. *Epilepsia* 1986; **27**:43–50.

47 Glantz MJ, Cole BF, Forsyth PA et al.: Practice parameter: anticonvulsant prophylaxis in patients with newly diagnosed brain tumor: report of the Quality Standards Subcommittee of the American Academy of Neurology. *Neurology* 2000; **54(10)**:1886–1893.

48 Sirven JI, Wingerchuk DM, Drazkowski JF et al.: Seizure prophylaxis in patients with brain tumors: a meta-analysis. *Mayo Clin Proc* 2004; **79**:1489–1494.

49 Glauser T, Ben-Menachem E, Bourgeois B et al.: ILAE treatment guidelines: evidence-based analysis of antiepileptic drug efficacy and effectiveness as initial monotherapy for epileptic seizures and syndromes. *Epilepsia* 2006; **47**:1094–1120.

50 Karceski S, Morrell MJ, Carpenter D: Treatment of epilepsy in adults: expert opinion, 2005. *Epilepsy Behav* 2005; **7**: S1–64.

51 Arif H, Buchsbaum R, Pierro J et al.: *Arch Neurol* 2010; **67(4)**:408–415.

52 Perucca E, Berlowitz D, Birnbaum A et al.: Pharmacological and clinical aspects of antiepileptic drug use in the elderly. *Epilepsy Res* 2006; **68(Suppl. 1)**:S49–S63.

53 Gurwitz JH, Field TS, Avorn J et al.: Incidence and preventability of adverse drug events in nursing homes. *Am J Med* 2000; **109**:87–94.

54 Gurwitz JH, Field TS, Harrold LR et al.: Incidnece and preventability of adverse drug events among older patients in the ambulatory setting. *JAMA* 2003; **289**:1107–1116.

55 Brodie MJ, Overstall PW, Giorgi L, UK Lamotrigine Elderly Study Group: Multicentre, double-blind, randomized comparison between lamotrigine and carbamazepine in elderly patients with newly diagnosed epilepsy. *Epilepsy Res* 1999; **37**:81–87.

56 Giorgi L, Gomez G, O'Neill F et al.: The tolerability of lamotrigine in elderly patients with epilepsy. *Drugs Aging* 2001; **18**:621–630.

57 Ferrendelli JA, French J, Leppik I et al.: Use of levetiracetam in a population of patients aged 65 years and older: a subset analysis of the KEEPER trial. *Epilepsy Behav* 2003; **4**:702–709.

58 Patsals PN, Froscher W, Pisani F, van Rijn CM: The importance of drug interactions in epilepsy therapy. *Epilepsia* 2002; **43**:365–385.

59 McLean MJ: New Antiepiletic medications: pharmacokinetic and mechanistic considerations in the treatment of seizures and epilepsy in the elderly. In: Rowan AJ, Ramsey RE (eds):

Seizures and Epilepsy in the Elderly. Butterworth-Heinemann, Boston, MA, 1997, pp. 239–307.

60 Cloyd JC, Lackner TE, Leppik IE: Antiepileptics in the elderly: pharmacoepidemiology and pharmacokinetics. *Arch Fam Med* 1994; **3**:589–598.

61 Birnbaum A, Hardie NA, Leppik IE et al.: Variability of total phenytoin serum concentrations within elderly nursing home residents. *Neurology* 2003; **60**:555–559.

62 Tallis R. Treatment of epilepsy in the elderly patient. In: Shorvon S, Dreifuss D, Fish D, Thomas D (eds): *The Treatment of Epilepsy*. Blackwell Science, London, 1996, pp. 227–237.

63 Vestergaard P, Tigaran S, Rejnmark L, Tigaran C: Fracture risk in epilepsy. *Acta Neurol Scand* 1999; **99**:269–275.

64 Souverein P, Webb DJ, Petri H et al.: Incidence of fractures among epilepsy patients: a population based prospective cohort study in the general practice research database. *Epilepsia* 2005; **46**:304–310.

65 Sirven JI, Fife TD, Wingerchuk DM, Drazkowski JF: Second generation antiepileptic drugs' impact on balance: a meta-analysis. *Mayo Clin Proc* 2007; **82**:40–47.

66 Pack AM, Gidal B, Vasquez B: Bone disease associated with antiepileptic drugs. *Clev Clin J Med* 2004; **71(Suppl. 2)**: S42–S48.

67 Pack AM, Olarte LS, Morrell MJ et al.: Bone mineral density in an outpatient population receiving enzyme inducing antiepileptic drugs. *Epilepsy Behav* 2003; **4**:169–174.

68 Farhat G, Yamout B, Mikati A et al.: Effect of antiepileptic drugs on bone density in ambulatory patients. *Neurology* 2002; **58**:1348–1353.

69 Sirven JI, VNS in the Elderly Group. Vagus nerve stimulation therapy for epilepsy in older adults. *Neurology* 2000; **54(5)**:1179–1182.

70 Sperling MR, O'Connor MJ, Saykin AJ et al.: Temporal lobectomy for refractory epilepsy. *JAMA* 1996; **276**: 470–475.

71 Wiebe S, Blume WT, Girvin JP, Eliaszsiw M: A randomized controlled trial of surgery for temporal lobe epilepsy. *N Engl J Med* 2001; **345**:311–318.

72 McLachlan RS, Chovaz CJ, Blume WT et al.: Temporal lobectomy for intractable epilepsy in patients over age 45 years. *Neurology* 1992; **42**:662–665.

73 Cascino GD, Sharbrough FW, Hirschorn KA, Marsh WR: Surgery for focal epilepsy in the older patient. *Neurology* 1991; **41**:1415–1417.

74 Boling W, Andermann F, Reutens D et al.: Surgery for temporal lobe epilepsy in older patients. *J Neurosurg* 2001; **95**:242–248.

75 Grivas A, Schramm J, Kral T et al.: Surgical treatment for refractory temporal lobe epilepsy in the elderly: seizure outcome and neuropsychological sequels compared with a younger cohort. *Epilepsia* 2006; **47(8)**:1364–1372.

76 Sirven JI, Malamut BL, O'Connor MJ, Sperling MR: Temporal lobectomy outcome in older versus younger adults. *Neurology* 2000; **54(11)**:2166–2170.

77 Martin R, Vogtle L, Gilliam F, Faught E: What are the concerns of older adults living with epilepsy? *Epilepsy Behav* 2005; **7**:297–300.

CHAPTER 19

Balance disorders and falls in epilepsy

Sandra J. Petty,[1] Keith D. Hill,[2] and John D. Wark[3]

[1] *The Florey Institute of Neuroscience and Mental Health, Ormond College, and Department of Medicine, Royal Melbourne Hospital, University of Melbourne, Australia*

[2] *School of Physiotherapy and Exercise Science, Curtin University and Department of Allied Health, La Trobe University, Northern Health and National Ageing Research Institute, Australia*

[3] *Department of Medicine, University of Melbourne and Bone & Mineral Medicine, Royal Melbourne Hospital, Australia*

Introduction

The increased rate of bone fractures seen in epilepsy [1–3] may be explained not only by bone disease but also by increased falls, either during seizures or at other times [4]. Patients with epilepsy taking antiepileptic drugs (AEDs) frequently complain of gait unsteadiness [5]. However, the effects of epilepsy and its treatment upon balance remain underinvestigated. The relationship of fractures to seizure events in patients with epilepsy has varied across studies [1,2,6–8] but probably points to the importance of both seizure- and non-seizure-related etiologies.

A fall is defined as "an unexpected event in which the participant comes to rest on the ground, floor, or lower level" [9]. Injury from falls can lead to morbidity and mortality, particularly in the case of hip fracture in older individuals [10]. Falls during seizures are of obvious importance as a potential cause of injury in the epilepsy population. Balance involves "maintaining, achieving or restoring the body's centre of mass within the base of support" [11] and is a complex function mediated by somatosensory, vestibular, and visual inputs and the integration of these factors via the central nervous system into motor outputs to maintain posture and stability. Impaired balance is an important risk factor for falls. A survey of falls and fractures in patients with epilepsy that included assessment of awareness of risk revealed that less than 30% of patients were aware of the increased falls and fracture risk in epilepsy;

improving patient education and reporting of falls is recommended [12].

This chapter reviews the epidemiology of falls and balance dysfunction in AED users and examines potential mechanisms contributing to them. It also describes some methods by which practitioners can identify and minimize risk for fractures, falls, and balance dysfunction.

Epidemiology

Balance dysfunction and falls appear to be more common in people taking AEDs. Increased imbalance or ataxia was demonstrated in a pooled analysis of adjunctive second-generation AEDs [13], which showed evidence for a dose–response effect upon imbalance [13], with the relative risk of imbalance for all second-generation AEDs at any dose being 2.73 (95% CI 2.07–3.61) and at lowest dose being 1.76 (95% CI 1.26–2.46).

In our study of twins and siblings discordant for indication and use of AEDs (mean (SD) age = 44.9 (15.7) years), 27% (8 of 29) of AED users reported non-seizure-related falling in the preceding year (7 of the 8 were taking AED polytherapy), while 21% reported seizure-related falls [14]. In total, 41% of AED users reported falling during a seizure, at other times, or both. In comparison, 10% of age- and gender-matched AED non-user cotwins and siblings reported falls. Five AED users had a history of low-trauma fractures resulting from a fall (four forearm, one foot fracture),

---

Epilepsy and the Interictal State: Co-Morbidities and Quality of Life, First Edition.
Edited by Erik K. St. Louis, David M. Ficker, and Terence J. O'Brien.
© 2015 John Wiley & Sons, Ltd. Published 2015 by John Wiley & Sons, Ltd.

while no AED non-users had a fracture resulting from a simple trip or fall [14].

Pathophysiology

Risk factors for falls are generally categorized as intrinsic (related to the individual, including the effect of age, pathology affecting any of the systems involved in effective balance, and medications), extrinsic (related to the environment, including poor lighting, slippery or uneven surfaces, and tripping obstacles), and behavioral (related to performing an activity with an inherently high risk of falling). Many falls result from a combination of intrinsic and extrinsic risk factors [15].

The etiology of falls in the epilepsy patient population is likely to be multifactorial, with intrinsic contributory factors including seizures, postictal confusion, drowsiness related to seizure activity or medication, ataxia, dizziness associated with medications, and neurological deficits superimposed on the many risk factors for falls in the general population, such as reduced vision, peripheral neuropathy, reduced muscle strength, polypharmacy, and the use of medications associated with increased falls, such as psychotropic medications. There is also a lower rate of sports and exercise participation in patients with epilepsy [16–19], which may result in lower levels of fitness and increased muscle deconditioning, further increasing fall risk in this population.

In a study of older women receiving central nervous system (CNS)-active medications, patients receiving antiepileptic medication had a multivariate odds ratio (MOR) for falling in the next year of 2.56 compared to non-users, higher than that of benzodiazepine- and antidepressant-treated women [4]. Benzodiazepines are also commonly used in the treatment of epilepsy and are associated with increased sway, contributing to an increase in fall risk [20–22]. Polypharmacy and concomitant treatment with other medications associated with increased fall risk, including antidepressants [23], may also be a factor in fall risk in patients treated for epilepsy. A meta-analysis of 16 studies showed that all of the second-generation AEDs were associated with an increased risk ratio for reports of imbalance at standard dosages, with the exception of gabapentin and levetiracetam [13]. A dose effect was also reported [13].

Cerebellar atrophy is associated with AED usage and epilepsy [24]. Whether this pathology is a dose-dependent drug side effect for patients taking phenytoin [25], a result of chronic seizures [26], or related to duration of epilepsy or AED therapy remains to be definitively established. The cerebellum is important in the coordination of movement, including eyes, trunk, limbs, and speech, and has an additional possible role in emotion and cognition [27]. Interestingly, cerebellar volumes may be reduced in temporal-lobe epilepsy (TLE) [28], although this has not been a consistent finding and may be associated with the number of generalized tonic–clonic seizures [29]. Whether epilepsy, underlying causes, or treatment with AEDs causes cerebellar degeneration, thereby impacting balance and increasing fall risk, requires further investigation.

Recent research also highlights the important role of vitamin D in falls and fall injury risk. Vitamin D has a role in neuromuscular function [30] and muscle tissue via both genomic and nongenomic actions [31]. Muscular weakness is seen in association with vitamin D deficiency states [32] and vitamin D level is predictive of physical performance in older people [33]. Hypovitaminosis D has been shown to correlate with increased postural sway, measured by Lord's Balance Test [34], and with falls [35]. In a study of older hostel and nursing home residents, a multivariate analysis of patients aged 65–90 years showed that serum intact parathyroid hormone (iPTH) predicted time to first fall, independent of serum 25-hydroxyvitamin D (25OHD) levels [36]. Whether low vitamin D or elevated PTH levels in AED users [8,37–39] are associated with neuromuscular and balance impairments has not been clearly demonstrated [14,40]. Vitamin D (with or without calcium) replacement improves balance performance [41] and reduces fall risk in older, frail, nonepileptic populations [42].

Etiology

Few studies of patients receiving AEDs have used detailed balance assessments to quantify balance impairments. Studies examining balance function in patients with epilepsy have generally been limited by small sample sizes and a lack of appropriate control groups. Whether the etiology of balance dysfunction in epilepsy relates to the type of medication used, epilepsy type, or a contribution of neurological lesions requires further study [14,43].

One study of 16 patients showed that those receiving AEDs, particularly in polytherapy (as compared to monotherapy), had impaired balance function when tested by posturography using a pedoscope, which assesses movement of the center of gravity [44], suggesting that this may be a useful technique for assessing balance impairments in this patient population. Two other studies analyzed the effect of antiepileptic medication in adult patients. In 30 patients aged over 50 receiving AED monotherapy for idiopathic or generalized epilepsy (10 on gabapentin, 10 on lamotrigine, and 10 on carbamazepine), there were no differences in balance confidence or Berg Balance Scale scores, but patients receiving lamotrigine were able to sustain balance on the Fregly ataxia balance tests longer than those on carbamazepine, indicating differential medication effects upon balance function and fall risk [45]. No vestibular dysfunction was seen in any subgroup. Limitations of this study included a small sample size and a potential ceiling effect of the Berg Balance Scale, which may not be sensitive enough to adequately identify participants with mild balance impairments [45]. In another study, 25 adults presenting to hospital with generalized tonic–clonic seizure (including 19 treated with therapeutic levels of an AED) and 11 healthy controls were studied with computerized dynamic platform posturography [46]. Postural sway index (SI, higher score indicating poorer balance performance) was nonsignificantly higher in epilepsy patients than in controls. A lower SI (indicating better balance performance) was seen in those with less than three seizures, a short disease duration (<1 year), and generalized rather than localized (focal) epilepsy. In contrast, another recent study showed significantly increased SI for left single-leg stance in patients with epilepsy compared to controls and higher SI in patients with generalized rather than localized epilepsy in right single-leg stance [43]. Further research into the etiology of falls and balance impairment in patients with epilepsy is necessary. Analysis of balance function and MRI findings, such as cerebellar volume and lesion type and location, may provide further insights into fall risk in patients with epilepsy.

Diagnosis/evaluation

Important considerations for a falls intervention program include evaluation for epilepsy type, underlying neurologic lesions, seizure control, cardiovascular health, and exercise capacity. A full fall risk assessment also includes medication recording and assessment of bone health, including bone mineral density (BMD; discussed in detail in Chapter 20).

An evaluation of fall history, fall risk, and balance performance is essential for anyone at an increased risk of falling. These factors should be assessed when commencing antiepileptic medications, and monitoring for change of these parameters over time in longitudinally treated epilepsy patients is reasonable given growing evidence of an increased risk of balance impairment and falls in people receiving antiepileptic medications.

Following review of the appropriate definition of a fall with the patient (as given in the Introduction to this chapter), a fall history should be part of the assessment. All instances meeting the definition of a fall should be explored in order to ascertain factors involved in falls (see Box 19.1). A patient's self-report of fall history is valuable and can provide an understanding of contributory factors. Older people report environmental factors as being the major factor in many falls [47]. Detailed clinical examination focused on balance performance often identifies major intrinsic factors contributing to an individual's fall risk as well.

Box 19.1 Important historical factors involved in falls.

- Location.
- Activity prior to a fall.
- Any precipitating sensations (dizziness, vertigo, palpitations, aura, weakness, or sensory disturbance).
- Potential obstacles involved in slipping or tripping.
- Loss of consciousness.
- Ability to get up after a fall.
- Loss of confidence in mobility after a fall.
- Resultant injuries and whether medical attention was sought.

Since balance is multidimensional, detailed assessment requires a number of tests assessing different domains. Many tests of balance performance have been validated [48] but no individual test is capable of assessing all aspects [49,50]. Clinical balance scales such as the Berg Balance Scale are limited by ceiling effects for milder levels of balance impairment in higher-functioning individuals [45]. A brief but comprehensive balance-assessment battery includes static stance with sensory challenge, a dynamic bilateral stance test, a dynamic single-limb stance test, and functional mobility.

Static stance with sensory challenge involves standing with feet together and eyes closed. Healthy older people can perform this maneuver for a minimum of 30 seconds [51]. The dynamic bilateral stance test (functional reach test) assesses the maximum amount of forward reach in standing. Scores for healthy older males (mean ± sd) are 33.4 ± 3.9 cm and for females are 26.6 ± 9.0 cm [52]. The dynamic single-limb stance test (step test) counts the number of steps taken on and off a 7.5 cm block in 15 seconds with one leg stepping. Scores for healthy older people are 18.2 ± 4.0 steps [53]. The functional mobility test (timed up and go) measures the time taken to stand up from a chair and walk at a comfortable speed for 3 m, turn, and return to sit in the chair. Scores for healthy older people aged 70–79 years are 9 ± 2 seconds [54].

Each of these tests requires minimal equipment and training and is quick to perform. All have been shown to have high reliability and to be responsive to change [52,53,55] and all are useful in monitoring performance over time. Fall prevention interventions should be considered when scores on any of these tests fall outside of normative limits.

The Balance Outcome Measure for Elder Rehabilitation (BOOMER) is a recently reported combined set of clinical balance tests, including a static-stance task, functional reach, timed up and go, and the step test. BOOMER categorizes the scores for each test into quintiles and aggregates them into an overall balance performance score [56].

Posturography is a sensitive tool for measuring balance, allowing identification of milder balance dysfunction elicited by a range of test conditions, as reflected by the results of three studies of community-dwelling patients receiving antiepileptic medications [14,43,46]. While this is a useful tool in research, it is generally not available to most clinicians.

Patients requiring AED therapy may also have a range of other fall risk factors that magnify risk. Assessment for other risk factors such as impaired vision, neuropathy, medication, foot pathology, footwear choice, gait disturbance, cognitive assessment, incontinence, and dizziness should be included. A fall risk screening tool is a useful way of determining an individual's overall risk. Examples of validated tools that can be performed quickly in a clinical setting include the Falls Risk for Older People – Community Setting screening tool (FROP-Com; see http://www.mednwh.unimelb.edu.au /nari_research/pdf_docs/FropCom2009/FROP-Com -Screen-Guidelines-Dec09.pdf, last accessed July 15, 2014) [57] and the Elderly Fall Screening Test (EFST) [58]. For patients identified as having an increased risk on a screening tool, a detailed fall risk assessment is recommended, in order to identify individual risk factors that can inform the management plan. Examples of validated fall risk assessment tools that are useful in the clinical setting include the full FROP-Com [59] and the Falls Risk Assessment Tool (FRAT) for primary care [60], which includes both a screening and a more detailed assessment and management section. The Physiological Profile Assessment (PPA) is a well-validated fall risk assessment that objectively quantifies fall risk on five physiological risk factors: balance, muscle strength, reaction time, lower limb proprioception, and vision [34]. Environmental factors within or around the home may contribute to a patient's risk of falling. Where there is a history of falls or near falls due to home environmental hazards, a detailed home assessment by a trained health professional such as an occupational therapist and appropriate home modifications to increase safety can reduce risk of future falls [61]. The Home Falls and Accidents Screening Tool (HOME FAST) is useful for assessing the home environment and the patient's interaction with it, and has been shown to identify risk of falls and to be responsive to change [62].

A commonly overlooked consequence of a fall is loss of confidence, or reduced fall efficacy. Loss of confidence may result in curtailed activity, which further increases muscle weakness and reduces balance and therefore further increases risk of future falls. A brief assessment tool, the Falls Efficacy Scale – International (FES-I), has been shown to have high retest reliability and responsiveness to change and is available in a number of languages [63,64]. The FES-I is available from the Prevention of Falls Network Europe (ProFaNE) Web site: www.profane.eu.org (last accessed July 15, 2014).

Management

There is level I and II evidence that a range of single interventions, including exercise, medication review, psychotropic medication reduction, home assessment,

Table 19.1 Factors to consider when managing fall risk in patients with epilepsy.

Fall risk factors in epilepsy	Duration of antiepileptic medication therapy
	Polytherapy with antiepileptic therapy
	Concomitant medications that increase fall risk
	Epilepsy type or underlying neurologic lesions
	Poorly controlled epilepsy
Investigations	AED levels (avoid acute toxicity)
	Vitamin D status
	Neuroimaging (excluding neurologic lesion)
	Appropriate screening for injury
	Fall screening and scales
	Balance and mobility assessment
Management strategies	Optimization of seizure control
	Patient education: reduction of falls risk
	Allied health assessment and management, including balance exercise programs and home safety assessment and modification
	Bone health assessment
	Rationalization of medications, where possible

modification for at-risk older people, and vitamin D supplementation when appropriate, as well as multifactorial interventions (combining two or more interventions, often based on a fall risk assessment), can be effective in reducing falls in the general at-risk population [65,66]. However, there are currently no published trials of falls and balance retraining in patients with epilepsy. Where possible, optimization of seizure control and reduction of AED toxicity and polypharmacy [4] may also be of value in preventing falls and related injuries. Table 19.1 lists factors to consider in the investigation and management of falls in patients with epilepsy. Exercise programs, particularly those with a focus on balance retraining [67], have been shown to be effective in community-dwelling older people and are likely to have positive benefits for those taking AEDs. Exercise approaches that have been shown to be effective in reducing falls in older people include individualized balance- and strength-training home programs prescribed by a physiotherapist or other trained health professional [68]; group exercise programs incorporating balance, strength, and fitness exercises [69]; and tai chi programs [70]. Periodic monitoring for

vitamin D deficiency or insufficiency, with treatment as required to ensure optimal levels, is prudent, although there are no published clinical trials of vitamin D treatment and its effect on balance function in patients with epilepsy. Involvement of balance clinics [71] and allied health staff with falls-prevention and neurological experience may be indicated in patients at risk of falls or with a history of falling. Treatment of underlying bone health problems is logical and may also be useful in the prevention of fractures, but there is a lack of evidence on the benefit of specific bone-active therapy to injuries associated with falls in the epilepsy population.

Conclusion

Patients with epilepsy receiving AEDs have increased fall risk, both during seizures and at other times. While data remain limited, factors such as chronic AED use, dose effects, and polytherapy may contribute to increased fall risk. The role of underlying epilepsy type and neurologic lesions should also be assessed. In addition, any history of falls, bone disease, balance problems, or neurologic impairments should be considered in the management of fall risk in patients with epilepsy. While there are no randomized trials investigating fall prevention approaches in people taking AEDs, treatment options for patients with identified increased risk of falls or fractures should include general approaches shown to be effective in improving balance and reducing falls in at-risk people, including exercise, medication review, and home environment assessment and modification.

References

1 Vestergaard P, Tigaran S, Rejnmark L et al.: Fracture risk is increased in epilepsy. *Acta Neurol Scand* 1999; **99(5)**: 269–275.

2 Vestergaard P: Epilepsy, osteoporosis and fracture risk: a meta-analysis. *Acta Neurol Scand* 2005; **112(5)**:277–286.

3 Mattson RH, Gidal BE: Fractures, epilepsy, and antiepileptic drugs. *Epilepsy Behav* 2004; **5(Suppl. 2)**:S36–S40.

4 Ensrud KE, Blackwell TL, Mangione CM et al.: Central nervous system-active medications and risk for falls in older women. *J Am Geriatr Soc* 2002; **50(10)**:1629–1637.

5 Tugendhaft P. [The follow-up of antiepileptic drugs.] *J Pharm Belg* 2004; **59(3)**:80–82.

6 Cummings SR, Nevitt MC, Browner WS et al.: Risk factors for hip fracture in white women. Study of Osteoporotic Fractures Research Group. *N Engl J Med* 1995; **332(12)**: 767–773.

7 Desai KB, Ribbans WJ, Taylor GJ: Incidence of five common fracture types in an institutional epileptic population. *Injury* 1996; **27(2)**:97–100.

8 Kulak CA, Borba VZ, Bilezikian JP et al.: Bone mineral density and serum levels of 25 OH vitamin D in chronic users of antiepileptic drugs. *Arq Neuropsiquiatr* 2004; **62(4)**:940–948.

9 Hauer K, Lamb SE, Jorstad EC et al.: Systematic review of definitions and methods of measuring falls in randomised controlled fall prevention trials. *Age Ageing* 2006; **35(1)**:5–10.

10 Grisso JA, Kelsey JL, Strom BL et al.: Risk factors for falls as a cause of hip fracture in women: The Northeast Hip Fracture Study Group. *N Engl J Med* 1991; **324(19)**:1326–1331.

11 Mancini M, Horak FB: The relevance of clinical balance assessment tools to differentiate balance deficits. *Eur J Phys Rehabil Med* 2010; **46(2)**:239–248.

12 Shiek Ahmad B, Hill KD, O'Brien TJ et al.: Falls and fractures in patients chronically treated with antiepileptic drugs. *Neurology* 2012; **79(2)**:145–151.

13 Sirven JI, Fife TD, Wingerchuk DM, Drazkowski JF: Second-generation antiepileptic drugs' impact on balance: a meta-analysis. *Mayo Clin Proc* 2007; **82(1)**:40–47.

14 Petty SJ, Hill KD, Haber NE et al.: Balance impairment in chronic antiepileptic drug users: a twin and sibling study. *Epilepsia* 2010; **51(2)**:280–288.

15 Tinetti ME, Gordon C, Sogolow E et al.: Fall-risk evaluation and management: challenges in adopting geriatric care practices. *Gerontologist* 2006; **46(6)**:717–725.

16 Howard GM, Radloff M, Sevier TL: Epilepsy and sports participation. *Curr Sports Med Rep* 2004; **3(1)**:15–19.

17 Steinhoff BJ, Neususs K, Thegeder H, Reimers CD: Leisure time activity and physical fitness in patients with epilepsy. *Epilepsia* 1996; **37(12)**:1221–1227.

18 Wong J, Wirrell E: Physical activity in children/teens with epilepsy compared with that in their siblings without epilepsy. *Epilepsia* 2006; **47(3)**:631–639.

19 Elliott JO, Lu B, Moore JL et al.: Exercise, diet, health behaviors, and risk factors among persons with epilepsy based on the California Health Interview Survey, 2005. *Epilepsy Behav* 2008; **13(2)**:307–315.

20 Swift CG: Postural instability as a measure of sedative drug response. *Br J Clin Pharmacol* 1984; **18(Suppl. 1)**:S87–S90.

21 Swift CG, Ewen JM, Clarke P, Stevenson IH: Responsiveness to oral diazepam in the elderly: relationship to total and free plasma concentrations. *Br J Clin Pharmacol* 1985; **20(2)**:111–118.

22 Swift CG, Swift MR, Ankier SI et al.: Single dose pharmacokinetics and pharmacodynamics of oral loprazolam in the elderly. *Br J Clin Pharmacol* 1985; **20(2)**:119–128.

23 Boyle N, Naganathan V, Cumming RG: Medication and falls: risk and optimization. *Clin Geriatr Med* 2010; **26(4)**: 583–605.

24 Botez MI, Attig E, Vezina JL: Cerebellar atrophy in epileptic patients. *Can J Neurol Sci* 1988; **15(3)**:299–303.

25 De Marcos FA, Ghizoni E, Kobayashi E et al.: Cerebellar volume and long-term use of phenytoin. *Seizure* 2003; **12(5)**:312–315.

26 Specht U, May TW, Rohde M et al.: Cerebellar atrophy decreases the threshold of carbamazepine toxicity in patients with chronic focal epilepsy. *Arch Neurol* 1997; **54(4)**:427–431.

27 Frings M, Maschke M, Timmann D: Cerebellum and cognition: viewed from philosophy of mind. *Cerebellum* 2007; **12**:1–7.

28 Sandok EK, O'Brien TJ, Jack CR, So EL: Significance of cerebellar atrophy in intractable temporal lobe epilepsy: a quantitative MRI study. *Epilepsia* 2000; **41(10)**: 1315–1320.

29 Szabo CA, Lancaster JL, Lee S et al.: MR imaging volumetry of subcortical structures and cerebellar hemispheres in temporal lobe epilepsy. *AJNR Am J Neuroradiol* 2006; **27(10)**:2155–2160.

30 Perez-Lopez FR: Vitamin D and its implications for musculoskeletal health in women: an update. *Maturitas* 2007; **58(2)**:117–137.

31 Pfeifer M, Begerow B, Minne HW: Vitamin D and muscle function. *Osteoporos Int* 2002; **13(3)**:187–194.

32 Eriksen EF, Glerup H: Vitamin D deficiency and aging: implications for general health and osteoporosis. *Biogerontology* 2002; **3(1–2)**:73–77.

33 Wicherts IS, van Schoor NM, Boeke AJ et al.: Vitamin D status predicts physical performance and its decline in older persons. *J Clin Endocrinol Metab* 2007; **92(6)**:2058–2065.

34 Lord SR, Menz HB, Tiedemann A: A physiological profile approach to falls risk assessment and prevention. *Phys Ther* 2003; **83(3)**:237–252.

35 Pfeifer M, Begerow B, Minne HW et al.: Vitamin D status, trunk muscle strength, body sway, falls, and fractures among 237 postmenopausal women with osteoporosis. *Exp Clin Endocrinol Diabetes* 2001; **109(2)**:87–92.

36 Sambrook PN, Chen JS, March LM et al.: Serum parathyroid hormone predicts time to fall independent of vitamin D status in a frail elderly population. *J Clin Endocrinol Metab* 2004; **89(4)**:1572–1576.

37 Hahn TJ, Shires R, Halstead LR: Serum dihydroxyvitamin D metabolite concentrations in patients on chronic anticonvulsant drug therapy: response to pharmacologic doses of vitamin D2. *Metab Bone Dis Relat Res* 1983; **5(1)**:1–6.

38 Nettekoven S, Strohle A, Trunz B et al.: Effects of antiepileptic drug therapy on vitamin D status and biochemical markers of bone turnover in children with epilepsy. *Eur J Pediatr* 2008; **167(12)**:1369–1377.

39 Pack AM, Morrell MJ, Randall A et al.: Bone health in young women with epilepsy after one year of antiepileptic drug monotherapy. *Neurology* 2008; **70(18)**:1586–1593.

40 Gerdhem P, Ringsberg KA, Obrant KJ, Akesson K: Association between 25-hydroxy vitamin D levels, physical activity, muscle strength and fractures in the prospective population-based OPRA Study of Elderly Women. *Osteoporos Int* 2005; **16(11)**:1425–1431.

41 Dhesi JK, Jackson SH, Bearne LM et al.: Vitamin D supplementation improves neuromuscular function in older people who fall. *Age Ageing* 2004; **33(6)**:589–595.

42 Bischoff-Ferrari HA, Conzelmann M, Stahelin HB et al.: Is fall prevention by vitamin D mediated by a change in postural or dynamic balance? *Osteoporos Int* 2006; **17(5)**:656–663.

43 Yahalom G, Blatt I, Neufeld MY et al.: Epilepsy syndrome-associated balance dysfunction assessed by static posturography. *Seizure* 2011; **20(3)**:214–217.

44 Arima K, Kitamura J, Onuma T et al.: Analysis of the swaying of center of gravity in standing posture of patients with antiepileptic drugs. *Jpn J Psychiatry Neurol* 1990; **44(2)**:371–373.

45 Southard V, Dave M, Davis MG et al.: The Multiple Tasks Test as a predictor of falls in older adults. *Gait Posture* 2005; **22(4)**:351–355.

46 Gandelman-Marton R, Arlazoroff A, Dvir Z: Balance performance in adult epilepsy patients. *Seizure* 2006; **15(8)**:582–589.

47 Braun BL. Knowledge and perception of fall-related risk factors and fall-reduction techniques among community-dwelling elderly individuals. *Phys Ther* 1998; **78(12)**:1262–1276.

48 Huxham FE, Goldie PA, Patla AE: Theoretical considerations in balance assessment. *Aust J Physiother* 2001; **47(2)**:89–100.

49 Winter DA, Patla AE, Frank JS: Assessment of balance control in humans. *Med Prog Technol* 1990; **16(1–2)**:31–51.

50 Muir SW, Berg K, Chesworth B et al.: Balance impairment as a risk factor for falls in community-dwelling older adults who are high functioning: a prospective study. *Phys Ther* 2010; **90(3)**:338–347.

51 Cohen H, Blatchly CA, Gombash LL: A study of the clinical test of sensory interaction and balance. *Phys Ther* 1993; **73(6)**:346–51; disc. 51–54.

52 Duncan PW, Weiner DK, Chandler J, Studenski S: Functional reach: a new clinical measure of balance. *J Gerontol* 1990; **45(6)**:M192–M197.

53 Hill K, Bernhardt J, McGann A et al.: A new test of dynamic standing balance for stroke patients: reliability, validity, and comparison with healthy elderly. *Physiother Can* 1996; **48**:257–262.

54 Steffen TM, Hacker TA, Mollinger L: Age- and gender-related test performance in community-dwelling elderly people: Six-Minute Walk Test, Berg Balance Scale, Timed Up & Go Test, and gait speeds. *Phys Ther* 2002; **82(2)**:128–137.

55 Podsiadlo D, Richardson S: The timed "Up & Go": a test of basic functional mobility for frail elderly persons. *J Am Geriatr Soc* 1991; **39(2)**:142–148.

56 Haines T, Kuys SS, Morrison G et al.: Development and validation of the balance outcome measure for elder rehabilitation. *Arch Phys Med Rehabil* 2007; **88(12)**:1614–1621.

57 Russell MA, Hill KD, Day LM et al.: Development of the Falls Risk for Older People in the Community (FROP-Com) screening tool. *Age Ageing* 2009; **38(1)**:40–46.

58 Cwikel JG, Fried A, Biderman A, Galinsky D: Validation of a fall-risk screening test, the Elderly Fall Screening Test (EFST), for community-dwelling elderly. *Disabil Rehabil* 1998; **20(5)**:161–167.

59 Russell MA, Hill KD, Blackberry I et al.: The reliability and predictive accuracy of the falls risk for older people in the community assessment (FROP-Com) tool. *Age Ageing* 2008; **37(6)**:634–639.

60 Nandy S, Parsons S, Cryer C et al.: Development and preliminary examination of the predictive validity of the Falls Risk Assessment Tool (FRAT) for use in primary care. *J Public Health (Oxf)* 2004; **26(2)**:138–143.

61 Cumming RG, Thomas M, Szonyi G et al.: Home visits by an occupational therapist for assessment and modification of environmental hazards: a randomized trial of falls prevention. *J Am Geriatr Soc* 1999; **47(12)**:1397–1402.

62 Mackenzie L, Byles J, D'Este C: Longitudinal study of the Home Falls and Accidents Screening Tool in identifying older people at increased risk of falls. *Australas J Ageing* 2009; **28(2)**:64–69.

63 Kempen GI, Yardley L, van Haastregt JC et al.: The Short FES-I: a shortened version of the falls efficacy scale-international to assess fear of falling. *Age Ageing* 2008; **37(1)**:45–50.

64 Ruggiero C, Mariani T, Gugliotta R et al.: Validation of the Italian version of the falls efficacy scale international (FES-I)

and the short FES-I in community-dwelling older persons. *Arch Gerontol Geriatr* 2009; **49(Suppl. 1)**:211–219.

65 AGS/BGS: Summary of the Updated American Geriatrics Society/British Geriatrics Society clinical practice guideline for prevention of falls in older persons. *J Am Geriatr Soc* 2011; **59(1)**:148–157.

66 Gillespie LD, Robertson MC, Gillespie WJ et al.: Interventions for preventing falls in older people living in the community. *Cochrane Database Syst Rev* 2012; **9**:CD007146.

67 Sherrington C, Tiedemann A, Fairhall N et al.: Exercise to prevent falls in older adults: an updated meta-analysis and best practice recommendations. *NSW Public Health Bull* 2011; **22(3–4)**:78–83.

68 Robertson MC, Campbell AJ, Gardner MM, Devlin N: Preventing injuries in older people by preventing falls:

a meta-analysis of individual-level data. *J Am Geriatr Soc* 2002; **50(5)**:905–911.

69 Day L, Fildes B, Gordon I et al.: Randomised factorial trial of falls prevention among older people living in their own homes. *BMJ* 2002; **325(7356)**:128.

70 Li F, Harmer P, Fisher KJ et al.: Tai chi and fall reductions in older adults: a randomized controlled trial. *J Gerontol A Biol Sci Med Sci* 2005; **60(2)**:187–194.

71 Hill KD, Moore KJ, Dorevitch MI, Day LML: Effectiveness of falls clinics: an evaluation of outcomes and client adherence to recommended interventions. *J Am Geriatr Soc* 2008; **56(4)**:600–608.

CHAPTER 20

Bone health in epilepsy

Sandra J. Petty,[1] and John D. Wark[2]

[1] The Florey Institute of Neuroscience and Mental Health, Ormond College, and Department of Medicine, Royal Melbourne Hospital, University of Melbourne, Australia

[2] Department of Medicine, University of Melbourne and Bone & Mineral Medicine, Royal Melbourne Hospital, Australia

Introduction

Patients with epilepsy have at least twice the fracture risk of the general community [1]. The problems of fractures and related issues in epilepsy were first reported in the medical literature in the 1950s. However, by 2001, a relatively low proportion of neurologists were assessing or treating fractures or referring patients to specialists for bone health review and management [2]. This apparent underrecognition of bone health problems in epilepsy could potentially relate to a number of factors, including limitations in the available literature and conflicting study results (earlier data predominantly being derived from institutionalized patients with multiple potential fracture risk confounders), uncertainty about the clinical relevance of older information for contemporary ambulatory patients with epilepsy and newer antiepileptic drugs (AEDs), and the lack of consensus and guidelines in the management of bone health in patients with epilepsy. There is also a general lack of awareness of bone health issues among patients with epilepsy [3].

Fracture rates

The magnitude of reduction in bone mineral density (BMD) seen in several studies does not appear to satisfactorily explain the observed increase in fracture risk. Moreover, increased fracture rates may be explained more by the underlying epilepsy disorder and seizure severity than by adverse effects of medications [4]. Factors likely to contribute to fracture risk in epilepsy include trauma from falls during seizures, fractures due to seizure biomechanics, impaired balance leading to increased falls risk [5], and associations with epilepsy as a disorder and AED use with impairment of BMD or bone quality [6]. The broadening of indications for prescription of antiepileptic medications, including chronic pain, migraine, and bipolar affective disorder, further raises the importance of defining the pathophysiology of fracture risk in those treated with AEDs and the development of appropriate practice guidelines for investigating and managing bone health in patients who receive these medications for prolonged periods of time. Whether all patients are likely to be equally affected or whether some specific risk factors for bone disease or fracture exist that may provide an opportunity for tailoring screening and treatment strategies requires careful study. The observed fracture rates and mechanisms of fracture vary across studies; in a meta-analysis including 11 studies of fracture risk, 35% of fractures occurred during seizures and relative risk (RR) of fractures at the hip (RR 5.3), spine (RR 6.2), and forearm (RR 1.7) was increased [1].

There are currently no formal guidelines for clinicians to refer to when managing bone health issues in patients with epilepsy. In the pediatric age group, possible associations or effects of epilepsy/AED on growth and peak bone mass are under investigation. However, the results of further longitudinal study are required to compile evidence to guide bone health management in this important age group. Indeed, further research to supply supporting evidence for detection, monitoring, and management of bone health in epilepsy across all age groups is required.

Epilepsy and the Interictal State: Co-Morbidities and Quality of Life, First Edition.
Edited by Erik K. St. Louis, David M. Ficker, and Terence J. O'Brien.
© 2015 John Wiley & Sons, Ltd. Published 2015 by John Wiley & Sons, Ltd.

Epidemiology

The incidence rate of fractures in patients with epilepsy was 241.9 per 10 000 person years in a study based on information from the UK General Practice Research Database (GPRD), which gave an age- and gender-adjusted incidence density ratio of 1.89 compared to the control cohort [7].

Fractures may be sustained during seizures, due to related mechanical forces or a resultant fall, or at other times, due to bone disease such as osteomalacia or osteoporosis. Most likely, a combination of these intrinsic bone and extrinsic biomechanical factors will determine fracture risk in epilepsy. The proportion of fractures related to seizures or occurring at other times varies widely across studies. An excess of pathological fractures (fractures occurring in areas of bone affected by disease) has been noted across all age groups in epilepsy; such fractures can occur at a younger age than is generally observed in the community [8]. Gender and age differences in fracture etiology have been described, with distribution of traumatic/seizure-related and pathological fractures: in a retrospective analysis utilizing ICD-9 codes for patients with epilepsy sustaining a fracture over a 7-year period, 39% of fractures were classified as pathological (clinically diagnosed osteoporosis or osteomalacia); the remainder were categorized as due either to seizures or to trauma in the absence of formally diagnosed bone disease. Whether the relatively high rate of pathological fractures at a younger age (56% of pathological fractures were recorded in patients aged under 50 years) was potentially underestimated due to noninclusion of osteopenia in the pathological fracture category was queried and whether bone disease was specifically searched for in all patients presenting with fracture in time to be included in the coding was not commented upon. Younger males and older females were more likely to fracture; for males, the proportion of pathological fractures peaked in this study in the 20–29-year-old group, whereas for females it peaked in the 70–79-year-old group [8].

Several studies in the pediatric age group have been performed. Results across studies have varied in terms of observed associations of epilepsy and/or AED use with reduced BMD [9]. Whether there is an effect on growth or an age at which patients are more susceptible to bone health problems – including failure to attain peak bone mass – requires further longitudinal study,

as does the association between duration of epilepsy, epilepsy treatments, and bone health [10]. Children treated with a combination of valproate and lamotrigine were found to have lower BMD and shorter stature, although reduced physical activity rather than medication effects may have been responsible for these findings [11]. The ketogenic diet is associated with progressive bone loss, although the mechanism remains to be established [10,12]. Developmental disorders associated with epilepsy and decreased mobility [13] may also be associated with impaired bone health.

Pathophysiology

The pathophysiology of fractures in epilepsy is likely to be multifactorial. Different factors may be relatively more important in selected patients (e.g., gender, age, menopausal status [14], vitamin D status, epilepsy syndrome type and comorbidities, and fall risk factors; see Chapter 19 for further discussion).

Potential mechanisms for bone disease associated with epilepsy/AED usage include cytochrome p450 inducer AEDs, vitamin D metabolism [15], and direct bone remodeling effects of AEDs demonstrated *in vitro*. In a rat model, phenobarbital and phenytoin produced inhibition of gastrointestinal calcium absorption [16]; carbamazepine and phenytoin have been shown to inhibit proliferation of human osteoblast-like cells at therapeutic dose levels [17]. Calcium homeostasis alterations and secondary hyperparathyroidism have also been observed in some patients treated with phenytoin [18]. Hormonal changes have been associated with epilepsy and AED treatments [19], resulting in secondary effects on bone health.

There may also be central nervous system (CNS) effects on bone health. The "brain–bone axis" could affect the neuro–osseous axis in bone, allowing medication or seizures to impact on the hypothalamus, leading to secondary effects on bone health [20]. Direct bone cell side effects, such as the action of histone deacetylases (Hdac), also play a role in bone remodeling and maintenance of bone mass. Valproate is a known Hdac inhibitor [21]. *In vitro*, valproate may also potentially contribute to osteomalacia via increased expression of CYP24, leading to accelerated catabolism of 1alpha,25(OH)(2)-vitamin D3 (VD3) [22]. A vitamin D receptor (VDR) BsmI restriction fragment polymorphism previously, although not universally, associated with reduced BMD has also been shown in one study to be associated with reduced BMD where at least one B allele is present [23]. Whether there is also a role for vitamin D and VDR in epileptogenesis requires further study [24–26].

General bone health risk factors may be increased in some patients with epilepsy, including smoking, excessive alcohol use, reduced exercise, dietary factors, and low vitamin D levels [27]. Whether there are any direct factors related to the type of epilepsy itself is not well described. Underlying neurologic disease, associations with epilepsy genetics, and factors involved in epileptogenesis that could have an impact on bone health require further study.

Potential mechanisms for fractures and bone disease associated with epilepsy/AED usage include bone health impairment (osteomalacia: reduced bone density or quality), falls during seizures, biomechanical stress during seizures, and balance impairment leading to increased fall risk [5], due either to medication usage or to the underlying epilepsy diagnosis [28]. Acute AED side effects, including ataxia and reduced alertness, as well as potential chronic toxicity and cerebellar atrophy [29], may also lead to balance impairment.

Diagnosis and evaluation

Screening of bone health in epilepsy is recommended [30]. However, limitations of the available data and conflicting study results have restricted the development of formal guidelines for clinicians. Patient and physician awareness of the potential increased fracture risk associated with epilepsy is necessary in order to make an assessment of risk factors for bone disease and create a monitoring and management plan.

Standard risk factors for osteoporosis should be assessed and modifiable factors optimized. Relevant risk factors include age, gender, family history of osteoporosis, smoking, alcohol intake, nutritional status and calcium intake, low body weight, vitamin D status, hypogonadism, delayed puberty, oligoamenorrhea, menopausal age and status, and immobility or lack of physical activity. Assessment for other medical conditions or medications which might be associated with osteoporosis is also important, such as renal disease, liver disease, malabsorption syndromes, primary

hyperparathyroidism, and glucocorticoid use. Relevant investigations should be tailored for each patient. Blood tests such as biochemistries; urea and electrolytes to assess renal function; calcium, magnesium, and phosphate levels; liver function tests; and serum protein electrophoresis for exclusion of other causes of bone disease or osteoporosis can be carried out. The optimal serum 25-OH vitamin D required to maintain bone health in patients with epilepsy has not been specifically determined, but in the general community a vitamin D level of >75 nmol/L has been proposed as optimal to maintain bone health, although further review of this level is in progress [31]. Hormone assays such as intact parathyroid hormone (iPTH), relevant sex steroid hormones (e.g., testosterone, estradiol, progesterone), sex hormone binding globulin (SHBG), and thyroid-stimulating hormone (TSH), as well as investigation for Cushing syndrome, may also be appropriate in selected patients.

Bone turnover markers in the serum and urine are listed in Table 20.1. Selected bone turnover markers may be useful in determining the etiology of bone disease and monitoring therapy, but a clinical role for measurement of these markers in AED-treated individuals has not yet been established. Currently, measurement of serum procollagen type 1 N-terminal propeptide (P1NP) and of either N-terminal telopeptide (NTX) or C-terminal telopeptide (CTX) is favored for the assessment of bone formation and bone resorption, respectively.

A recent review of current clinical and research imaging strategies for quantitative bone health assessment is available [32]. In all patients, the risk/benefit ratio of repeated exposure to radiation should be considered by the clinician and patient, although these techniques involve only low-level exposure to ionizing radiation compared with conventional radiography. Currently utilized quantitative bone health techniques include dual-energy X-ray absorptiometry (DXA), peripheral quantitative computerized tomography (pQCT), and quantitative ultrasound (QUS). DXA is currently a clinical gold-standard tool but is not universally accessible or reimbursable for the patient and involves use of low-dose radiation. This test should not be performed during pregnancy. While predominantly a research tool, pQCT offers advantages in analysis of bone health over the DXA scan in terms of assessment of trabecular and cortical bone compartments and stress–strain index, but it can be used only at peripheral bone sites. QUS is

Table 20.1 Bone turnover markers.

Bone formation markers in serum	Bone resorption markers in urine
Alkaline phosphatase (AP)	Hydroxyproline
Bone-specific alkaline phosphatase (BSAP)	Total pyridinoline (PYD)
Osteocalcin	Free deoxypyridinoline (DPD)
Type 1 procollagen (C-terminal/N-terminal): C1NP or P1NP	Collagen type 1 crosslinked N-telopeptide (NTX)[a]
	Collagen type 1 crosslinked C-telopeptide (CTX)[a]
	Bone sialoprotein (BSP)
	Tartrate-resistant acid phosphatase 5b (TRAP5b)

[a]May also be done in serum.

often used as a screening tool, having the advantage of no radiation exposure, and has been applied to some studies of bone health in epilepsy [33]. Axial QCT (spine, plus hip in a few centers) is still used in some centers but is limited by low accuracy and precision in non-expert hands and by relatively high radiation exposure (and cost). Bone biopsy is usually reserved for circumstances when clinical uncertainty remains after other clinical and laboratory investigation of established fractures proves inconclusive regarding the nature of underlying bone disease.

Management

Patients should be aware of general and specific measures for optimizing bone health. They should not smoke and should limit alcohol intake. Where possible, they should partake in regular exercise (within the limitations of any neurologic or other medical conditions). They should have an adequate source of vitamin D (diet and possibly sensible sunlight exposure, taking into account the risks of UV exposure on the skin; authorities in many countries publish guidelines for reasonable sun exposure). A good dietary calcium intake should be maintained. WHO recommendations for daily calcium intake are widely available [34] but there are some current controversies regarding calcium intake and supplementation that should be considered, which still require further study (see http://www.iom .edu/Reports/2010/Dietary-Reference-Intakes-for -Calcium-and-Vitamin-D.aspx, last accessed July 15, 2014).

Achieving optimal control of the epilepsy may reduce the risk of falls, injury, and fracture [4]. There is currently no published evidence to suggest that changing AEDs might be useful for fall reduction, but alteration of the AED regiment may be considered if seizures are poorly controlled and the AED prescribed is known to be associated with reduced BMD. In some situations, supplementation with vitamin D with or without calcium may be necessary. The prevalence of vitamin D deficiency in patients treated for epilepsy is high and treatment of vitamin D deficiency is recommended [35]. There is published evidence of a positive treatment response to supplementation of vitamin D [36,37]. However, in a recent retrospective study of calcium and vitamin D supplementation in patients with epilepsy receiving AEDs, no statistically significant fracture prevention benefit was seen [38], but this study was retrospective, patients taking supplementation with vitamin D and calcium were older, and supplements may have been prescribed to those patients seen to be at higher risk of fracture [38].

Data regarding the use of specific osteoporosis medications such as antiresorptive bisphosphonates in patients with epilepsy and low bone density or fractures are limited. One recent study reported that the use of calcium and vitamin D supplements improved BMD at the lumbar spine and that calcium, vitamin D, and the antiresorptive agent risedronate improved BMD and prevented new-onset vertebral fracture in older male patients compared to a group given placebo [39]. Treatment with such agents may be required but should be guided by a physician experienced in managing bone health. Most clinical trials of antiresorptive medications were performed in older postmenopausal female populations and long-term safety profiles should be considered, particularly in prescribing to younger age groups.

There is no published evidence for balance retraining in epilepsy patients at risk for falls. However, if a patient is identified to have increased fall risk, this may be a useful strategy [40] (see Chapter 19).

Prognosis

The impact of fractures in epilepsy has not been specifically studied but the general morbidity and mortality of injuries from seizures and from fractures in the community is well established [41]. Improved awareness of bone health by clinicians and patients should enable the development of optimal approaches toward evaluation and management of bone health, including bone health monitoring, translational research into mechanisms, and development and optimization of subsequent treatments to prevent fractures in patients with epilepsy. Further research in this field is necessary in order to establish both pathophysiology and well-targeted treatment strategies.

References

1 Vestergaard P: Epilepsy, osteoporosis and fracture risk: a meta-analysis. *Acta Neurol Scand* 2005; **112(5)**:277–286.
2 Valmadrid C, Voorhees C, Litt B, Schneyer CR: Practice patterns of neurologists regarding bone and mineral effects of antiepileptic drug therapy. *Arch Neurol* 2001; **58(9)**:1369–1374.
3 Shiek Ahmad B, Hill KD, O'Brien TJ et al.: Falls and fractures in patients chronically treated with antiepileptic drugs. *Neurology* 2012; **79(2)**:145–151.
4 Vestergaard P: Changes in bone turnover, bone mineral and fracture risk induced by drugs used to treat epilepsy. *Curr Drug Saf* 2008; **3(3)**:168–172.
5 Petty SJ, Hill KD, Haber NE et al.: Balance impairment in chronic antiepileptic drug users: a twin and sibling study. *Epilepsia* 2010; **51(2)**:280–288.
6 Pack AM, Morrell MJ: Adverse effects of antiepileptic drugs on bone structure: epidemiology, mechanisms and therapeutic implications. *CNS Drugs* 2001; **15(8)**:633–642.
7 Souverein P, Webb DJ, Petri H et al.: Incidence of fractures among epilepsy patients: a population-based retrospective

cohort study in the general practice research database. *Epilepsia* 2005; **46(2)**:304–310.
8 Sheth RD, Gidal BE, Hermann BP: Pathological fractures in epilepsy. *Epilepsy Behav* 2006; **9(4)**:601–605.
9 Gissel T, Poulsen CS, Vestergaard P: Adverse effects of antiepileptic drugs on bone mineral density in children. *Expert Opin Drug Saf* 2007; **6(3)**:267–278.
10 Sheth RD, Binkley N, Hermann BP: Progressive bone deficit in epilepsy. *Neurology* 2008; **70(3)**:170–176.
11 Guo CY, Ronen GM, Atkinson SA: Long-term valproate and lamotrigine treatment may be a marker for reduced growth and bone mass in children with epilepsy. *Epilepsia* 2001; **42(9)**:1141–1147.
12 Bergqvist AG, Schall JI, Stallings VA, Zemel BS: Progressive bone mineral content loss in children with intractable epilepsy treated with the ketogenic diet. *Am J Clin Nutr* 2008; **88(6)**:1678–1684.
13 Coppola G, Fortunato D, Auricchio G et al.: Bone mineral density in children, adolescents, and young adults with epilepsy. *Epilepsia* 2009; **50(9)**:2140–2146.
14 Petty SJ, Paton LM, O'Brien TJ et al.: Effect of antiepileptic medication on bone mineral measures. *Neurology* 2005; **65(9)**:1358–1365.
15 Pack AM, Olarte LS, Morrell MJ et al.: Bone mineral density in an outpatient population receiving enzyme-inducing antiepileptic drugs. *Epilepsy Behav* 2003; **4(2)**:169–174.
16 Koch HU, Kraft D, von Herrath D, Schaefer K: Influence of diphenylhydantoin and phenobarbital on intestinal calcium transport in the rat. *Epilepsia* 1972; **13(6)**:829–834.
17 Feldkamp J, Becker A, Witte OW et al.: Long-term anticonvulsant therapy leads to low bone mineral density: evidence for direct drug effects of phenytoin and carbamazepine on human osteoblast-like cells. *Exp Clin Endocrinol Diabetes* 2000; **108(1)**:37–43.
18 Pack AM, Morrell MJ, Randall A et al.: Bone health in young women with epilepsy after one year of antiepileptic drug monotherapy. *Neurology* 2008; **70(18)**:1586–1593.
19 Bauer J, Cooper-Mahkorn D: Reproductive dysfunction in women with epilepsy: menstrual cycle abnormalities, fertility, and polycystic ovary syndrome. *Int Rev Neurobiol* 2008; **83**:135–155.
20 Luef G, Rauchenzauner M: Epilepsy and hormones: a critical review. *Epilepsy Behav* 2009; **15(1)**:73–77.
21 McGee-Lawrence ME, Westendorf JJ: Histone deacetylases in skeletal development and bone mass maintenance. *Gene* 2011; **474(1–2)**:1–11.
22 Vrzal R, Doricakova A, Novotna A et al.: Valproic acid augments vitamin D receptor-mediated induction of CYP24 by vitamin D3: a possible cause of valproic acid-induced osteomalacia? *Toxicol Lett* 2011; **200(3)**:146–153.
23 Lambrinoudaki I, Kaparos G, Armeni E et al.: BsmI vitamin D receptor's polymorphism and bone mineral density in men

and premenopausal women on long-term antiepileptic therapy. *Eur J Neurol* 2011; **18(1)**:93–98.

24 Fernandes de Abreu DA, Eyles D, Feron F: Vitamin D, a neuro-immunomodulator: implications for neurodegenerative and autoimmune diseases. *Psychoneuroendocrinology* 2009; **34(Suppl. 1)**:S265–S277.

25 Janjoppi L, Katayama MH, Scorza FA et al.: Expression of vitamin D receptor mRNA in the hippocampal formation of rats submitted to a model of temporal lobe epilepsy induced by pilocarpine. *Brain Res Bull* 2008; **76(5)**:480–484.

26 Kalueff AV, Minasyan A, Keisala T et al.: Increased severity of chemically induced seizures in mice with partially deleted vitamin D receptor gene. *Neurosci Lett* 2006; **394(1)**: 69–73.

27 Petty SJ, O'Brien TJ, Wark JD: Anti-epileptic medication and bone health. *Osteoporos Int* 2007; **18(2)**:129–142.

28 Yahalom G, Blatt I, Neufeld MY et al.: Epilepsy syndrome-associated balance dysfunction assessed by static posturography. *Seizure* 2011; **20(3)**:214–217.

29 Sandok EK, O'Brien TJ, Jack CR, So EL: Significance of cerebellar atrophy in intractable temporal lobe epilepsy: a quantitative MRI study. *Epilepsia* 2000; **41(10)**:1315–1320.

30 Sheth RD, Harden CL: Screening for bone health in epilepsy. *Epilepsia* 2007; **48(Suppl. 9)**:39–41.

31 Bischoff-Ferrari H. Vitamin D: what is an adequate vitamin D level and how much supplementation is necessary? *Best Pract Res Clin Rheumatol* 2009; **23(6)**:789–795.

32 Ito M. Recent progress in bone imaging for osteoporosis research. *J Bone Miner Metab* 2011; **29(2)**:131–140.

33 Song XQ, Wang ZP, Bao KR et al.: [Effect of carbamazepine and valproate on bone metabolism in children with epilepsy.] *Zhonghua Er Ke Za Zhi* 2005; **43(10)**:728–732.

34 World Health Organization. *Vitamin and Mineral Requirements in Human Nutrition*, 2 edn. World Health Organization, Geneva, 2004.

35 Nettekoven S, Strohle A, Trunz B et al.: Effects of antiepileptic drug therapy on vitamin D status and biochemical markers of bone turnover in children with epilepsy. *Eur J Pediatr* 2008; **167(12)**:1369–1377.

36 Pedrera JD, Canal ML, Carvajal J et al.: Influence of vitamin D administration on bone ultrasound measurements in patients on anticonvulsant therapy. *Eur J Clin Invest* 2000; **30(10)**:895–899.

37 Mikati MA, Dib L, Yamout B et al.: Two randomized vitamin D trials in ambulatory patients on anticonvulsants: impact on bone. *Neurology* 2006; **67(11)**:2005–2014.

38 Espinosa PS, Perez DL, Abner E, Ryan M: Association of antiepileptic drugs, vitamin D, and calcium supplementation with bone fracture occurrence in epilepsy patients. *Clin Neurol Neurosurg* 2011; **113(7)**:548–551.

39 Lazzari AA, Dussault PM, Thakore-James M et al.: Prevention of bone loss and vertebral fractures in patients with chronic epilepsy – antiepileptic drug and osteoporosis prevention trial. *Epilepsia* 2013; **54(11)**:1997–2004.

40 Gardner MM, Buchner DM, Robertson MC, Campbell AJ: Practical implementation of an exercise-based falls prevention programme. *Age Ageing* 2001; **30(1)**:77–83.

41 Bliuc D, Nguyen ND, Milch VE et al.: Mortality risk associated with low-trauma osteoporotic fracture and subsequent fracture in men and women. *JAMA* 2009; **301(5)**:513–521.

CHAPTER 21

Sleep and epilepsy

Irakli Kaolani and Erik K. St. Louis
Department of Neurology, Mayo Clinic, USA

Introduction

Parallels between sleep and epilepsy have been recognized since antiquity. Philosophers and theologians from Aristotle to Aquinas believed that states of altered consciousness, including sleep and seizures, allowed dissociation of the soul and the body, freeing the mind to prophesy the future [1]. While others speculated about the relationship between seizures and sleep, the first major scientific study to examine this relationship was conducted in the 19th century, when Gowers [2] found that approximately 20% of persons with epilepsy experienced their seizures solely during sleep. Then, in the 20th century, when EEG was developed for clinical use, Gibbs and Gibbs recognized that epileptiform activity was often significantly increased during sleep [3]. Since that time, the obtaining of sleep and sleep deprivation prior to EEG have been used as standard laboratory activating techniques for EEG recordings. Janz [4] noted that 45% of patients with generalized tonic–clonic seizures had nocturnal predominance. Aside from these earlier clinical observations, few systematic studies of the influence of sleep on seizures were performed until recently, but over the last 2 decades sleep has been shown to affect both the tendency toward seizure onset and seizure type in sleep-related epilepsies (those with preferential occurrence during sleep or following arousal), particularly for frontal- and temporal-lobe partial epilepsies, benign epilepsy of childhood with centrotemporal spikes (benign rolandic epilepsy, BRE), and juvenile myoclonic epilepsy (JME) in children and adolescents. The relationship between sleep and epilepsy also seems reciprocal, as comorbid sleep disorders are more frequent in patients with epilepsy, particularly obstructive sleep apnea (OSA) in patients with refractory epilepsy, which may aggravate seizure burden, while treatment with nasal continuous positive airway pressure (CPAP) often improves seizure frequency and insomnia. Differentiating nocturnal seizures from primary sleep disorders is essential for determining appropriate therapy and recognizing coexistent sleep disorders in patients with epilepsy may improve their seizure burden and quality of life (QOL).

Pathophysiology

Sleep clearly influences the expression of interictal epileptiform discharges (IEDs) and epileptic seizures. In general, IEDs and seizures are facilitated during non-REM (NREM) sleep and relatively inhibited during REM sleep [5–7] (see Figure 21.1). NREM sleep is a state reflecting a progressive increase in synchronized neuronal discharges, with maximal synchronicity in slow-wave sleep (stages 3 and 4, now known as N3) [8]. The density of IEDs also increases with descending sleep depth, reaching its peak during N3 sleep, although no further increase is observed in the hour before seizure onset [9].

In contrast to IEDs, which are most prevalent in N3, seizures occur more frequently in lighter stages of NREM sleep (stages N1 and N2) [10,11]. Over one-third of partial seizures arise from sleep and nocturnal complex partial seizures are more likely than awake complex partial seizures to propagate and undergo secondary generalization [10,11]. Besides the well-known dichotomy between the different sleep stages, epileptic

Epilepsy and the Interictal State: Co-Morbidities and Quality of Life, First Edition.
Edited by Erik K. St. Louis, David M. Ficker, and Terence J. O'Brien.
© 2015 John Wiley & Sons, Ltd. Published 2015 by John Wiley & Sons, Ltd.

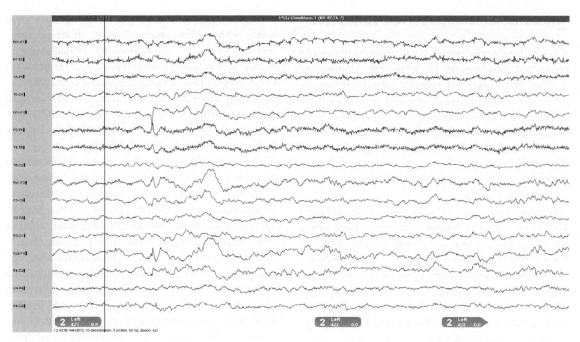

Figure 21.1 EEG in a 35-year-old man, showing a right temporal interictal epileptiform discharge (IED) during N2 sleep, in the form of a spike with maximal electronegativity at F8.

phenomena are also sensitive to the state of arousal [12]. Fluctuating, unstable arousal propensity during NREM sleep, characterized by K complexes and transient EEG rhythms of NREM sleep microarchitecture known as the cyclic alternating pattern (CAP), appears to be quite favorable toward the activation of nocturnal seizures, particularly phase A of CAP [12–14].

About 80% of pure sleep epilepsies are focal epilepsies [15]. Interestingly, frontal-lobe seizures have a strong preponderance to occur during sleep and occur much more commonly during sleep than do temporal-lobe seizures [10,16]. Nocturnal focal seizures also tend to correlate with medical intractability, while generalized tonic–clonic seizures without focality carry a more benign prognosis [17]. From the electrographic perspective, NREM sleep is an effective facilitator of focal IEDs in focal epilepsies, resulting in more frequent IEDs with a more extensive field of distribution [6]. In contrast, REM sleep IEDs are more restricted in electrical field and thus more localizing to the epileptic focus [6].

Some seizures occur only during sleep, while others appear to be activated by arousal. The prototypical idiopathic primary generalized epilepsy syndromes of adolescent onset, such as JME and the similar syndrome of generalized tonic–clonic seizures upon awakening, often produce myoclonic or generalized tonic–clonic seizures within the first hour after awakening [4].

Normal sleep or its disruption may also significantly impact the occurrence of both IEDs and seizures. Primary sleep disorders, common in these patients, may worsen seizure control by increasing seizure frequency or severity. Although sleep deprivation may activate IEDs, seizure frequency does not appear to be substantially impacted by sleep deprivation in patients undergoing inpatient video-EEG monitoring [18], despite the common persisting use of this technique in epilepsy monitoring unit practices.

While many studies have presented evidence that sleep deprivation can exacerbate several seizure types, circadian mechanisms also play a significant role in the timing of seizure occurrence. Several recent studies have confirmed day or night patterns for seizure periodicity, varying by lobe of onset in the partial epilepsies, with most suggesting either an afternoon or a bimodal morning and afternoon peak for temporal-lobe seizures and an evening peak for frontal-lobe seizures [19–23].

The common sleep-related epilepsies

Some representative epilepsy syndromes with a clearly recognized relationship to sleep are summarized in Table 21.1. Nocturnal epileptic seizures frequently arise outside the temporal lobe and may initially be misdiagnosed as psychogenic, given the lack of obvious EEG change, variably preserved consciousness, bizarre movements, and lack of a postictal state. However, stereotypic spells arising directly out of sleep that occur multiple times per night should be considered epileptic until proven otherwise.

BRE or benign epilepsy with centrotemporal spikes (BECTS) is the most common and most characteristic form of idiopathic focal epilepsy of childhood. It features partial seizures with hemifacial tonic contractions, hypersalivation, and secondary generalized tonic–clonic seizure activity, occurring exclusively during sleep in 70–80% of cases. Mean age of onset is approximately 7. Males are more commonly affected [24]. Family history is common. In its usual presentation, children enjoy normal development and only those with particularly frequent attacks or generalized seizures may need treatment, until midadolescene, when seizures most often remit and seizure tendency is typically outgrown. Antiepileptic drugs (AEDs) effective in partial epilepsy syndromes are generally used, such as carbamazepine, oxcarbazepine, gabapentin, or levetiracetam. On EEG, the IEDs of BECTS are often infrequent or absent during wakefulness but are markedly activated during drowsiness and light NREM sleep, manifested by high-voltage spike–wave discharges over the centrotemporal region, although discharges may occur contralaterally or bilaterally [2].

Landau–Kleffner syndrome (LKS) presents with subacutely progressive language regression with verbal and auditory agnosia in children between ages 1 and 8 years who previously had normal development [26]. EEG in LKS is characterized by spike and slow-wave discharges, most often in the temporal regions bilaterally, frequently with electrical status epilepticus during sleep. Treatment with traditional AEDs or immunosuppressive therapy may stop seizures but aphasia is often persistent. Although the prognosis in LKS is guarded, in selected patients early and aggressive treatment with multiple subpial transections (MSTs) in the active epileptogenic site has resulted in complete or partial language recovery [27,28].

Lennox–Gastaut syndrome (LGS) is one of the most severe epileptic encephalopathies of childhood onset and is commonly characterized by a triad of signs, including multiple seizure types, slow spike–wave complexes on EEG, and impairment of cognitive function [29]. The optimum treatment for LGS remains uncertain, with best evidence for valproate, rufinamide, lamotrigine, topiramate, and felbamate. Clobazam may be helpful for atonic/astatic (drop) seizures.

Most nocturnal epileptic phenomena with prominent motor features are extratemporal partial-onset seizures, of which frontal-lobe onset is most common. Nocturnal frontal-lobe epilepsy (NFLE) may be characterized by varying phenotypes, including paroxysmal arousals with brief hypermotor movements, motor attacks with complex dystonic and dyskinetic features, and episodic nocturnal wandering mimicking sleepwalking [30–33]. NFLE predominates in males, often with onset in childhood, and 6–40% of cases are familial. Video-EEG polysomnography is necessary for definitive diagnosis, confirming abrupt awakening, stereotyped motor behavior with vocalization, and violent or dystonic–dyskinetic movements. Response to carbamazepine and other AEDs is usually excellent, although up to one-third of patients may prove medically intractable [30–33].

Supplementary sensorimotor area (SSMA) epilepsy is another distinctive subtype of frontal-lobe epilepsy. SSMA seizures typically begin with somatosensory auras and then rapidly evolve to asymmetric tonic posturing of the upper extremities, with speech arrest or vocalizations and flailing, thrashing limb movements.

Sleep-related temporal-lobe seizures are quite frequent, representing approximately one-third of overall temporal-lobe seizures recorded during epilepsy monitoring [11]. Nocturnal temporal-lobe epilepsy (NTLE) is a subtype of medically refractory temporal-lobe epilepsy (TLE) in which seizures occur nearly exclusively at nighttime [34]. Approximately 70% of patients may awaken from sleep with an aura then progress to a complex partial (focal dyscognitive) seizure involving amnesia and automatisms. Episodic nocturnal wandering mimicking sleepwalking may also occur. Most patients also have secondary generalized tonic–clonic seizures, with seizures generalizing more frequently during sleep than wakefulness in mesial TLE.

JME is an idiopathic generalized epilepsy syndrome appearing around the time of puberty. Myoclonic

Table 21.1 The common sleep-related epilepsies.

Epilepsy syndrome	Classification	Age of onset	Genetics	Seizure types	EEG characteristics	Neuroimaging characteristics	Usual AED treatment options
Benign Rolandic epilepsy	Focal	First decade	Autosomal dominant	Focal	Centrotemporal spikes	Normal	CBZ, GBP, LEV, OXC
Landau–Kleffner syndrome	Unknown	First decade	Usually sporadic	Focal or generalized	Focal, generalized continuous spike–wave in sleep	Normal or lesional	Any partial
Lennox–Gastaut syndrome	Generalized	First decade to teenage years	Usually sporadic	Focal or generalized	Slow spike–wave discharges	Normal or lesional	VPA, CLBZ, RFM, TPM, LTG
Juvenile myoclonic epilepsy	Generalized	Teenage to young adulthood	Autosomal dominant	Generalized	Generalized spikes	Normal	VPA, LTG, TPM, ZNS
Autosomal dominant nocturnal frontal-lobe epilepsy	Focal	Childhood or adulthood	Autosomal dominant	Focal	Normal or focal frontal spikes	Normal	Any partial
Nocturnal temporal-lobe epilepsy	Focal	Childhood or adulthood	Autosomal dominant or recessive	Focal	Anterior or midtemporal spikes	Normal or hippocampal sclerosis	Any partial

CBZ=carbamazepine; CLBZ=clobazam; GBP=gabapentin; LTG=lamotrigine; LEV=levetiracetam; OXC=oxcarbazepine; RFM=rufinamide; TPM=topiramate; VPA=valproate; ZNS=zonisamide seizures involving bilateral arm jerks often occur shortly after arousal [4,34]. EEG typically demonstrates primary generalized IEDs. In general, 80–90% of patients can achieve complete seizure control with appropriate AED therapy, but lifelong treatment may be required. A closely related primary generalized epilepsy syndrome, generalized tonic–clonic seizures on awakening, has a similar pattern of convulsions but lacks myoclonic seizures.

Evaluation and differential diagnosis

The sleep state has a significant influence on epilepsy, but the converse is also true, as epilepsy and AEDs also impact sleep in people with epilepsy. Excessive daytime sleepiness (EDS) is the most commonly identified sleep-related symptom in patients with epilepsy and can be related to nocturnal seizures, sedative effects of AEDs, poor sleep hygiene, and comorbid primary sleep disorders [35,36].

Seizures, both diurnal and nocturnal, may disrupt sleep. Treating epilepsy may thus improve sleep architecture [8,36]. Patients with nocturnal seizures show reduced sleep efficiency and increased REM latency and patients with diurnal seizures show reduced REM and NREM sleep during the night following seizures [37]. Polysomnography may show significantly reduced REM, N2, and slow-wave sleep and objective sleepiness has been shown in epilepsy patients on a modified Maintenance of Wakefulness Test (MWT) [37]. People with TLE tend to have more altered and severe disorganization of sleep than those with extratemporal foci [30,38].

In addition to seizures, independent effects of AEDs on sleep have been observed. All of the older and some newer AEDs have important modulatory effects on sleep physiology. Most of the older AEDs reduce REM and slow-wave sleep, shorten sleep latency, and increase the percentage of light NREM sleep [39]. Following initiation, carbamazepine transiently reduces REM sleep, but otherwise it has little effect on sleep architecture [40]. Lamotrigine reduces slow-wave sleep and increases N2 but is also associated with reduced arousals and stage shifts and usually increases REM without significant subjective insomnia [41], although in some individuals the drug may be relatively activating. Whether AEDs have any specific or independent

effects on sleep-disordered breathing remains unknown and is in need of study.

While epilepsy and antiepileptic therapies have been shown to affect sleep, clinicians should not assume that nocturnal seizures or AED toxicity explain excessive daytime sleepiness, since underlying primary sleep disorders need to be aggressively sought and treated in order to achieve optimal management in patients with epilepsy and somnolence [42–45]. Sleep-disordered breathing may exacerbate seizure burden in as many as one-third of patients with medically intractable epilepsy undergoing presurgical evaluation and may be a particularly important and treatable problem in elderly patients with refractory seizure disorders [44–46]. OSA is the most common cause of sleep-disordered breathing and is particularly important to identify given the risk of injury from driving while sleepy, in addition to potential cardiovascular and general health complications. Polysomnography is the test of choice for investigation of sleep-disordered breathing, although home portable oximetry may be helpful for initial screening of patients who lack typical symptoms of snoring or daytime sleepiness. Several retrospective and prospective studies have demonstrated the benefit of nasal CPAP therapy for seizure reduction in patients with refractory epilepsy and comorbid OSA [47–49]. In fact, one recent study suggests that the level of benefit toward seizure reduction provided by nasal CPAP treatment in epilepsy patients with comorbid OSA is comparable to that of an adjunctive AED for seizure treatment, with approximately 50% of patients experiencing a 50% or greater seizure reduction [49].

The differentiation of nocturnal epilepsy from other nonepileptic dissociated states of wakefulness and sleep is also of extreme importance. Many parasomnias are easily confused with seizures by their similar clinical phenomenology of episodic confusion and abnormal sleep-related motor activity or sleepwalking. (see Table 21.2). Clinical features of multiple recurrences within a single sleep episode, relative stereotypy, postictal behavior, and rhythmic EEG abnormalities are more commonly seen with epileptic events but video-EEG polysomnography is often necessary to distinguish nocturnal events when the diagnosis is unclear on clinical grounds.

Differential diagnosis of nocturnal events includes REM sleep behavior disorder (RBD), NREM parasomnias, non-state-dependent parasomnias, periodic

Table 21.2 Distinguishing features of nocturnal events.

	Premonitory symptoms	Behavioral characteristics	Duration	EEG/PSG frequency	Findings
NREM parasomnias					
Night terrors	None	Inconsolable screaming	Minutes	1 or less nightly	Arousal from N2 to N3
Confusional arousals	None	Confused, amnestic	Seconds to minutes	1 or less nightly	Arousal from N3 to N2
Sleepwalking	None	Ambulation, amnesia	Minutes	1 or less nightly	Arousal from N3 to N2
REM parasomnias					
Nightmares	Dream recall	Arousal, fright, palpitations	Seconds	Generally, 1 nightly	Arousal from REM
REM sleep behavior disorder (RBD)	Variable dream recall	Thrashing, complex motor behavior	Seconds to minutes	More than 1 nightly, second > first half	REM sleep without atonia
Non-state-dependent parasomnias					
Rhythmic movement disorder (RMD)	None	Head banging, body rocking, bruxism	Seconds to minutes	Several times nightly	Any sleep stage, movement artifact
Sleep-related epilepsies					
Benign epilepsy of childhood with centrotemporal spikes (BECTS)	Facial twitching, hypersalivation	Focal motor or GTC, postictal	Seconds to minutes	More than 1 nightly	Arousal from NREM, IEDs, ictal EEG pattern
Autosomal dominant nocturnal frontal-lobe epilepsy (ADNFLE)	Bizarre stereotyped motor behavior	Focal motor, bizarre motor	Seconds to less than 1 minute	1 or multiple attacks nightly	Arousal from N2
Temporal-lobe epilepsy (TLE)	Aura variable	CPS, postictal	1–2 minutes	1 or multiple attacks nightly	Arousal from N2
Physiologic/psychogenic nocturnal events					
Physiologic/"hypnic" myoclonus	None	Brief body/limb jerks	Seconds	1 or multiple nightly at sleep onset or awakening	Sleep–wake transition movement artifact
Periodic leg movements	None, variable	Leg/arm movements, restless legs while awake	Seconds, recurrent	Multiple/night	Typically, NREM sleep predominance
Psychogenic spells	Variable	Variable	Often >5 minutes	1 or multiple attacks nightly	Normal awake EEG
Nocturnal panic	None	Arousal, feeling of panic/ anxiousness, fear, doom, diaphoresis, palpitations	Seconds to1 minute	Generally, 1 nightly	Arousal from N1 to N2

EEG, electroencephalogram; PSG, polysomnogram; NREM, non-rapid-eye-movement sleep; REM, rapid-eye-movement sleep; IED, interictal epileptiform discharge; N1, stage 1 NREM sleep; N2, stage 2 NREM sleep; N3, stage 3 NREM sleep.

limb movements of sleep, and nocturnal panic attacks. Disorders arising from REM sleep include nightmares and RBD. Nightmares usually occur during REM sleep and may awaken the sleeper. Dream recall is a common feature and patients are alert, coherent, and well oriented. Night terrors of NREM sleep, in contrast, involve a confusional arousal that may include prominent vocalization and movement, mimicking a complex partial (focal dyscognitive) seizure type but unaccompanied by EEG changes other than arousal from sleep.

RBD is characterized by complex, often violent dream enactment behaviors, occurring most commonly in the second half of the night, when REM sleep is most prevalent, accompanied by polysomongraphic REM sleep without atonia (loss of the normal REM atonia, with consequent abnormally elevated phasic or tonic muscle activity during REM) [50]. Recalled dream mentation often involves a theme of defense against attack or being chased by animals or people, accompanied by screaming, shouting, punching, or kicking motor behaviors that are often dramatic and extreme, leading some clinicians to initially errantly suspect a psychogenic cause. Making the diagnosis of RBD is imperative given the risk for injury, and

video-EEG polysomnography may support a clinical diagnosis of RBD, even if clinical spells are not captured, by documenting features of REM sleep without atonia (Figure 21.2). The importance of accurately diagnosing RBD is also crucial prognostically, since recent long-term follow-up studies of idiopathic RBD patients have confirmed a high risk of later eventual development of overt synucleinopathy neurodegenerative disorders including Parkinson's disease, dementia with Lewy bodies, and multiple-system atrophy.

The NREM parasomnias are a continuum of behavioral disorders associated with abnormal arousal from NREM sleep, particularly slow-wave sleep. They are thus often seen between 60 and 90 minutes after sleep onset. NREM parasomnias are more common in children than adults. While the pathophysiology of NREM arousal disorders remains poorly understood, maturational factors are felt to be important and hereditary factors likely play an important role, since familial history is frequent. The range of behavior seen with NREM parasomnias includes night terrors, confusional arousals, sleepwalking, and sleep-eating syndrome. Events are frequently nonstereotyped and video-EEG polysomnography most often shows generalized or

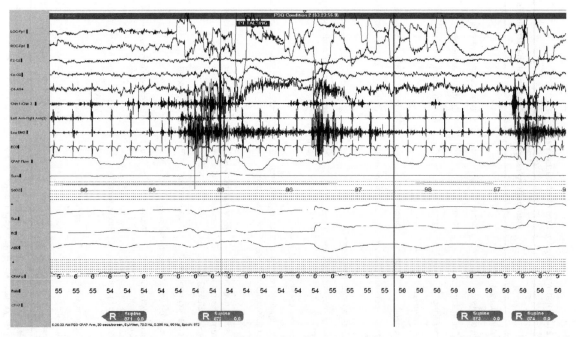

Figure 21.2 REM sleep without atonia in a 72-year-old man with parkinsonism and dream-enactment behavior. Note the elevated muscle tone in the chin, arm, and leg EMG leads (channels 6-8, 30-second epoch).

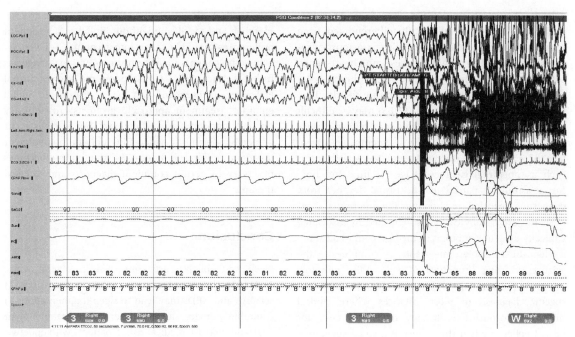

Figure 21.3 Hypersynchronous delta activity accompanying a confusion arousal in a 55-year-old woman.

bifrontal rhythmic delta, theta, or alpha activity on EEG immediately preceding and briefly persisting following arousal (see Figure 21.3). Stereotypy, multiple episodes per night, prolonged postictal confusion, incontinence, and focally abnormal ictal EEG recording would favor an epileptic etiology.

Rhythmic movement disorder (RMD) consists of stereotyped, semirhythmic movements of large muscle groups characterized by head banging or body rocking. RMD is most frequently seen in cognitively disabled individuals. It may occur during any stage of sleep or wakefulness and is unaccompanied by a change in the EEG background, other than muscle and movement artifact.

A rare and unusual nocturnal parasomnia of children is benign nocturnal alternating hemiplegia of childhood (BNAHC). Clinical features include early life onset and episodic attacks of hemiplegia lasting 5–20 minutes, which may occur several times per month [51]. There is a frequent family history of migraine. One difference from classic alternating hemiplegia of childhood (AHC), which has diurnal attacks, is that patients with exclusively nocturnal attacks are unlikely to evolve developmental regression of motor or cognitive function.

Another nocturnal event that may be confused with nocturnal epilepsy is complex visual hallucinations, which typically involve visual hallucinations persisting following awakening, with nearby objects often initially mistaken for a person or other object (e.g., a robe on a hanger initially errantly seen as a person standing in the closet). Underlying visual and/or mild cognitive impairment is often present in patients having complex visual hallucinations in Charles Bonnet syndrome.

Periodic limb movements of sleep (PLMS) may be normal if limited in number, but if associated with frequent arousals may present as a primary sleep disorder associated with excessive daytime sleepiness. Sleep starts (also known as sensory starts or hypnic myoclonic jerks) may occur at the transition between sleep and wakefulness. Other sleep-related movements that may rarely be seen include abnormal motor phenomena associated with severe sleep-disordered breathing and propriospinal myoclonus, a sleep–wake transition disorder characterized by single or briefly repetitive axial myoclonic jerks [52].

Although unusual, psychogenic or functional disturbances may arise from sleep. Nocturnal panic attacks are common among those with diurnal panic disorder but may occur as a distinctive and isolated nighttime episode of arousal from NREM sleep [53]. Nocturnal panic attacks are typically easily differentiated from seizures on clinical grounds by their characteristic features of panic and anxiety, diaphoresis, and heart-racing palpitations at the time of arousal, seen either in isolation or, often, with similar attacks during the daytime. Psychogenic nonepileptic spells (PNES) may be difficult to distinguish from a true epileptic seizure; eye closure and nonphysiologic spread of movements (e.g., from face to leg to opposite arm) are typical. Medical disorders such as nocturnal gastroesophageal reflux and nocturnal asthma or paroxysmal nocturnal dyspnea from congestive heart failure also enter the differential diagnosis but are usually easily distinguished by associated clinically evident symptoms or medical comorbidities.

Video-EEG polysomnography combines the seizure-localizing properties of video-EEG monitoring with polysomnography and allows for confident specific diagnosis in most instances where clinical history is inconclusive. It may reveal evidence for partial epilepsy when the history is instead suggestive of nonepileptic parasomnias [54]. Formal diagnostic assessment should be pursued for any nocturnal spell involving potentially injurious behavior or disturbance of the patient or their partner's sleep, or when the diagnosis is unclear on clinical grounds.

Treatment

Treatment of nocturnal epilepsies follows similar tenets to the treatment of all epilepsies. The electroclinical epilepsy syndrome is a primary consideration, with either narrow- or broad-spectrum AED therapy chosen as appropriate and patient characteristics, comorbid conditions, and comedications then taken into consideration in arriving at the most appropriate individual medication choice. Patients with refractory nocturnal epilepsies should receive prompt consideration for appropriate nonpharmacological therapies, including epilepsy surgery, neurostimulation, and dietary therapy, to reduce the likelihood of psychosocial morbidity and QOL impairment, injury, and status epilepticus or sudden unexpected death in epilepsy (SUDEP). In nocturnal TLE or lesional extratemporal epilepsies, surgical outcomes are similar to those for focal epilepsies overall. Some patients with pure sleep epilepsies may be reluctant to pursue aggressive treatment measures if they reside in areas that allow them to continue driving, working, and socializing without limitations, so patient preferences should be taken into account.

In some patients for whom the provisional diagnosis includes either NREM arousal parasomnias or nocturnal epilepsies, clonazepam can be a reasonable initial empirical treatment approach, given its cross-efficacy for both parasomnias and epilepsy, but if spells recur or persist, diagnostic video-EEG polysomnography or inpatient prolonged video-EEG monitoring becomes necessary to permit confident diagnosis and directed therapy.

Conclusion

Sleep and epilepsy are connected in several ways: 1) NREM sleep may activate spikes and seizures; 2) seizures and AEDs may lead to sleep fragmentation; 3) comorbid primary sleep disorders may further impair QOL and increase medical risk in patients with epilepsy; and 4) the parasomnias may mimic epileptic seizures, leading to diagnostic challenges.

Recognizing and effectively treating primary sleep disorders in patients with epilepsy may frequently improve seizure frequency and overall functioning. The diagnostic evaluation of nocturnal events benefits from a collaborative approach by epilepsy and sleep specialists and from utilization of video-EEG polysomnography for confident and accurate diagnosis. Epilepsy and sleep are interwoven in many respects, leading to many fascinating intersections between these disciplines.

References

1 Temkin O: *The Falling Sickness: A History of Epilepsy from the Greeks to the Beginnings of Modern Neurology.* Johns Hopkins University Press, Baltimore, MD and London, 1971.

2 Gowers WR: *Epilepsy and Other Chronic Convulsive Diseases.* William Wood, New York, NY, 1885.

3 Lennox WG: *Epilepsy and Related Disorders.* Little, Brown, Boston, MA, 1960, pp. 509–512.

4 Janz D: The grand mal epilepsies and the sleeping-waking cycle. *Epilepsia* 1962; **3**:69–109.

5 Malow BA, Lin X, Kushwaha R, Aldrich MS: Interictal spiking increases with sleep depth in temporal lobe epilepsy. *Epilepsia* 1998; **39**:1309–1316.

6 Sammaritano M, Gigli GL, Gotman J: Interictal spiking during wakefulness and sleep and the localization of foci in temporal lobe epilepsy. *Neurology* 1991; **41**:290–297.

7 Kumar P, Raju TR: Seizure susceptibility decreases with enhancement of rapid eye movement sleep. *Brain Res* 2001; **922(2)**:299–304.

8 Derry CP, Duncan S: Sleep and epilepsy. *Epilepsy Behav* 2013; **26(3)**:394–404.

9 Natarajan A, Marzec ML, Lin X et al.: Interictal epileptiform discharges do not change before seizures during sleep. *Epilepsia* 2002; **43(1)**:46–51.

10 Herman ST, Walczak TS, Bazil CW: Distribution of partial seizures during the sleep-wake cycle: differences by seizure onset site. *Neurology* 2001; **56(11)**:1453–1459.

11 St. Louis EK, Genilo P, Granner MA, Zimmerman B: Sleep-onset mesial temporal seizures arise from light NREM sleep. *Epilepsia* 2004; **45(Suppl. 7)**:86–87.

12 Parrino L, Smerieri A, Spaggiari MC, Terzano MG: Cyclic alternating pattern (CAP) and epilepsy during sleep: how a physiological rhythm modulates a pathological event. *Clin Neurophysiol* 2000; **111(Suppl. 2)**:S39–S46.

13 Parrino L, Halasz P, Tassinari CA, Terzano MG: CAP, epilepsy and motor events during sleep: the unifying role of arousal. *Sleep Med Rev* 2006; **10(4)**:267–285.

14 Parrino L, Smerieri A, Terzano MG: Combined influence of cyclic arousability and EEG synchrony on generalized interictal discharges within the sleep cycle. *Epilepsy Res* 2001; **44(1)**:7–18.

15 Yaqub BA, Waheed G, Kabiraj MM: Nocturnal epilepsies in adults. *Seizure* 1997; **6(2)**:145–149.

16 Crespel A, Baldy-Moulinier M, Coubes P: The relationship between sleep and epilepsy in frontal and temporal lobe epilepsies: practical and physiopathologic considerations. *Epilepsia* 1998; **39**:150–157.

17 Park SA, Lee BI, Park SC et al.: Clinical course of pure sleep epilepsies. *Seizure* 1998; **7(5)**:369–377.

18 Malow BA, Passaro E, Milling C et al.: Sleep deprivation does not affect seizure frequency during inpatient video-EEG monitoring. *Neurology* 2002; **59(9)**:1371–1374.

19 Duckrow RB, Tcheng TK: Daily variation in an intracranial EEG feature in humans detected by a responsive neurostimulator system. *Epilepsia* 2007; **48(8)**:1614–1620.

20 Durazzo TS, Spencer SS, Duckrow RB et al.: Temporal distributions of seizure occurrence from various epileptogenic regions. *Neurology* 2008; **70(15)**:1265–1271.

21 Hofstra WA, Gordijn MC, van der Palen J et al.: Timing of temporal and frontal seizures in relation to the circadian phase: a prospective pilot study. *Epilepsy Res* 2011; **94(3)**:158–162.

22 Karafin M, St Louis EK, Zimmerman MB et al.: Bimodal ultradian seizure periodicity in human mesial temporal lobe epilepsy. *Seizure* 2010; **19(6)**:347–351.

23 Zarowski M, Loddenkemper T, Vendrame M et al.: Circadian distribution and sleep/wake patterns of generalized seizures in children. *Epilepsia* 2011; **52(6)**:1076–1083.

24 Bouma PAD, Bovenkerk AC, Westendorp RGJ, Brouwer OF: The course of benign partial epilepsy of childhood with centrotemporal spikes: a meta-analysis. *Neurology* 1997; **48**:430–437.

25 Guerrini R, Pellacini S: Benign childhood focal epilepsies. *Epilepsia* 2012; **53(Suppl. 4)**:9–18.

26 Camfield P, Camfield C: Epileptic syndromes in childhood: clinical features, outcomes, and treatment. *Epilepsia* 2002; **43(Suppl. 3)**:27–32.

27 Morrell F, Whisler WW, Smith MC et al.: Landau-Kleffner syndrome: treatment with subpial intracortical transection. *Brain* 1995; **118**:1529–1546.

28 Nass R, Gross A, Wisoff J et al.: Outcome of multiple subpial transactions for autistic epileptiform regression. *Pediatr Neurol* 1999; **21**:464–470.

29 Arzimanoglou A, French J, Blume WT et al.: Lennox-Gastaut syndrome: a consensus approach on diagnosis, assessment, management, and trial methodology. *Lancet Neurol* 2009; **8(1)**:82–93.

30 Provini F, Plazzi G, Tinuper P et al.: Nocturnal frontal lobe epilepsy: a clinical and polygraphic overview of 100 consecutive cases. *Brain* 1999; **122(6)**:1017–1031.

31 Provini F, Plazzi G, Lugaresi E: From nocturnal paroxysmal dystonia to nocturnal frontal lobe epilepsy. *Clin Neurophysiol* 2000; **111(Suppl. 2)**:S2–S8.

32 Oldani A, Zucconi M, Ferini-Strarnbi L et al.: Autosomal dominant nocturnal frontal lobe epilepsy: electroclinical picture. *Epilepsia* 1996; **37(10)**:964–976.

33 Oldani A, Zucconi M, Asselta R et al.: Autosomal dominant nocturnal frontal lobe epilepsy: a video-polysomnographic and genetic appraisal of 40 patients and delineation of the epileptic syndrome. *Brain* 1998; **121(2)**:S20–S23.

34 Bernasconi A, Andermann F, Cendes F et al.: Nocturnal temporal lobe epilepsy. *Neurology* 1998; **50**:1772–1777.

35 Foldvary N. Sleep and epilepsy. *Curr Treat Options Neurol* 2002; **4(2)**:129–135.

36 Malow BA, Bowes RJ, Lin X: Predictors of sleepiness in epilepsy patients. *Sleep* 1997; **20(12)**:1105–1110.

37 Bazil CW, Castro LH, Walczak TS: Reduction of rapid eye movement sleep by diurnal and nocturnal seizures in temporal lobe epilepsy. *Arch Neurol* 2000; **57(3)**:363–368.

38 Matos G, Andersen ML, do Valle AC, Tufik S: The relationship between sleep and epilepsy: evidence from clinical trials and animal models. *J Neurol Sci* 2010; **295(1–2)**:1–7.

39 Sammaritano MR, Sherwin AL: Effects of anticonvulsants on sleep. In: Bazil C, Malow B, Sammaritano M (eds): *Sleep and Epilepsy: The Clinical Spectrum*. Elsevier, Amsterdam, 2002, pp. 187–194.

40 Gigli GL, Placidi F, Diomedi M et al.: Nocturnal sleep and daytime somnolence in untreated patients with temporal lobe epilepsy: changes after treatment with controlled-released carbamazepine. *Epilepsia* 1997; **38(6)**:696–701.

41 Foldvary N, Perry M, Lee J et al.: The effects of lamotrigine on sleep in patients with epilepsy. *Epilepsia* 2001; **42(12)**:1569–1573.

42 Bassetti CL, Gugger M: Sleep disordered breathing in neurological disorders. *Swiss Med Wkly* 2002; **132(9–10)**:109–15.

43 Vaughn BV, D'Cruz OF: Obstructive sleep apnea in epilepsy. *Clin Chest Med* 2003; **24(2)**:239–248.

44 Malow BA, Levy K, Maturen K, Bowes R: Obstructive sleep apnea is common in medically refractory epilepsy patients. *Neurology* 2000; **55(7)**:1002–1007.

45 Chihorek AM, Abou-Khalil B, Malow BA: Obstructive sleep apnea is associated with seizure occurrence in older adults with epilepsy. *Neurology* 2007; **69(19)**:1823–1827.

46 Berth W, St. Louis EK, Zimmerman MB et al.: Predictors of co-morbid obstructive sleep apnea in epilepsy. *Neurology* 2011; **76(Suppl. 4)**:A337.

47 Malow BA, Foldvary-Schaefer N, Vaughn BV et al.: Treating obstructive sleep apnea in adults with epilepsy: a randomized pilot trial. *Neurology* 2008; **71(8)**:572–577.

48 Vendrame M, Auerbach S, Loddenkemper T et al.: Effect of continuous positive airway pressure treatment on seizure control in patients with obstructive sleep apnea and epilepsy. *Epilepsia* 2011; **52(11)**:e168–e171.

49 St. Louis EK, Berth W, Granner MA et al.: Seizure reduction following nasal continuous positive airway pressure therapy for co-morbid obstructive sleep apnea in epilepsy. *Neurology* 2011; **76(Suppl. 4)**:A453.

50 Boeve BF: REM sleep behavior disorder: updated review of the core features, the REM sleep behavior disorder-neurodegenerative disease association, evolving concepts, controversies, and future directions. *Ann NY Acad Sci* 2010; **1184**:15–54.

51 Chaves-Vischer V, Picard F, Andermann E et al.: Benign nocturnal alternating hemiplegia of childhood: six patients and long-term follow-up. *Neurology* 2001; **57(8)**:1491–1493.

52 Roze E, Bounolleau P, Ducreux D et al.: Propriospinal myoclonus revisited: clinical, neurophysiologic, and neuroradiologic findings. *Neurology* 2009; **72(15)**:1301–1309.

53 Craske MG, Tsao JC: Assessment and treatment of nocturnal panic attacks. *Sleep Med Rev* 2005; **9(3)**:173–184.

54 Dyken ME, Yamada T, Lin-Dyken DC: Polysomnographic assessment of spells in sleep: nocturnal seizures versus parasomnias. *Semin Neurol* 2001; **21(4)**:377–390.

CHAPTER 22

Use of complementary and alternative medicine in epilepsy

Dana Ekstein[1] and Steven C. Schachter[2,3]

[1] Epilepsy Center, Department of Neurology, Hadassah University Medical Center, Israel
[2] Departments of Neurology, Beth Israel Deaconess Medical Center, Massachusetts General Hospital
[3] Harvard Medical School, Consortia for Improving Medicine with Innovation and Technology, Boston, MA

Introduction

Approximately one-third of people with epilepsy continue to have drug-resistant seizures despite the introduction of many new antiepileptic drugs (AEDs) over the last 2 decades [1,2]. Although the newer AEDs can offer a better Adverse Events Profile (AEP) than the older generation, they may still have significant undesired systemic and central nervous system (CNS) effects, such as decreased cognitive abilities and psychiatric complications [3]. Surgery is highly effective and safe for selected patients with treatment-resistant focal epilepsy [4,5] but is still underused [6]. Other treatment strategies are primarily palliative (vagus nerve stimulation, VNS) or still under investigation (closed-loop cortical stimulation) [7]. Therefore, new treatments with efficacy against drug-resistant seizures, favorable AEP, and, if possible, low costs to patients and high worldwide availability, are clearly needed. The cognitive, psychological, and social consequences of epilepsy are now considered an integral part of this disease [8]. In addition, neuropsychiatric conditions (anxiety, depression, bipolar disorder, attention deficit/hyperactivity disorder (ADHD), sleep disorder/apnea, and movement disorder/tremor), pain syndromes (migraine headache, chronic pain, fibromyalgia, and neuropathic pain) and asthma are recognized as significant comorbidities in people with epilepsy [9]. People with epilepsy, whether their seizures are controlled by medications or not, may benefit from special consideration and treatment of these consequences and comorbidities.

Complementary and alternative medicine (CAM) is defined by the National Center for Complementary and Alternative Medicine (NCCAM) as a group of diverse medical and health care systems, practices, and products that are not generally considered part of conventional medicine as practiced in the West (e.g., the United States) [10]. Four domains of practice are recognized: mind–body medicine (meditation, prayer, mental healing, art, music, dance), biologically-based practices (use of substances found in nature, such as herbs, foods, vitamins, animal compounds), manipulative and body-based practices (chiropractic or osteopathic manipulation, massage), and energy medicine (biofield and bioelectromagnetic therapies). Separately recognized are whole medical systems such as homeopathy, naturopathy, ayurveda, and traditional Chinese medicine (TCM), each of them characterized by a complex and unique system of diagnostics and therapeutics.

Although they have a long history of successful traditional use in various regions of the world, the efficacy of different CAM interventions for epilepsy has not been adequately proved in clinical trials. For example, three Cochrane reviews evaluated the published data on the use of acupuncture [11], yoga [12], and TCM [13] for epilepsy and none found sufficient evidence of efficacy for any of these techniques. However, some CAM treatments may be effective against conditions commonly encountered in people with epilepsy, such as psychiatric comorbidities and headaches. This chapter reviews current knowledge on the use of CAM in people

Epilepsy and the Interictal State: Co-Morbidities and Quality of Life, First Edition.
Edited by Erik K. St. Louis, David M. Ficker, and Terence J. O'Brien.
© 2015 John Wiley & Sons, Ltd. Published 2015 by John Wiley & Sons, Ltd.

with epilepsy and in conditions of relevance for people with epilepsy.

Use of CAM by people with epilepsy in Western countries

While CAM treatments have for centuries provided the main form of medical therapy in certain areas of the world, such as East Asia, Africa, and Latin America, the use of CAM in Western countries has only developed over the last few decades, but it keeps increasing. In the 2007 American National Health Interview Survey (NHIS) of 23 393 adults and 9417 children, 38.3% of adults and 11.8% of children reported using CAM therapies [14]. These therapies were used more frequently by people with higher levels of education, women, and the Native American population. In addition, people with chronic medical conditions may have a greater tendency to use CAM. For example, CAM treatments were used by 42% of the adults who had been hospitalized during the 12 months prior to the survey, 53% of those who had visited their doctors 10 or more times in the same period, and 54% of those with six or more predefined health conditions. The most commonly utilized form of CAM was natural products, which were used by 17.7% of surveyed adults, with fish oil/omega-3 fatty acids the most widely consumed. The next most common forms were deep-breathing exercises (12.7%), meditation (9.4%), chiropractic or osteopathic manipulation (8.6%), and massage (8.3%) [14]. In a Canadian survey performed in 2001–05, 12% of those surveyed had visited a CAM practitioner within the previous 12 months [15]. The most frequently sought type of CAM was massage therapy (63%), followed by acupuncture (18%), homeopathy (18%), chiropractic care (11%), and herbal therapy (5%). While people with asthma and migraine were found to use CAM more than the general population, about 10% of people with epilepsy visited CAM practitioners (not significantly different than the general population) [15]. The distribution of use of CAM services by people with epilepsy was not significantly different than the general population.

A subanalysis of the 2007 NHIS found that 44% of adults with common neurological conditions (regular headaches, migraines, back pain with sciatica, strokes, dementia, seizures, or memory loss) used CAM [16]. CAM was used significantly more frequently by this population than by those without neurological conditions, even after adjusting for sociodemographics, illness burden, access to care, and health habits. While natural products were the most commonly used form of CAM in the general surveyed population [14], mind–body therapies were the most commonly used by adults with neurological conditions, who had higher rates of mind–body therapy use than the rest of the US population [16].

Several population- and hospital-based studies have investigated CAM use by adults [17–24] and children [25–27] with epilepsy in high-income countries (Table 22.1). According to these studies, 24–56% of adult patients and 12–32% of children have used CAM therapies at some time. Some of the differences in the frequency of CAM use between studies may pertain to differences in the definition and types of CAM in each study. However, another possible factor could be inclusion of patients with different ethnicities and cultural backgrounds, as exemplified by studies of patients originating from South Asia in the United Kingdom [28] and an ethnically diverse population in Brooklyn, New York [29]. Ethnic and cultural differences may influence both frequency and type of CAM use [30]. The use of CAM in this patient population was not always associated with the same factors as in the general population.

Because of the risk of aggravation of seizures and of pharmacokinetic interactions with AEDs [31], it is concerning that many people with epilepsy do not inform their physicians about their use of natural products [17,18,20–22]. Only 2–44% of the patients in the reviewed studies reported using CAM products specifically for control of seizures. However, the reasons noted by many patients may be relevant to known comorbidities of epilepsy such as depression or to common AED adverse events such as impaired memory. The efficacy of CAM for the control of seizures cannot be accurately assessed from the available studies because of their significant methodological shortcomings. However, patients typically report overall subjective benefit in these studies; whether this is consistent with the general population's view of CAM as "natural" and therefore beneficial requires further study.

Mind–body medicine

These are techniques designed to enhance the mind's capacity to affect bodily function and symptoms, including meditation, prayer, mental healing, art, music, and dance. They aim to modulate the stress and relaxation responses of the organism [32].

As mentioned earlier, mind–body medicine was found to be the most commonly used form of CAM by adults with chronic neurological conditions [16]. The age–sex-adjusted prevalence of mind–body use varied across conditions: 22.9% with seizures and regular headaches, 25.4% with sciatic back pain, 27.5% with migraines, and 27.8% with memory loss used mind–body therapies. For comparison, the prevalence of the use of mind–body medicine in the general adult American population, as reported by the 2007 NHIS, was 19.2% [14]. Of the mind–body therapies, deep-breathing exercises, meditation, and yoga were the most common among those with neurological conditions (19, 13, and 7%, respectively) [33].

A Cochrane review comprehensively assessed the evidence for efficacy of various mind–body therapies in people with epilepsy [34]. Trials of psychological interventions such as relaxation therapy, cognitive behavioral therapy (CBT), biofeedback, and educational interventions for reduction of seizure frequency and improvement of quality of life (QOL) in people with epilepsy were sought. The authors found three trials of relaxation therapy, which did not show a significant reduction in seizure frequency. One trial of CBT found statistically significant reduction in seizure frequency and duration but one of group cognitive therapy found no significant effect on seizure frequency. Two out of three trials found that CBT was effective in reducing depression among people with epilepsy with a depressed affect and another two trials of CBT found improvement in QOL scores. Two trials of combined relaxation and behavior therapy, one of EEG biofeedback, and four of educational interventions did not provide sufficient information to assess their effect on seizure frequency. One study of galvanic skin-response biofeedback reported significant reduction in seizure frequency. Combined use of relaxation and behavior modification was found to be beneficial for anxiety and adjustment in one study. In one study, EEG biofeedback was found to improve cognitive and motor functions in those individuals with the greatest seizure reduction. Educational interventions were found to be beneficial in improving knowledge and understanding of epilepsy, coping with epilepsy, compliance with medication, and social competencies. Overall, due to methodological

limitations and the small number of available studies, not enough evidence was found in this Cochrane review to support the use of any of these mind–body therapies in patients with epilepsy.

Similarly, despite some reports of beneficial effects on seizures [35], a Cochrane review concluded that no reliable conclusions can be drawn regarding the efficacy of yoga as a treatment for epilepsy [12]. However, yoga may be beneficial for amelioration of depression [36] and mindfulness-based stress reduction may enhance sleep [37]. Also, relaxation techniques were reported to be more effective at reducing self-rated depressive symptoms than no or minimal treatment, but not as effective as psychological treatment [38]. Neurofeedback was reported in a meta-analysis to be effective and specific for treatment of inattention and impulsivity in patients with attention-deficit disorder and to have a medium effect on hyperactivity [39]. However, a more recent sham-controlled double-blind trial, designed to assess whether EEG biofeedback enhances attention and decreases impulsive behavior in students with attention-deficit disorder, was ceased after interim data analysis due to lack of a trend for efficacy, despite successful blinding of participants [40].

Biologically-based practices

These practices include use of substances found in nature such as herbs, foods, vitamins, and animal compounds. In the 2007 NHIS, this was the most commonly utilized form of CAM [14].

Herbal remedies

Despite the abundant available data on the efficacy of herbal-derived remedies in animal models of epilepsy and against molecular mechanisms known to underlie seizure activity, publications of clinical trials of botanicals in epilepsy, especially well-designed ones, are extremely scarce. There are no English-language publications of randomized clinical trials of herbal medicines for treatment of epilepsy. The authors of a Cochrane review on TCM for epilepsy found seven Chinese trials comparing herbal products with AEDs (phenytoin, valproic acid, and phenobarbital) for the treatment of epilepsy, diagnosed according to the International League Against Epilepsy (ILAE) classifications [13]. The herbal products assessed in these trials were xaxingci

Table 22.1 Publications reporting use of complementary and alternative medicine (CAM) by people with epilepsy.

Publication	Population studied	Percentage using CAM	Associations	Doctor's knowledge	Most common CAM (in descending order, where known)	Reasons for use	Outcome measures
Easterford et al. [17]	377 adults with epilepsy in Manchester, United Kingdom	34.6%	Higher education	37%	NA	11.1% epilepsy	No significant effect on seizure frequency CAM was cheap
Gidal et al. [18]	465 adults with epilepsy from nine regions in the United States	31%, within previous year	Associated with high-school education or less No influence of age, gender, seizure type	33%	Ginkgo biloba, vitamins (55%), relaxation (45%), ginseng, St. John's wort	13% epilepsy (relaxation, vitamins, herbals, homeopathy), 28% general health/cold prevention, 11% mood difficulties, 5% cognition, 4% fatigue	NA
Kaiboriboon et al. [19]	187 adults with epilepsy at UCSF medical center, United States (only use of herbs and dietary supplements was studied)	56% (current use)	Partial epilepsy and Caucasian race No association with gender, age, level of education, income, duration of epilepsy, or seizure frequency	71%	Multivitamins and minerals, folic acid, ginseng, Ginkgo biloba, glucosamine and chondroitin, St. John's wort, black cohosh, Echinacea, evening primrose, ephedra, caffeine, melatonin, milk thistle, omega-3, kava, skullcap, valerian, grapefruit juice, glutamine, clover/nettles, parsley leaf, DHEA, coenzyme Q10, ginger, fish oil, garlic, grape seed, L-lysine	6 epilepsy (kava, skullcap, valerian, folic acid, vitamin B6, vitamin E, multivitamins, minerals), 35 general health, 13 physician's recommendation, 13 improve bone density, 10 increase energy, 10 boost immune system, 7 improve memory	9 patients reported adverse events that they attributed to these products; none reported aggravation of seizures 88% of patients spent less than $50 a month and only 5% spent more than $100
Liow et al. [20]	228 adults with epilepsy in US Midwest	39%	No association with education level	49%	Prayer/spirituality, megavitamins, chiropractic, stress management	57 (25%) epilepsy, 33 prayer/spirituality, 14 megavitamins, 11 chiropractic, 11 stress management	Subjective benefit of 74% of 57 Only a few side effects Increased seizures in diet pills, chiropractic, ketogenic diet, Atkin's megavitamins
Murphy et al. [21]	671 adults with neurological conditions in Ireland (189 with epilepsy)	47.6% of patients with epilepsy (63.3% of all conditions)	NA	25% for all conditions	Massage, acupuncture, vitamins, reflexology, yoga, evening primrose/starflower oil, chiropractic, homeopathy (for all conditions)	NA	Most had subjective benefit Annual cost €1170.32

Study	Population	CAM use	Associations	Disclosure	Types of CAM	Reasons	Notes
Peebles et al. [22]	92 adults with epilepsy in Ohio, United States	24%	No significant association with education level, sex, ethnicity, age	31%	Massage (50%), herbs/supplements (41%), music therapy, meditation, art therapy, aromatherapy, acupuncture	2% epilepsy (massage, acupuncture and meditation), pain, muscle tension, stress, low energy, cold, depression	NA
Plunkett et al. [23]	187 adults with epilepsy in San Francisco area, United States	56%	No association with seizure frequency or with having adverse events from AEDs	68%	Vitamins or minerals supplements	3% epilepsy or AED adverse events, general health, diet supplementation, physician's recommendation	NA (19% used products with cyp450 activity, 14% used potentially epileptogenic agents)
Sirven et al. [24]	425 adults with epilepsy in Arizona, United States	44% for epilepsy 42% for other conditions	No association with education level	93% would tell	Prayer, stress management, botanicals, chiropractic (specifically for epilepsy)	44% epilepsy, 42% other conditions	Stress management, yoga, and botanicals subjectively most beneficial 43% using botanicals for epilepsy had increased seizure frequency; three had major side effects (intracranial hemorrhage with ephedra)
Gross-Tsur et al. [25]	115 children with epilepsy in Israel (compared with children with ADHD and control)	32%	In general: higher education, prior use For epilepsy and ADHD: longer disease duration, less satisfaction with conventional therapy	NA	Dietary interventions, followed by homeopathy, biofeedback, acupuncture, Reike, reflexology, shiatsu, chiropractic (in all groups)	NA	NA
Waaler et al. [26]	198 children with active epilepsy in Norway	11.6%	Additional neurological deficits	NA	Homeopathy	NA	NA
Yuncker et al. [27]	350 children with neurological conditions (60% with epilepsy) in Pennsylvania, United States	28% of children with epilepsy (37% of all conditions)	Diagnosed for less than 1 year	69%	NA	NA	87% overall felt CAM was effective and similar to conventional therapy 40% knew possible side effects

CAM, complementary and alternative medicine; NA, not available; ADHD, attention deficit/hyperactivity disorder; AED, antiepileptic drug.

granule, dianxianning, tianmadingxian, zhixian, xifeng capsule, and antiepilepsy capsule. Variation in the baseline patient characteristics, herbal formulations, and AEDs between the studies precluded meta-analysis of the results. Although the studies did report some benefit, no reliable conclusion on the effect of TCM for epilepsy could be drawn due to methodological limitations and, therefore, a high probability of selection, detection, and performance bias [13]. Three Chinese articles in which botanicals (alkaline extract of *Euphorbia fisheriana*, Ningxian capsule, and *Ginkgo biloba*) were used in conjunction with AEDs will be included in the update of the Cochrane review [13].

A planned phase II randomized, placebo-controlled, double-blind, crossover clinical trial, initiated by Dr. Siegward Elsas of Oregon Health and Science University, aimed to be completed in 2011, will test the safety and potential anticonvulsant efficacy of a botanical extract from *Passiflora incarnata* in patients with partial-onset epilepsy [41]. The investigators intend to randomize approximately 25 people with active focal-onset epilepsy to take either one or two conventional AEDs for two crossover arms of treatment or placebo (11 weeks for each). The primary outcome measure will be seizure frequency and the secondary outcome measures will be anxiety, cognitive function, and QOL. Screening for adverse effects will be performed. Upon completion, this trial will provide a high level of evidence for the efficacy of *Passiflora* in the treatment of epilepsy.

No publication has specifically studied the efficacy of herbal medicines for comorbidities in the epilepsy patient population. However, a search of planned clinical trials of herbal products in patients with epilepsy revealed a trial intended to be completed in 2011, whose primary investigator is Wang Xin, from China [42]. This study will evaluate the efficacy and safety of add-on therapy of wuling capsule in epilepsy patients with depression. It is a multicenter, randomized, double-blinded, placebo-controlled superiority clinical trial, taking place in eight centers from four different cities in China, aiming to enroll 230 patients with epilepsy and depression and to randomize them to either treatment or placebo for 3 months. The primary outcome is improvement in depression and the secondary outcomes are frequency and severity of seizures, sleeping condition, and QOL. Current evidence supports the use of St. John's wort in treating mild to moderate

depression [43] and the use of kava in treatment of generalized anxiety [43,44]. Passionflower extracts may also be effective as anxiolytics [45]. Rosenroot was found to improve attention in cognitive function in fatigue, to have antifatigue effect in physical, emotional, and mental exhaustion, to treat mild depression, and to improve mental performance [46]. There is not yet enough evidence for the use of other herbal remedies in psychiatric disorders [47] or insomnia [48] or as adjuvants to conventional antidepressants, mood stabilizers, or benzodiazepines [49]. Natural products and especially herbal-derived compounds, together with weight-bearing exercise, may improve bone health, which is sometimes negatively affected by chronic use of AEDs [50].

In general, herbal medicines are considered relatively safe and indeed only minimal gastrointestinal discomfort was reported in the available clinical trials of herbal products for treatment of epilepsy [13]. While many botanicals are known to affect the CNS, only case reports of an association between use of herbal products and seizures have been published in humans. These involved mainly ephedra, caffeine, *Gingko biloba* seeds, star anise, star fruit, and evening primrose [31,51]. A review of the 65 cases of dietary supplement-associated seizures reported to the FDA between 1993 and 1999 concluded that 20 seizures were probably related to the dietary supplement (19 of them involved ephedra consumption and 14 caffeine), 13 were possibly related (7 involved ephedra, 5 caffeine; creatine, St. John's wort, and *Ginkgo biloba* were also implicated), and 10 were unrelated [52]. Five cases were not seizures and seventeen provided insufficient information.

Although multiple interactions between botanicals and AEDs may be assumed from knowledge of the effects of herbal products on motility of the intestines, absorption, and liver enzymes and from animal trials, very few works have directly studied these interactions in humans [31,51,53,54]. The best available evidence for interaction between a herbal medicine and AEDs was provided by a study showing that piperine coadministration significantly increased the mean plasma concentration of two different doses of phenytoin at steady state in 20 patients with uncontrolled epilepsy [55]. This finding was further supported by a trial showing a similarly significant raise in the concentration of phenytoin after its coadministration with piperine in six healthy volunteers [56]. Similarly, grapefruit juice increased the bioavailability of carbamazepine at steady state in patients with epilepsy [57] and increased the concentration of diazepam in healthy subjects [58]. Chronic treatment with St. John's wort was found to decrease the bioavailability of benzodiazepines in healthy subjects, presumably through its effects on the cytochrome P450 system [59–61]. Interestingly, this decrease in the plasma concentration did not induce pharmacodynamic effects in one of the studies [60]. In one case report of fatal seizures accompanied by low plasma concentrations of phenytoin and valproic acid in an epilepsy patient who had been using herbal supplements that contained *Gingko biloba*, it was assumed that gingko might decrease the bioavailability of these AEDs [62]. Many herbal remedies that contain high fiber concentrations may theoretically interfere with the absorption of concomitantly ingested drugs, including AEDs. However, this theory has only been tested in humans in regard to psyllium, which was found to decrease the plasma concentration of carbamazepine when taken together by four healthy subjects [63].

Despite reporting on generally encouraging outcomes, trials assessing treatment with botanicals are limited by serious methodological caveats. Many do not adequately randomize study subjects or use proper controls, while others are not blinded or do not rigorously monitor the results of the interventions. While the requirements of evidence-based medicine have become familiar to conventional/Western practitioners, implementing these principles into trials of other medical systems is problematic because these systems may involve a holistic, personalized approach to treating patients rather than one that is disease-focused and therefore applied in the same way to all patients characterized by a specific disease. In addition, there are cultural differences between Western and traditional populations that raise ethical issues which make the incorporation of evidence-based principles for randomized clinical trials even harder [64]. The Consolidated Standards of Reporting Trials (CONSORT) statement, based on a 22-item checklist, guides authors, readers, reviewers, and editors on the essential information required in reports of two-group parallel randomized clinical trials [65,66]. In 2006, specific recommendations for reporting randomized clinical trials of herbal medicines were issued by a group of individuals with international expertise in clinical trial methodology, pharmacognosy, and herbal products [67]. Nine items of

the CONSORT statement were elaborated for relevance to randomized clinical trials of herbal medicines. Further recommendations for reporting of randomized clinical trials of TCM interventions [68], outcomes [69], and adverse events [70] were than proposed by Chinese researchers. A follow-up work that looked at the implementation of the herbal medicine CONSORT recommendations in 406 randomized clinical trials up to the end of 2007 found that although only 38% of the required information was reported, the reports were better in the more recent years [71]. Future studies will undoubtedly be able to provide proper evidence for the use of herbal medicines in epilepsy and conditions commonly associated with it.

Other natural products

Omega-3 fatty acids were the most common type of biologically-based products used by Americans according to the 2007 NHIS [14], most probably due to their beneficial effects on cardiac disorders [72,73]. Omega-3 polyunsaturated fatty acids may also have antiseizure properties [74], decrease the risk of sudden unexpected death in epilepsy [75,76], and ameliorate depression [77]. Combinations of L-lysine and L-arginine and magnesium-containing supplements may be beneficial for the treatment of anxiety symptoms and disorders [45].

Energy medicine

This domain of CAM includes practices such as therapeutic touch, reiki, and acupuncture. The medical efficacy of acupuncture is the most widely studied among these techniques. Its efficacy in treating epilepsy was summarized in a Cochrane review [11] that included 11 trials with 914 participants. Although some data were found for a higher likelihood of achieving 75% or more reduction in seizure frequency in the acupuncture groups in comparison to phenytoin or valproic acid, the general conclusion of this review was that there is not enough evidence to support acupuncture for treatment of epilepsy. There are no studies that specifically assessed the effect of acupuncture on comorbidities in patients with epilepsy. Although a Cochrane review of the effect of acupuncture on depression concluded that in general there is not enough evidence to support this form of treatment, it did find significant

Table 22.2 Types of complementary and alternative medicine (CAM) interventions that may be used for various health issues in patients with epilepsy.

Health issue	Types of CAM
Epilepsy	There is no evidence for efficacy of any CAM practice. Cognitive behavioral therapy, biofeedback, yoga, botanicals, omega-3 fatty acids, and acupuncture may have some beneficial effects
Depression and anxiety	There is evidence that depression can be efficaciously treated with St. John's wort (mild to moderate depression) and acupuncture (stroke-related depression) and that Kava improves symptoms of anxiety. Cognitive behavioral therapy, relaxation, yoga, passionflower (anxiety), omega-3 (depression), and acupuncture may also have some beneficial effects
Cognitive decline	There is evidence for the use of rosenroot to improve mental performance. Biofeedback may also have some beneficial effect
ADHD	There is contradictory evidence for the efficacy of biofeedback
Sleep	Relaxation and acupuncture may have some beneficial effects
Pain and headache	There is evidence for the use of acupuncture in the treatment of pain and tension-type and chronic headache and the prevention of migraine headache

evidence for acupuncture as treatment of depression in patients with stroke [78]. There is proven evidence for efficacy of acupuncture in treatment of pain [79], specifically in tension-type headache [80,81], chronic headache [82], and prophylaxis of migraine [83]. The evidence for the efficacy of acupuncture in treatment of insomnia [84] and of generalized anxiety disorder (GAD) or anxiety neurosis [85] is still insufficient. Pregnancy in women with epilepsy requires special consideration and careful management, due to potential harmful effects of seizures and AEDs on mother and fetus. Acupuncture may relieve nausea, back pain, and labor pain [86] without significant adverse events.

Whole medical systems

Traditional medical systems, such as TCM and ayurveda, have been practiced for thousands of years in certain regions of the world. However, treatments offered as part of these systems have only recently started to be evaluated according to the modern requirements of evidence-based medicine. Indeed, even in regard to TCM, which is the most widely studied medical system, there is still no compelling evidence to support its use in clinical practice [87]. More specifically, there is not enough of a base of evidence for the use of TCM in

epilepsy [13]. There is also no evidence for a general clinical benefit of homeopathy [88], particularly in the treatment of ADHD [89] or cognitive impairment [90]. Bach flower treatment is commonly used for psychological problems and pain. However, the currently available evidence indicates that Bach flowers are not more efficacious than a placebo intervention for anxiety and ADHD but are probably safe [91].

Conclusion

While there is no compelling evidence that any CAM practices effectively treat epilepsy, some interventions may be beneficial for common comorbidities and cognitive and psychological consequences of epilepsy or its treatments (Table 22.2). For example, herbal remedies may assist in the alleviation of anxiety and depression and acupuncture may help to treat ADHD, pain, and depression. Further studies, especially of the complementary use of CAM to improve QOL and comorbid conditions in people with epilepsy, are clearly needed.

References

1 Kwan P, Arzimanoglou A, Berg AT et al.: Definition of drug resistant epilepsy: consensus proposal by the ad hoc Task

Force of the ILAE Commission on Therapeutic Strategies. *Epilepsia* 2010; **51(6)**:1069–1077.

2 Kwan P, Brodie MJ: Early identification of refractory epilepsy. *N Engl J Med* 2000; **342(5)**:314–319.

3 Schmidt D: Drug treatment of epilepsy: options and limitations. *Epilepsy Behav* 2009; **15(1)**:56–65.

4 Choi H, Sell RL, Lenert L et al.: Epilepsy surgery for pharmacoresistant temporal lobe epilepsy: a decision analysis. *JAMA* 2008; **300(21)**:2497–2505.

5 Engel J Jr , Wiebe S, French J et al.: Practice parameter: temporal lobe and localized neocortical resections for epilepsy: report of the Quality Standards Subcommittee of the American Academy of Neurology, in association with the American Epilepsy Society and the American Association of Neurological Surgeons. *Neurology* 2003; **60(4)**:538–547.

6 Engel J Jr : Surgical treatment for epilepsy: too little, too late? *JAMA* 2008; **300(21)**:2548–2550.

7 Boon P, Raedt R, de Herdt V et al.: Electrical stimulation for the treatment of epilepsy. *Neurotherapeutics* 2009; **6(2)**: 218–227.

8 Fisher RS, van Emde Boas W, Blume W et al.: Epileptic seizures and epilepsy: definitions proposed by the International League Against Epilepsy (ILAE) and the International Bureau for Epilepsy (IBE). *Epilepsia* 2005; **46(4)**:470–472.

9 Ottman R, Lipton RB, Ettinger AB et al.: Comorbidities of epilepsy: results from the Epilepsy Comorbidities and Health (EPIC) survey. *Epilepsia* 2011; **52(2)**:308–315.

10 National Center for Complementary and Alternative Medicine: nccam.nih.gov (last accessed July 15, 2014).

11 Cheuk DK, Wong V: Acupuncture for epilepsy. *Cochrane Database Syst Rev* 2008; **4**:CD005062.

12 Ramaratnam S, Sridharan K: Yoga for epilepsy. *Cochrane Database Syst Rev* 2000; **2**:CD001524.

13 Li Q, Chen X, He L, Zhou D: Traditional Chinese medicine for epilepsy. *Cochrane Database Syst Rev* 2009; **3**:CD006454.

14 Barnes PM, Bloom B, Nahin RL: Complementary and alternative medicine use among adults and children: United States, 2007. *Natl Health Stat Report* 2008; **10(12)**:1–23.

15 Metcalfe A, Williams J, McChesney J et al.: Use of complementary and alternative medicine by those with a chronic disease and the general population: results of a national population based survey. *BMC Complement Altern Med* 2010; **10**:58.

16 Wells RE, Phillips RS, Schachter SC, McCarthy EP: Complementary and alternative medicine use among US adults with common neurological conditions. *J Neurol* 2010; **257(11)**:1822–1831.

17 Easterford K, Clough P, Comish S et al.: The use of complementary medicines and alternative practitioners in a cohort of patients with epilepsy. *Epilepsy Behav* 2005; **6(1)**:59–62.

18 Gidal BE, Sheth RD, Bainbridge J et al.: Alternative medicine (AM) use in epilepsy: results of a national, multicenter survey. *Epilepsia* 1999; **40**:107–108.

19 Kaiboriboon K, Guevara M, Alldredge BK: Understanding herb and dietary supplement use in patients with epilepsy. *Epilepsia* 2009; **50(8)**:1927–1932.

20 Liow K, Ablah E, Nguyen JC et al.: Pattern and frequency of use of complementary and alternative medicine among patients with epilepsy in the Midwestern United States. *Epilepsy Behav* 2007; **10(4)**:576–582.

21 Murphy SM, Rogers A, Hutchinson M, Tubridy N: Counting the cost of complementary and alternative therapies in an Irish neurological clinic. *Eur J Neurol* 2008; **15(12)**:1380–1383.

22 Peebles CT, McAuley JW, Roach J et al.: Alternative medicine use by patients with epilepsy. *Epilepsy Behav* 2000; **1(1)**:74–77.

23 Plunkett MV, Klein EW, Alldredge BK: Use of complementary and alternative medicine products by persons with epilepsy. *Epilepsia* 2004; **45**:148–149.

24 Sirven JI, Drazkowski JF, Zimmerman RS et al.: Complementary/alternative medicine for epilepsy in Arizona. *Neurology* 2003; **61(4)**:576–577.

25 Gross-Tsur V, Lahad A, Shalev RS: Use of complementary medicine in children with attention deficit hyperactivity disorder and epilepsy. *Pediatr Neurol* 2003; **29(1)**:53–55.

26 Waaler PE, Blom BH, Skeidsvoll H, Mykletun A: Prevalence, classification, and severity of epilepsy in children in western Norway. *Epilepsia* 2000; **41(7)**:802–810.

27 Yuncker LA, Kerszberg S, Hunt SL et al.: The use of alternative/complementary therapies in children with epilepsy and other neurologic disorders. *Epilepsia* 2004; **45**:326–327.

28 Rhodes PJ, Small N, Ismail H, Wright JP: The use of biomedicine, complementary and alternative medicine, and ethnomedicine for the treatment of epilepsy among people of South Asian origin in the UK. *BMC Complement Altern Med* 2008; **8**:7.

29 Prus N, Grant AC: Patient beliefs about epilepsy and brain surgery in a multicultural urban population. *Epilepsy Behav* 2010; **17(1)**:46–49.

30 Cohen MH: Regulation, religious experience, and epilepsy: a lens on complementary therapies. *Epilepsy Behav* 2003; **4(6)**:602–606.

31 Samuels N, Finkelstein Y, Singer SR, Oberbaum M: Herbal medicine and epilepsy: proconvulsive effects and interactions with antiepileptic drugs. *Epilepsia* 2008; **49(3)**: 373–380.

32 Dusek JA, Benson H: Mind-body medicine: a model of the comparative clinical impact of the acute stress and relaxation responses. *Minn Med* 2009; **92(5)**:47–50.

33 Wells RE, Phillips RS, McCarthy EP: Patterns of mind-body therapies in adults with common neurological conditions. *Neuroepidemiol* 2011; **36**:46–51.

34 Ramaratnam S, Baker GA, Goldstein LH: Psychological treatments for epilepsy. *Cochrane Database Syst Rev* 2008; **3**:CD002029.

35 Wahbeh H, Elsas SM, Oken BS: Mind-body interventions: applications in neurology. *Neurology* 2008; **70(24)**: 2321–2328.

36 Pilkington K, Kirkwood G, Rampes H, Richardson J: Yoga for depression: the research evidence. *J Affect Disord* 2005; **89(1–3)**:13–24.

37 Winbush NY, Gross CR, Kreitzer MJ: The effects of mindfulness-based stress reduction on sleep disturbance: a systematic review. *Explore (NY)* 2007; **3(6)**:585–591.

38 Jorm AF, Morgan AJ, Hetrick SE: Relaxation for depression. *Cochrane Database Syst Rev* 2008; **4**:CD007142.

39 Arns M, de Ridder S, Strehl U et al.: Efficacy of neurofeedback treatment in ADHD: the effects on inattention, impulsivity and hyperactivity: a meta-analysis. *Clin EEG Neurosci* 2009; **40(3)**:180–189.

40 Logemann HN, Lansbergen MM, Van Os TW et al.: The effectiveness of EEG-feedback on attention, impulsivity and EEG: a sham feedback controlled study. *Neurosci Lett* 2010; **479(1)**:49–53.

41 Oregon Health and Science University: Safety and anticonvulsant efficacy of *Passiflora incarnate* extract in patients with partial epilepsy. Available from: http://clinicaltrials.gov /ct2/show/NCT00982787?term=epilepsy&rank=85 (last accessed July 15, 2014).

42 Shanghai Zhongshan Hospital: A study to evaluate the efficacy and safety of add-on therapy of Wuling capsule in epilepsy patients with depression. Available from: http: //clinicaltrials.gov/ct2/show/NCT01125241?term=epilepsy &rank=96 (last accessed July 15, 2014).

43 Sarris J, Kavanagh DJ: Kava and StJohn's wort : current evidence for use in mood and anxiety disorders. *J Altern Complement Med* 2009; **15(8)**:827–836.

44 Sarris J, LaPorte E, Schweitzer I: Kava: a comprehensive review of efficacy, safety, and psychopharmacology. *Aust NZ J Psychiatry* 2011; **45(1)**:27–35.

45 Lakhan SE, Vieira KF: Nutritional and herbal supplements for anxiety and anxiety-related disorders: systematic review. *Nutr J* 2010; **9**:42.

46 Panossian A, Wikman G, Sarris J: Rosenroot (*Rhodiola rosea*): traditional use, chemical composition, pharmacology and clinical efficacy. *Phytomedicine* 2010; **17(7)**:481–493.

47 Sarris J: Herbal medicines in the treatment of psychiatric disorders: a systematic review. *Phytother Res* 2007; **21(8)**: 703–716.

48 Sarris J, Byrne GJ: A systematic review of insomnia and complementary medicine. *Sleep Med Rev* 2011; **15(2)**: 99–106.

49 Sarris J, Kavanagh DJ, Byrne G: Adjuvant use of nutritional and herbal medicines with antidepressants, mood stabilizers and benzodiazepines. *J Psychiatr Res* 2010; **44(1)**:32–41.

50 Putnam SE, Scutt AM, Bicknell K et al.: Natural products as alternative treatments for metabolic bone disorders and for maintenance of bone health. *Phytother Res* 2007; **21(2)**:99–112.

51 Ulbricht C, Basch E, Weissner W, Hackman D: An evidence-based systematic review of herb and supplement interactions by the Natural Standard Research Collaboration. *Expert Opin Drug Saf* 2006; **5(5)**:719–728.

52 Haller CA, Meier KH, Olson KR: Seizures reported in association with use of dietary supplements. *Clin Toxicol (Phila)* 2005; **43(1)**:23–30.

53 Izzo AA, Ernst E: Interactions between herbal medicines and prescribed drugs: an updated systematic review. *Drugs* 2009; **69(13)**:1777–1798.

54 Ulbricht C, Chao W, Costa D et al.: Clinical evidence of herb-drug interactions: a systematic review by the natural standard research collaboration. *Curr Drug Metab* 2008; **9(10)**:1063–1120.

55 Pattanaik S, Hota D, Prabhakar S et al.: Effect of piperine on the steady-state pharmacokinetics of phenytoin in patients with epilepsy. *Phytother Res* 2006; **20(8)**:683–686.

56 Velpandian T, Jasuja R, Bhardwaj RK et al.: Piperine in food: interference in the pharmacokinetics of phenytoin. *Eur J Drug Metab Pharmacokinet* 2001; **26(4)**:241–247.

57 Garg SK, Kumar N, Bhargava VK, Prabhakar SK: Effect of grapefruit juice on carbamazepine bioavailability in patients with epilepsy. *Clin Pharmacol Ther* 1998; **64(3)**:286–288.

58 Ozdemir M, Aktan Y, Boydag BS et al.: Interaction between grapefruit juice and diazepam in humans. *Eur J Drug Metab Pharmacokinet* 1998; **23(1)**:55–59.

59 Dresser GK, Schwarz UI, Wilkinson GR, Kim RB: Coordinate induction of both cytochrome P4503A and MDR1 by St John's wort in healthy subjects. *Clin Pharmacol Ther* 2003; **73(1)**:41–50.

60 Kawaguchi A, Ohmori M, Tsuruoka S et al.: Drug interaction between St John's wort and quazepam. *Br J Clin Pharmacol* 2004; **58(4)**:403–410.

61 Wang Z, Gorski JC, Hamman MA et al.: The effects of St John's wort (*Hypericum perforatum*) on human cytochrome P450 activity. *Clin Pharmacol Ther* 2001; **70(4)**:317–326.

62 Kupiec T, Raj V: Fatal seizures due to potential herb-drug interactions with *Ginkgo biloba*. *J Anal Toxicol* 2005; **29(7)**:755–758.

63 Etman MA: Effect of a bulk forming laxative on the bioavailability of carbamazepine in man. *Drug Dev Ind Pharm* 1995; **21(16)**:1901–1906.

64 Zaslawski C: Ethical considerations for acupuncture and Chinese herbal medicine clinical trials: a cross-cultural perspective. Evid Based Complement Alternat Med 2010; **7(3)**:295–301.

65 Begg C, Cho M, Eastwood S et al.: Improving the quality of reporting of randomized controlled trials: the CONSORT statement. *JAMA* 1996; **276(8)**:637–639.

66 Moher D, Schulz KF, Altman D: The CONSORT statement: revised recommendations for improving the quality of reports of parallel-group randomized trials. *JAMA* 2001; **285(15)**:1987–1991.

67 Gagnier JJ, Boon H, Rochon P et al.: Reporting randomized, controlled trials of herbal interventions: an elaborated CONSORT statement. *Ann Intern Med* 2006; **144(5)**:364–367.

68 Bian Z, Moher D, Li Y et al.: Precise reporting of traditional Chinese medicine interventions in randomized controlled trials. *J Chinese Integrative Med* 2008; **6(7)**:661–667.

69 Bian Z, Moher D, Li Y et al.: Appropriately selecting and concisely reporting the outcome measures of randomized controlled trials of traditional Chinese medicine. *J Chinese Integrative Med* 2008; **6(8)**:771–775.

70 Cheng C, Bian Z, Li Y et al.: Transparently reporting adverse effects of traditional Chinese medicine interventions in randomized controlled trial. *J Chinese Integrative Med* 2008; **6(9)**:881–886.

71 Gagnier JJ, Moher D, Boon H et al.: Randomized controlled trials of herbal interventions underreport important details of the intervention. *J Clin Epidemiol* 2011; **64(7)**:760–769.

72 Filion KB, El Khoury F, Bielinski M et al.: Omega-3 fatty acids in high-risk cardiovascular patients: a meta-analysis of randomized controlled trials. *BMC Cardiovasc Disord* 2010; **10**:24.

73 Patel JV, Tracey I, Hughes EA, Lip GY: Omega-3 polyunsaturated fatty acids: a necessity for a comprehensive secondary prevention strategy. *Vasc Health Risk Manag* 2009; **5**:801–810.

74 Taha AY, Burnham WM, Auvin S: Polyunsaturated fatty acids and epilepsy. *Epilepsia* 2010; **51(8)**:1348–1358.

75 DeGiorgio CM, Miller P: n-3 fatty acids (eicosapentanoic and docosahexanoic acids) in epilepsy and for the prevention of sudden unexpected death in epilepsy. *Epilepsy Behav* 2008; **13(4)**:712–713.

76 DeGiorgio CM, Miller P, Meymandi S, Gornbein JA: n-3 fatty acids (fish oil) for epilepsy, cardiac risk factors, and risk of SUDEP: clues from a pilot, double-blind, exploratory study. *Epilepsy Behav* 2008; **13(4)**:681–684.

77 Kraguljac NV, Montori VM, Pavuluri M et al.: Efficacy of omega-3 fatty acids in mood disorders: a systematic review and metaanalysis. *Psychopharmacol Bull* 2009; **42(3)**:39–54.

78 Smith CA, Hay PP, Macpherson H: Acupuncture for depression. *Cochrane Database Syst Rev* 2010; **1**:CD004046.

79 Hopton A, MacPherson H: Acupuncture for chronic pain: is acupuncture more than an effective placebo? A systematic review of pooled data from meta-analyses. *Pain Pract* 2010; **10(2)**:94–102.

80 Davis MA, Kononowech RW, Rolin SA, Spierings EL: Acupuncture for tension-type headache: a meta-analysis of randomized, controlled trials. *J Pain* 2008; **9(8)**:667–677.

81 Linde K, Allais G, Brinkhaus B et al.: Acupuncture for tension-type headache. *Cochrane Database Syst Rev* 2009; **1**:CD007587.

82 Sun Y, Gan TJ: Acupuncture for the management of chronic headache: a systematic review. *Anesth Analg* 2008; **107(6)**:2038–2047.

83 Linde K, Allais G, Brinkhaus B et al.: Acupuncture for migraine prophylaxis. *Cochrane Database Syst Rev* 2009; **1**:CD001218.

84 Cheuk DK, Yeung WF, Chung KF, Wong V: Acupuncture for insomnia. *Cochrane Database Syst Rev* 2007; **3**:CD005472.

85 Pilkington K, Kirkwood G, Rampes H et al.: Acupuncture for anxiety and anxiety disorders: a systematic literature review. *Acupunct Med* 2007; **25(1–2)**:1–10.

86 Smith CA, Cochrane S: Does acupuncture have a place as an adjunct treatment during pregnancy? A review of randomized controlled trials and systematic reviews. *Birth* 2009; **36(3)**:246–253.

87 Manheimer E, Wieland S, Kimbrough E et al.: Evidence from the Cochrane Collaboration for Traditional Chinese Medicine therapies. *J Altern Complement Med* 2009; **15(9)**:1001–1014.

88 Ernst E: Homeopathy: what does the "best" evidence tell us? *Med J Aust* 2010; **192(8)**:458–460.

89 Coulter MK, Dean ME: Homeopathy for attention deficit/hyperactivity disorder or hyperkinetic disorder. *Cochrane Database Syst Rev* 2007; **4**:CD005648.

90 McCarney R, Warner J, Fisher P, Van Haselen R: Homeopathy for dementia. *Cochrane Database Syst Rev* 2003; **1**:CD003803.

91 Thaler K, Kaminski A, Chapman A et al.: Bach flower remedies for psychological problems and pain: a systematic review. *BMC Complement Altern Med* 2009; **9**:16.

CHAPTER 23

Epilepsy and alcohol and substance abuse

Ekrem Kutluay and Jonathan C. Edwards
Department of Neurosciences, Medical University of South Carolina, USA

Introduction

As one of the most common neurological disorders, epilepsy is seen throughout the world and affects people of any age, race, nationality, religion, or gender. The relationship between epilepsy and alcohol or substance abuse is complex. In some cases, the abuse of substances can result in recurrent provoked [induced] seizures, leading to a misdiagnosis of epilepsy. In others, substance or alcohol abuse may increase the risk of developing epilepsy. Further, alcohol or drug use can lower the seizure threshold in a patient with preexisting epilepsy and the coexistence of a substance abuse history can delay the diagnosis of epilepsy, due to false assumptions that seizures were provoked. Because of the complex nature of the relationship between epilepsy and alcohol or substance abuse and the legal and health aspects surrounding the issue, well-controlled studies are lacking. However, the medical literature has numerous case series, case reports, and reports of survey data that give some insights into this complex relationship.

Alcohol

Alcohol consumption and dependency is one of the top five leading causes of the global burden of disease [1]. Excessive use of alcohol is a significant risk factor for several health problems, including stroke, hypertension, heart disease, and several cancers [1]. It is estimated that close to 2 million deaths per year are related to alcohol globally [1]. Additionally, alcohol abuse increases the risk of developing epilepsy [1].

Although most of the seizures reported as causally related to alcohol occur during the withdrawal phase, they can occur during intoxication or as the result of chronic effects of alcohol [2]. A study of 247 patients who had their first generalized seizure showed that alcohol abuse was one of the top four etiologies [3]. The prevalence of seizures in patients with alcohol dependency varies but numbers close to 15% have been reported [4,5]. However, most of these studies include alcohol withdrawal seizures; if these provoked seizures are excluded, the prevalence is estimated at 2–9% [5]. A general-population study in Sweden revealed a slight difference of seizure prevalence between genders in alcohol-dependent patients (7.5% male versus 6.6% female) [6]. Most dramatically, a retrospective chart review revealed that alcohol abuse was the only identifiable risk factor in almost 11% of the patients who presented to the emergency room with generalized convulsive status epilepticus [7]. In fact, in roughly half of those patients, status epilepticus was the first presentation of seizures. Alcohol abuse is considered one of the major causes of status epilepticus [6].

The majority of alcohol-related seizures are withdrawal seizures. The diagnosis is based on exclusion of other risk factors and the causal relationship to heavy daily alcohol intake and recent abstinence. These seizures typically occur 6–48 hours after a relative reduction or complete cessation of alcohol intake [6,8]. Although most are generalized tonic–clonic seizures, partial-onset seizures are also observed. The risk of alcohol-related seizures seems to be dose-related. A recent study showed that the risk starts with over 50 g alcohol intake per day and increases gradually up to 300 g/day [9]. The risk is up to 20 times higher in alcohol abusers consuming 200–300 g/day than in nondrinkers [9]. However, the study did not find further incremental increase in risk over 300 g/day consumption. Several

Epilepsy and the Interictal State: Co-Morbidities and Quality of Life, First Edition.
Edited by Erik K. St. Louis, David M. Ficker, and Terence J. O'Brien.
© 2015 John Wiley & Sons, Ltd. Published 2015 by John Wiley & Sons, Ltd.

confounding factors were also implicated in a subgroup of patients with increased risk factors, such as existing idiopathic generalized epilepsy, previous history of stroke, traumatic brain injury or tumor, other drug abuse, and alcohol-related metabolic changes [8]. It is well known that persons with alcohol dependency are more prone to having head trauma and traumatic brain injury as a result of falls, car accidents, or assaults [8]. Although there are no systematic human studies available for a pathophysiological explanation of alcohol withdrawal seizures, several animal studies provide some valuable insight. During the acute phase, alcohol seems to reduce glutamergic transmission by acting like an NMDA receptor antagonist [6,10,11]. However, chronic exposure leads to upregulation of NMDA receptors in the brain and increased binding of glutamate to NMDA receptors [6,10,11]. Similar changes occur in an opposite direction for GABA-A receptors. With chronic use, GABA-A receptors undergo downregulation and, despite some increase in CSF GABA levels during the withdrawal phase, disinhibition occurs [10]. Hence, increases in NMDA receptors and increased sensitivity of these receptors to glutamate lead to an excitatory state [6]. Also, chronic stimulation of NMDA receptors increases homocysteine levels, contributing to excitotoxicity during the withdrawal phase [11].

In addition to withdrawal seizures, unprovoked spontaneous seizures and epilepsy may also develop in chronic alcohol consumers. Samokhvalov et al. [12] performed a comprehensive review and meta-analysis of the association between alcohol consumption and epilepsy, summarizing their findings by stating that the risk of developing unprovoked seizures increases in a dose-dependent manner and is influenced by the duration of chronic heavy alcohol consumption. The risk of unprovoked seizures increases with 10 years or more of heavy consumption of alcohol ($\geq$50 g/day). Their meta-analysis also summarized several theories explaining the epileptogenesis in heavy alcohol users, including cerebral atrophy as a result of chronic alcohol use, increased incidence of traumatic brain injuries, possible kindling due to repeated withdrawals, and chronic changes in neurotransmitter systems, as described earlier [12].

EEG is usually of limited value in the evaluation of alcohol-related seizures. The presence of pathological slowing and interictal epileptiform activity may suggest that the seizures for a given patient are not solely alcohol-related [13]. However, the most common EEG finding in alcohol-related seizures is a normal EEG with low-amplitude alpha activity postictally [13].

The management of alcohol-related seizures is considerably similar to that of other provoked seizures. However, prolonged exposure to alcohol may lead to certain metabolic changes. Supplementation of thiamine and correction of possible hyponatremia and hypomagnesemia are especially important, particularly since both problems may further lower the seizure threshold [14]. Benzodiazepines are recommended for primary prevention of seizures during acute alcohol withdrawal [14]. Prophylactic use of antiepileptic agents is only warranted if a person has recurrent seizures unrelated to alcohol intake [14].

The use of alcohol in the epilepsy population

A fairly recent study of behavioral risk factors in persons with epilepsy was reported following a survey across 19 US states. The study was supported by the Centers for Disease Control and Prevention (CDC) as part of the Behavioral Risk Factor Surveillance System (BRFSS). The BRFSS is a random digit-dialed telephone survey of adults (aged 18 or older) in the United States. Core questions are asked of all participants, with additional questions about certain diseases asked in some states. Nineteen states elected to add questions about epilepsy, and twelve of those included all five epilepsy-related questions. In this study, 1.65% of adult participants reported having a history of epilepsy diagnosed by a doctor and 0.84% reported having "active epilepsy," defined as taking medication for epilepsy or having had a seizure within the last 3 months. Among the adults surveyed who had active epilepsy, 30.4% reported drinking alcohol within the past month. Further stratification to heavy versus light alcohol use was not available. While the use of alcohol was lower (at 30.4%) than for those without epilepsy (53.4%), it is important to note that although most clinicians recommend that patients with epilepsy avoid alcohol, one-third of adults with epilepsy do drink alcoholic beverages [15].

Marijuana

Marijuana is most commonly used as an illicit drug. According to the National Survey on Drug Use and

Health, 104 million Americans older than 12 years of age have tried marijuana at least once in their lifetime. Marijuana is usually smoked.

The effect of marijuana on seizures and epilepsy is not well known. Unfortunately, to date there have been no placebo-controlled clinical trials showing marijuana's anti- or proconvulsant effects. However, two studies, one case–control and the other based on a phone survey, have reported antiseizure affects of marijuana use. The case–control study, with 308 cases of new-onset seizures, suggested that marijuana use was protective for unprovoked seizures [16,17]. However, this effect was statistically significant only in men; the authors attributed this gender difference to the small number of women who were users [16]. The telephone survey study, from Canada, revealed that many patients with epilepsy believe marijuana helps them with their seizures [18]. Of the patients included in the study, 68% stated that marijuana improved their seizure severity, while 54% claimed their seizure frequency was decreased [18]. The predictors of marijuana use in this particular population were seizure frequency (more than once a month), longer duration of disease, and additional illicit drug use [18]. Challenges exist in designing and implementing blinded placebo-controlled trials to determine whether marijuana has an effect on seizures. Patients who would agree to enter a trial involving the use of marijuana might be inherently biased toward a particular result. Additionally, because of the recreational/euphoric effects of marijuana, blinding a trial is challenging, while legal issues pose practical problems. Nevertheless, epilepsy is one of the common indications cited for medical marijuana use and currently 20 US states and Washington, DC allow its use in this capacity.

The effect of marijuana on the central nervous system is not fully understood. It appears to be that the main psychoactive agent, Δ9-tetrahydocannabiol (THC), reduces GABA turnover at low doses and increases it at high doses [19]. Animal models of different epilepsy syndromes show that THC is effective in forms of partial and generalized seizures, whereas in genetic and absence epilepsies and in other models of partial epilepsy it is proconvulsant [20,21]. However, cannabinoid receptors (CB1) are found in different neuronal populations – both GABAergic and glutamergic – and activation of these receptors leads to a reduction of the release of neurotransmitters [22]. Therefore, since systemic application of THC or CB1 agonists may trigger neurotransmitter release from both inhibitory and excitatory neurons, this may not be a practical means of creating a selective protective effect [22]. As of now, although there is some evidence that marijuana can offer a protective effect against epileptic seizures, controversial data against this theory still exist.

Cocaine

Illicit drug use, especially with a CNS stimulant, may have a wide variety of adverse events on the central nervous system. Cocaine is one of the most commonly used illicit drugs on the street. It can be smoked, snorted, or injected.

Cocaine can provoke seizures in patients with no history of seizures and can lower the seizure threshold in patients with an existing seizure disorder. One retrospective study showed that the risk of cocaine-induced seizures is about 3% [23]. However, this study also included patients with preexisting seizure disorders, which made up about 20% of all patients with cocaine-induced seizures [23]. Cocaine-induced seizures are usually generalized tonic–clonic in semiology and are short in duration [24–26]. In one animal study comparing different stimulants, including cocaine and amphetamine derivatives, it was found that convulsive seizure duration was shortest for cocaine and longest for methamphetamine [24]. Although a single seizure is the most common seizure-related presentation after cocaine use, multiple episodes or status epilepticus (partial or generalized) may develop too [25,26]. Some cases of status epilepticus might be refractory to standard treatment options and require the use of a drug-induced coma [27]. Cocaine increases the risk for ischemic or hemorrhagic stroke, both of which can cause seizures and development of epilepsy [25,28].

Cocaine may cause temporary and permanent changes in the brain neurotransmitter system. The neuropsychological effects of cocaine are most likely related to its action on the dopaminergic system. Cocaine increases dopamine neurotransmission by inhibiting its uptake [25]. This effect is most likely responsible for cocaine's strong additive properties. The convulsive properties of cocaine are not very well understood.

Initial reports suggested that cocaine-induced seizures were mostly mediated by voltage-dependent Na channels; however, pharmacological studies show that sodium and calcium channel blockers are not very effective in blocking cocaine-induced seizures [29]. On the other hand, GABA-A receptor agonists and NMDA receptor antagonists do inhibit such seizures [29]. Cocaine has also shown to reduce inhibitory GABAergic currents in rat hippocampal neurons. This may contribute to its proconvulsant activity [30].

Heroin

Heroin is a powerful opioid and extremely addictive substance. Several papers have reported seizures that were most likely related to heroin use. In one of the first reports, Quattrini et al. [31] examined 33 drug users with multiple drug addictions, all including heroin. Seizures (either partial-onset or generalized) were found in five cases (15.1%), but since heroin was one of multiple drugs subjects, a clear determination of its role could not be made [31]. Aldredge et al. [27] reported five cases of heroin-associated seizures. However, they also commented that seizures might be triggered by heroin's convulsant effect, as well as by cerebral anoxia or other injected contaminants. On the other hand, heroin use was found to be significantly related to first seizures, either provoked or unprovoked [17]. Heroin use within 24 hours of hospitalization carried the highest risk [17]. Additionally, the same study made it clear that although seizures were reported after large doses of opioids, none of the study patients were admitted because of heroin overdose. The symptoms and sensations that heroin produces in abusers are most likely related to alteration in the endogenous opioid, beta endorphin [25]. However, how heroin triggers seizures is still not well understood.

Amphetamines, methamphetamine, and MDMA

The use of both methamphetamine and MDMA (ecstasy) has risen sharply over the last 2 decades [32,33]. Each of these drugs has been found to trigger seizures.

Amphetamines are typically taken in pill form. A recent study from Australia found that 4% of patients presenting with first seizures had amphetamine-associated seizures [34]. These included patients who had taken MDMA only, patients who had taken amphetamines only, and patients who had taken multiple amphetamines and/or amphetamine-related drugs. All patients experienced generalized tonic–clonic seizures, although some appeared to have been partial in onset. A significant number of patients (40%) with amphetamine-associated seizures had other epilepsy risk factors. At follow-up, 16% experienced seizure recurrence, which in most cases was associated with subsequent amphetamine use. A small number of patients (7%) with amphetamine-associated seizures developed epilepsy, and each of these has other epilepsy risk factors [34].

Methamphetamine (also known as "crystal meth" or "meth") is a synthetic stimulant made from pseudoephedrine that is highly addictive, with drug effects similar to those of cocaine. Methamphetamine use has been associated with numerous adverse health effects, including many consequences for neurological health. In addition to common ill effects such as confusion, motor slowing, memory loss, and impaired verbal learning, methamphetamine has been associated with significant risk for seizures [32].

MDMA (3,4-methylenedioxymethamphetamine, also known as "ecstasy" or "X") has both psychedelic and stimulant properties. It is typically taken by the oral or intranasal route. The 2004 National Survey on Drug Use and Health indicated that more than 11 million Americans have tried MDMA at least once. MDMA acts on several neurotransmitters in the brain, including serotonin, dopamine, and norepinephrine [35]. In addition to its effects on neurotransmitters, MDMA can also cause metabolic derangements, including hyperthermia and hyponatremia, which may trigger seizures [36].

Benzodiazepines and barbiturates

Although benzodiazepines and barbiturates are prescribed for the treatment of acute seizures and for epilepsy, both classes of medicine may be used as recreational drugs. Their recreational use revolves mostly around their sedating effect and both have potential for addiction. While their acute use is not typically associated with triggering seizures, it has been well established that seizures, including status epilepticus, may be caused by withdrawal from benzodiazepines or barbiturates [37].

Drug use in persons with preexisting epilepsy

The overall incidence of recreational drug use in persons with epilepsy is not well known. In clinical practice, active drug and alcohol use is not typically information that is readily disclosed by patients, unless specifically asked. Due to the complex nature of the interaction between seizures, drugs, and alcohol, it is important that clinicians be informed about drug and alcohol use in patients that have experienced seizures. A detailed social history, in the context of a trusting doctor–patient relationship, is essential.

Conclusion

Epileptic seizures can be triggered by the use of a variety of legal and illicit substances. Alcohol abuse is one of the leading causes of health problems in westernized countries. The prevalence of seizures is significantly higher in alcohol abusers than in the general population. Withdrawal from alcohol and acute intoxication or chronic heavy use can lead to seizures. Chronic use of alcohol leads to upregulation of NMDA receptors and downregulation of GABA-A receptors. This chronic excitatory state, as well cerebral atrophy, the high incidence of traumatic brain injuries, and the possibility of kindling caused by repeated withdrawals, are blamed for epileptogenesis in alcohol abuse.

Practical advice and pearls

- The majority of alcohol-related seizures are related to withdrawal. However, acute intoxication or chronic exposure to heavy use can also trigger them.
- Alcohol abuse is considered one of the major causes of status epilepticus.
- Withdrawal seizures typically occur 6–48 hours following cessation or relative reduction of use.

- Marijuana is the most commonly used illicit substance. Although there is some evidence that marijuana can show some protection against seizures, the exact effect is still not well known.
- Cocaine use is also associated with increased risk of seizures but the exact mechanism is not well understood. The associated risk of stroke – both ischemic and hemorrhagic – could play a role.
- How heroin produces convulsive effects is still unknown. Published case series fail to reveal whether seizures are triggered directly by heroin's convulsive effect or indirectly by cerebral anoxia or by other injected contaminants.
- Use of amphetamines and amphetamine derivatives is also associated with increased risk of seizures. These drugs pose a significant threat to general and neurological health.
- Benzodiazepines are generally used for prevention of withdrawal seizures. However, prophylactic use of antiepileptic medications is usually not necessary unless the patient has seizures unrelated to alcohol intake.

References

1 Ezzati M, Lopez AD, Rodgers A et al.: Selected major risk factors and global and regional burden of disease. *Lancet* 2002; **360**:1347–1360.
2 Mattoo SK, Singh SM, Bhardwaj R et al.: Prevalence and correlates of epileptic seizures in substance-abusing subjects. *Psych Clin Neurosci* 2009; **63**:580–582.
3 Tardy B, Lafond P, Convers P et al.: Adult first generalized seizure: etiology, biological tests, EEG, CT scan, in an ED. *Am J Emerg Med* 1995; **13**:1–5.
4 Hauser WA, Ng SK, Brust JC: Alcohol, seizures and epilepsy. *Epilepsia* 1988; **29(Suppl. 2)**:S66–S78.
5 Chan AW: Alcoholism and epilepsy. *Epilepsia* 1985; **26**: 323–333.
6 Hillbom M, Pieninkeroinen I, Leone M: Seizures in alcohol-dependent patients. *CNS Drugs* 2003; **17**:1013–1030.
7 Alldredge BK, Lowenstein DH: Status epilepticus related to alcohol abuse. *Epilepsia* 1993; **34**:1033–1037.
8 Rathlev NK, Ulrich AS, Delanty N, D'Onofrio G: Alcohol-related seizures. *J Emerg Med* 2006; **31**:157–163.
9 Ng SK, Hauser A, Brust JCM, Susser M: Alcohol consumption and withdrawal in new onset seizures. *N Engl J Med* 1988; **319**:666–673.
10 McKeon A, Frye MA, Delanty N: The alcohol withdrawal syndrome. *J Neurol Neurosurg Psychiatry* 2008; **79**:854–862.
11 Hughes JR: Alcohol withdrawal seizures. *Epilepsy Behav* 2009; **15**:92–97.

12 Samokhvalov AV, Irving H, Mohapatra S, Rehm J: Alcohol consumption, unprovoked seizures, and epilepsy: a systematic review and meta-analysis. *Epilepsia* 2010; **51**: 1177–1184.

13 Sand T, Brathen G, Michler R et al.: Clinical utility of EEG in alcohol-related seizures. *Acta Neurol Scand* 2002; **105**:18–24.

14 Bråthen G, Ben-Menachem E, Brodtkorb E et al.: EFNS guideline on the diagnosis and management of alcohol-related seizures: report of an EFNS task force. *Eur J Neurol* 2005; **12**:575–581.

15 Kobau R, Zahran H, Thurman D et al.: Epilepsy Surveillance among Adults – 19 States, Behavioral Risk Factor Surveillance System, 2005. Available from: http://www.cdc.gov/mmwr/pdf/ss/ss5706.pdf (last accessed July 15, 2014).

16 Brust JC, Ng SK, Hauser AW, Susser M: Marijuana use and the risk of new onset seizures. *Trans Am Clin Climatol Assoc* 1992; **103**:176–181.

17 Ng SK, Brust JC, Hauser WA, Susser M: Illicit drug use and the risk of new-onset seizures. *Am J Epidemiol* 1990; **132**: 47–57.

18 Gross DW, Hamm J, Ashworth NL, Quigley D: Marijuana use and epilepsy: prevalence in patients of a tertiary care epilepsy center. *Neurology* 2004; **62**:2095–2097.

19 Zagnoni PG, Albano C: Psychostimulants and epilepsy. *Epilepsia* 2002; **43(Suppl. 2)**:28–31.

20 Gordon E, Devinsky O: Alcohol and marijuana: effects on epilepsy and use by patients with epilepsy. *Epilepsia* 2001; **42**:1266–1272.

21 Wallace MJ, Blair RE, Felenski KW et al.: The endogenous cannabinoid system regulates seizure frequency and duration in a model of temporal epilepsy. *J Pharmacol Exp Ther* 2003; **307**:129–137.

22 Lutz B: On-demand activation of the endocannabinoid system in the control of neuronal excitability and epileptiform seizures. *Biochem Pharmacol* 2004; **68**:1691–1698.

23 Koppel BS, Samkoff L, Daras M: Relation of cocaine use to seizures and epilepsy. *Epilepsia* 1996; **37**:875–878.

24 Hanson GR, Jensen M, Johnson M, White HS: Distinct features of seizures induced by cocaine and amphetamine analogs. *Eur J Pharmacol* 1999; **377**:167–173.

25 Neiman J, Haapaniemi HM, Hillbom M: Neurological complications of drug abuse: pathophysiological mechanisms. *Eur J Neurol* 2000; **7**:595–606.

26 Pascual-Leone A, Dhuna A, Altafullah I, Anderson DC: Cocaine-induced seizures. *Neurology* 1990; **40**:404–407.

27 Allredge BK, Lowenstein DH, Simon RP: Seizures associated with recreational drug abuse. *Neurology* 1989; **39**: 1037–1039.

28 Nnadi CU, Mimiko OA, McCurtis HL, Cadet JL: Neuropsychiatric effects of cocaine use disorders. *J Natl Med Assoc* 2005; **97**:1504–1515.

29 Lason W: Neurochemical and pharmacological aspects of cocaine-induced seizures. *Pol J Pharmacol* 2001; **53**:57–60.

30 Ye JH, Ren J: Cocaine inhibition of GABA(A) current: role of dephosphorylation. *Crit Rev Neurobiol* 2006; **18**:85–94.

31 Quattrini A, Paggi A, Silvestri R et al.: Neurological complications in drug dependence with special reference to the development of epileptic syndromes. *Rev Patol Nerv Ment* 1982; **103**:262–270.

32 Winslow BT, Voorhes KI, Pehl KA: Methamphetamine abuse. *Am Fam Physician* 2007; **76**:1169–1174.

33 Maxwell JC, Rutkowski BA: The prevalence of methamphetamine and amphetamine abuse in North America: a review of indicators, 1992–2007. *Drug Alcohol Rev* 2008; **27**:229–235.

34 Brown JW, Dunne JW, Fatovic DM et al.: Amphetamine-associated seizures: clinical features and prognosis. *Epilepsia* 2011; **52(2)**:401–404.

35 Liechti ME, Vollenweider FX: Which neuroreceptors mediate the subjective effects of MDMA in humans? A summary of mechanistic studies. *Hum Psychopharmacol* 2001; **16**:589–598.

36 Holmes SB, Banerjee AK, Alexander WD: Hyponatraemia and seizures after ecstasy use. *Postgrad Med J* 1999; **75**: 32–34.

37 Devlin RJ, Henry JA: Major consequences of illicit drug consumption. *Crit Care* 2008; **12**:202.

CHAPTER 24

Driving, employment, and related issues in epilepsy

Kristine Ziemba and Joe Drazkowski

Department of Neurology, Mayo Clinic, USA

Introduction

People with epilepsy can face significant challenges with respect to functioning effectively in society. Quality of life (QOL) may be diminished by myriad social factors affected by the diagnosis, including interpersonal relationships, education, employment, and driving. Surveys have indicated that driving restriction is the number one QOL concern for people with epilepsy [1]. This chapter will focus primarily on driving restrictions and their impact on people with epilepsy but will also touch on other social consequences of epilepsy, including unemployment, underemployment, and limits on recreational activities.

Driving

The ability to drive a motor vehicle is paramount to social functioning and employment in many developed countries, especially where public transportation is limited. Collisions, sometimes with injuries and fatalities, are an unfortunate consequence of our dependence on motor vehicles. In the United States, 37 261 people were killed in motor vehicle crashes (MVCs) in 2008. This was a decline of nearly 10% from 2007, with total vehicle miles traveled declining only about 2% during the same time frame (2974 billion miles in 2008) [2]. There is a continuing downward trend in MVC fatalities in the United States since peaks reached in the early 1970s, attributed to significant vehicle and occupant safety regulations and programs enacted by the National

Highway Traffic Safety Administration (NHTSA) and governing bodies across the country [2].

Driving is a skilled activity that requires intact neurologic systems, including vision, motor control, coordination, maintenance of attention, and higher cognitive functioning. "Higher cognitive functioning" includes the ability to perceive and attend to external stimuli (potential hazards on the road), formulate and execute a plan of action (applying a brake, steering, accelerating to avoid danger), and monitor outcomes to determine the necessity for further action [3]. Most drivers are capable of carrying out these complex mental programs reflexively and quickly, but many medical, neurologic, and psychiatric disorders can impair these processes. Epilepsy is one paroxysmal disorder with the potential to decrease attention and awareness but other conditions also fall into this category, such as cardiac arrhythmias or dysautonomia leading to syncope, acute hypoglycemia, and excessive somnolence due to sleep disorders [3].

Restrictions

In order to protect the road-using public, driving limitations have been placed upon people with epilepsy ever since the automobile was introduced 100 years ago [4]. The nature and extent of current driving restrictions vary widely among different states and countries [5]. Health care professionals and epilepsy advocacy groups have published specific recommendations regarding driving laws applicable to people with epilepsy. Most are in agreement that some form of restriction is reasonable when seizures are poorly controlled [6]. Key

---

Epilepsy and the Interictal State: Co-Morbidities and Quality of Life, First Edition.
Edited by Erik K. St. Louis, David M. Ficker, and Terence J. O'Brien.
© 2015 John Wiley & Sons, Ltd. Published 2015 by John Wiley & Sons, Ltd.

recommendations were outlined after a 1991 meeting of representatives from the American Epilepsy Society (AES), American Academy of Neurology (AAN), and Epilepsy Foundation of America (EFA), including a 3-month seizure-free interval to restore driving rights and exemptions for those with purely nocturnal seizures, isolated events due to change in medication or acute illness, simple partial seizures that do not affect driving, or a consistent and prolonged aura. These representatives also recommended against required physician reporting of people with epilepsy to driving authorities and suggested treating physicians should be granted legal immunity regarding their decision to report or not report, assuming reporting decisions were made in good faith. Such immunity is considered necessary to protect the doctor–patient relationship and ensure honesty on the part of the patient when reporting seizure recurrence [6]. The American Medical Association (AMA) has joined the AES and AAN in voicing opposition to mandatory reporting of patients' medical conditions to the government [7]. Despite these recommendations, six states in the United States *do* require physicians to report persons with a neurologic disability (including epilepsy) that may impair driving: California, Delaware, Nevada, New Jersey, Oregon, and Pennsylvania [8].

The seizure-free interval (SFI) required to restore driving rights also varies from state to state, ranging from 3 to 12 months. The optimal SFI required to ensure public safety is still a matter of debate. Current state laws regarding SFI and other pertinent legal details for drivers with epilepsy may be found on the EFA's website, www.epilepsyfoundation.org (last accessed July 15, 2014) [9]. While some governing bodies equate longer SFIs (e.g., 1 year) to a lower incidence of seizure-related collisions, data do not support this stance. Collision and associated fatality rates were found to remain statistically stable following reduction of the legal SFI in Arizona from 12 to 3 months [10]. There was no statistically significant increase in injuries resulting from seizure-related crashes, although a trend toward increased injuries was seen. Another study similarly found that the fatality rate of seizure-related crashes was not affected by SFI length [11]. One retrospective case–control study suggested an association between higher collision rates and shorter SFIs (≤12 months), but this conclusion was limited by retrospective design and selection bias [12].

Risk

Driving restrictions for people with epilepsy are a fact of life but the actual risk posed by a driver with epilepsy on the road is uncertain. Data regarding drivers' specific medical conditions are not often collected or analyzed. The latest statistics compiled by the NHTSA (2009) reveal that 2.7% of fatal crashes were associated with drivers who were "drowsy, asleep, fatigued, ill, or blacked out" [2]. This category likely includes drivers who experienced a seizure, among other paroxysmal and sleep disorders. For comparison, drivers "under the influence of alcohol, drugs or medication" accounted for 15.4% and inattentive drivers (talking, eating, etc.) 9.3% of fatal crashes [2]. A population-based study in the United States between 1995 and 1997 found that an average of 0.2% of fatal crashes were seizure-related (86 out of 44 027 per year) [11], representing only 4.2% of fatal crashes due to medical conditions (86 out of 2030 per year). In contrast, cardiac and hypertensive disease caused an average of 1800 fatal crashes per year (4.1% of total fatal crashes or 89% of those related to a medical condition). However, when the prevalence of these conditions is considered, epilepsy does carry a higher risk of crashes, with a disease-specific fatal crash rate of 8.6 per 100 000 people with epilepsy, versus only 3.74 fatal crashes per 100 000 people with cardiac or hypertensive disease; people with epilepsy thus have an attributable hazard ratio of 2.3 compared to these other medical conditions [11]. A more recent population-based Canadian study comparing people with epilepsy to age-matched controls that adjusted for comorbid conditions such as cardiac arrhythmias and alcohol or drug abuse found that people with epilepsy did not crash more frequently than people with other chronic medical conditions [13].

The risk of an individual driver with epilepsy being involved in a crash depends partly on that person's risk of seizure recurrence. The risk of recurrence, in turn, depends on seizure etiology, medication compliance, stress, fatigue, and general health status. Medically refractory epilepsy patients with frequent seizures are likely to be at high risk but prediction of risk of seizure occurrence in a person with a single or controlled seizures is less clear. A large, multinational, randomized trial (the MRC Multicentre trial for Early Epilepsy and Single Seizures or MESS trial) [14,15] has quantified the risk for newly diagnosed seizure patients, which is especially important for drivers in the United Kingdom and other European Union states where licensing agencies use a risk-based approach to reinstating driving rights after a seizure. In the MESS trial, a prognostic model was developed that placed patients into low-, medium-, or high-risk categories. Factors determined to significantly impact risk of recurrence included the presence of a neurological disorder, an abnormal EEG, and a high number of seizures at presentation [14]. Patients falling into the low-risk category did not benefit from immediate initiation of antiepileptic drug (AED) treatment. Multivariate analysis of individual risk for seizure recurrence over 1 year following 6, 12, 18, or 24 month SFIs demonstrated that several factors impacted individual risk in an additive manner, including a remote symptomatic etiology, abnormal EEG, abnormal neuroimaging with CT or MRI, increasing duration of seizure freedom, and immediate or delayed AED therapy [15]. External validation will be necessary to confirm whether this prognostic model can guide development of driving policies based on individual risk. In the United Kingdom, risk for seizure recurrence must be less than 20% before a person can regain a noncommercial driver's license.

While seizures behind the wheel have been presumed to account for most driving mishaps for people with epilepsy, research indicates that interictal disturbances in cognition and vigilance may also play a significant role. A large cohort study conducted in the state of Wisconsin between 1985 and 1988 showed that drivers with epilepsy were more likely than healthy controls to receive moving violations due to "careless driving" (standardized mishap ratio (SMR) 1.57, 95% CI 1.05–2.25) and due to the influence of alcohol or drugs (SMR 2.75, 95% CI 1.50–4.62) [16]. Although not examined specifically in that study, contributors to "careless driving" were hypothesized to include lapses in concentration, consciousness, or bodily control that could be attributed to interictal abnormalities associated with epilepsy or side effects of antiepileptic medications. Why people with epilepsy had a disproportionate number of violations attributed to alcohol and drugs remains unclear and merits further study.

Awareness of driving regulation and requirements

Driving laws specific to people with epilepsy have been established in virtually every state and country despite significant persisting uncertainties about the

degree of risk posed by drivers with epilepsy and an optimal SFI that appropriately balances public safety with individual freedom. Problems arise when people with epilepsy are unaware of the restrictions dictated by their governing bodies. Since physicians are ultimately responsible for educating people with epilepsy about driving restrictions – whether in a "reporting" or a "nonreporting" state – a lack of knowledge on the part of people with epilepsy likely reflects lack of appropriate doctor–patient communication or, worse yet, lack of knowledge or awareness of issues and laws pertaining to driving and epilepsy by treating physicians. Unfortunately, this vacuum of communication and knowledge seems to be a widespread problem. Initial diagnosis of seizures is often made in an acute-care setting such as a hospital emergency department and this is where patient education should begin. A retrospective chart review of patients discharged from one Arizona hospital's emergency department after episodes of altered consciousness (seizures and other causes) revealed that only about 10% had been counseled about state driving restrictions [17]. State law in Arizona dictates that a person who experiences a seizure or other alteration in consciousness must promptly report this event to the motor vehicle division and relinquish driving privileges for 3 months. Patients were more likely to have been counseled about this law if they had been seen by a neurologist (34.5%) than if seen solely by the emergency-department physician (7.1%) and if their primary diagnosis was a seizure (30.4%) rather than altered level of consciousness (4.3%) or syncope (2.9%) [17].

The knowledge gap regarding driving laws for people with epilepsy may persist until referral to centers specializing in epilepsy care. One survey of patients newly referred to an epilepsy care center demonstrated a correct response rate of only 13.6% to questions on the legalities of driving with epilepsy [18]. A more recent survey of people with new-onset epilepsy presenting to epilepsy referral centers indicated that 50% or less had been counseled about driving laws at the time of seizure diagnosis, with fewer people having been counseled in New Jersey (37%, a mandatory reporting state) than in Arizona (52%, a voluntary reporting state) [19]. A similar lack of patient education was highlighted in a recent survey-based study of people with epilepsy attending a specialist-led epilepsy clinic in Ireland, with lowest scores on questions related to safety and legal issues, such as "How long do you have to be seizure-free to drive?" (34.6% correct, with answer being 12 months) [20].

For physicians providing epilepsy care, education concerning local driving laws and other related safety issues is necessary for each patient's best interests and is a metric of quality health care. The AAN deemed this an important enough issue to include driving and safety education as one of the eight final quality improvement measures approved by the AMA-convened Physician Consortium for Performance Improvement (PCPI) in 2010 [21]. These quality measures are to be integrated into practice modules for maintenance of certification requirements for neurologists and may be used in pay-for-performance programs in the near future.

Employment

A recent systematic review of disparities in epilepsy was published by the North American Commission of the International League Against Epilepsy (ILAE). This review of literature, spanning the years 1965–2007, confirmed disparities for people with epilepsy in education and employment, among other areas of concern [22]. One population-based study in the states of Georgia and Tennessee reported that people with epilepsy had lower educational attainment, higher unemployment rate, and lower household incomes when compared to similar adults without epilepsy [23]. A later study based on the 2002 National Health Interview Survey (NHIS) of over 30 000 adults across the United States also reflected lower levels of education and higher levels of unemployment among people with epilepsy [24]. Likewise, a Canadian study indicated that people with epilepsy had lower incomes than adults with other chronic illnesses and a multinational study across seven European countries revealed higher unemployment rates in people with epilepsy despite slightly *higher* levels of education [25,26]. Driving restrictions on people with epilepsy can dramatically limit their ability to obtain and maintain employment. In addition to transportation issues, several other potential barriers toward finding and keeping employment exist, including a lack of specific education and/or training, real or perceived stigma, and discrimination in the workplace.

Stigma associated with epilepsy is addressed in Chapter 3 but it is worth considering here given the direct impact of stigma on employment. People with epilepsy have a long history of marginalization and stigmatization across cultures and centuries and, unfortunately, continue to be stigmatized in modern developed societies. Stigma has been postulated to occur in two forms: "enacted" and "felt" stigma, the former referring to episodes of true public discrimination against people with epilepsy based on ignorance and negative attitudes and the latter to an internalized shame of having epilepsy and a *fear* of discrimination [27,28]. Whether felt or enacted stigma directly impacts low employment rates and incomes for people with epilepsy is uncertain, yet studies have shown that employers continue to hold discriminatory attitudes toward and negative perceptions of people with epilepsy. A recent survey of manufacturing, retail, and public service companies in the United Kingdom found that 21% of employers described hiring someone with epilepsy as a "major issue" and 44% felt epilepsy would cause them a "high level of concern" [29]. Epilepsy support groups around the world are actively campaigning on multiple fronts to reduce negative attitudes and move toward equality in the treatment of people with epilepsy in the workforce [30].

Laws protecting people with epilepsy

The Americans with Disabilities Act (ADA) was enacted in 1990 with the intent of ensuring equality in hiring, firing, and promotion decisions for people with disabilities. Such decisions were to be made based solely on an individual's ability to do a job, without reference to their impairment(s). The ADA broadly defined a *disability* as "A) a physical or mental impairment that substantially limits one or more major life activities … B) a record of such an impairment; or C) being regarded as having such an impairment" [31]. In the ensuing years, lawsuits have challenged the ADA and certain key court decisions have served to limit the scope and, arguably, negate the intent of the law [32]. One such decision was made by the Supreme Court in 1999, in the case of *Sutton v. United Airlines*. The court ruled that people whose impairments are successfully treated or controlled with medication or other "mitigating measures" are *not* protected by the ADA [33]. An additional Supreme Court case in 2002 ruled that the ADA only covers a disability that prevents a person from carrying out tasks "central to most people's daily lives" [34]. These limited interpretations of the ADA essentially stripped legal protections from people with epilepsy, whose condition may be well controlled on medications, such that they are quite "able" interictally – but when an employer becomes aware of their "hidden" diagnosis, may be the subject of discrimination.

Backlash against the Supreme Court's stepwise stripping of protections from the ADA led to reclarification of the law's intent with the ADA Amendments Act, which became effective January 1, 2009. In general, the amendments directed courts to interpret the ADA broadly, "To restore the intent and protections of the Americans with Disabilities Act of 1990" [35]. Specifically, the amendments clarified the meaning of "major life activities" to include manual tasks, standing, concentrating, and similar normal physiologic functions. Additionally, the amendments forbade consideration of "the ameliorative effects of mitigating measures" such as antiepileptic medications when considering whether a person has a disability and dictated that the episodic nature (or "remission") of epilepsy could not be used as an argument against its disabling nature, since a person is substantially "limited in life activities" during a seizure. And finally, the concept of being "regarded as" having a disability was spelled out, validating a person's claim that they had suffered discrimination based on a disability *whether or not* the person was actually impaired at the time of the act of discrimination [36]. These amendments serve to refocus the ADA toward the original intent of eliminating discrimination against employees based on irrational fears and misconceptions about conditions such as epilepsy (Table 24.1).

Part of a physician's role when caring for a person with epilepsy is to educate that person about the social implications of their diagnosis, including driving laws. In addition, people with epilepsy may not be familiar with legal protections pertaining to their diagnosis, such as the ADA. People with epilepsy may look to their physician for guidance regarding employment and whether and how to discuss issues pertaining to their diagnosis openly with their employers. People with epilepsy should be assured that they are not required to disclose their diagnosis of epilepsy to a prospective employer at the time of an interview, regardless of the type of work. For some jobs, however, the employer is within rights, once a conditional job offer has been made, to ask about medical conditions that could potentially impair a person's ability to carry out essential job functions safely (Table 24.2) [37].

Box 24.1 Examples of reasonable accommodations for people with epilepsy.

- Breaks to take medication.
- Leave to seek treatment or adjust to medication changes.
- A private area to rest after experiencing a seizure.
- Adjustments to work schedules to allow for adequate sleep or alternative transportation.
- Carpool assistance to get to work-related events.
- Ability to work at home.
  An employer may refuse to provide an accommodation if it would be an *undue hardship* to the company.

The person with epilepsy is also within their rights to request "reasonable accommodations" in order to be able to function on the job. Accommodations that do not cause undue hardship (financial or logistic) to the company should be made by the employer, according to the ADA (Box 24.1) [37]. People with well-controlled epilepsy working in jobs that would not be dangerous in the event of a seizure may choose not to disclose their diagnosis to their employers. People with epilepsy should be counseled that the decision to disclose their diagnosis to an employer is a personal one and involves consideration of the likelihood of a seizure, seizure type, and the potential impact of a seizure on the job, should one occur. People with epilepsy should feel comfortable in alerting employers and coworkers about potential seizures at their discretion, without fear of repercussions. Unfortunately, health care providers, families, and people with epilepsy may be challenged by these complex legal issues, especially as each individual may possess unique features or situations that are not specifically elucidated in the statute. Independent resources, including advocacy groups such as the AES, may be able to assist the person with epilepsy when questions arise, and occasionally direct and individual legal counsel may be needed.

Specific job restrictions

There are some jobs that are essentially off limits to people with epilepsy, such as commercial interstate driving and piloting airplanes. The US Department of Transportation (DOT) regulates interstate commerce and prohibits persons with epilepsy from driving in this capacity. Among many other medical disqualifications,

Table 24.1 When is epilepsy considered a disability according to the Americans with Disabilities Act (ADA)?

Definition of disability	Examples for people with epilepsy
The condition (or medications to control it) *substantially limits* one or more *major life activities*	Seizures or medication side effects may impair a person's ability to speak, perform manual tasks, think, concentrate, learn, or interact with others effectively
The condition *was* substantially limiting at some time in the past	Seizures may have been disabling in the past, even though they are now controlled with medications
Employers *regard* the person as having a disability	An employer may refuse to hire a person with epilepsy due to an *assumption* that their diagnosis limits them in some way

Table 24.2 Americans with Disabilities Act (ADA) Q&A for people with epilepsy. Adapted from http://www.eeoc.gov/laws/types/epilepsy.cfm (last accessed July 15, 2014).

The application process	
May an employer ask questions about medical conditions (such as epilepsy) or require a medical exam *prior to* making a conditional job offer?	No
Must a job applicant disclose their diagnosis of epilepsy *before accepting* a job offer?	No
If an applicant volunteers that they have epilepsy, may the employer ask follow-up questions?	*Only* regarding need for accommodations
May an employer ask questions about medical conditions (such as epilepsy) or require a medical exam *after* making a conditional job offer?	*Only as necessary* to determine the ability to perform job functions safely [a]

On the job	
When may an employer ask an employee if epilepsy might be affecting their ability to do a job, or to do it safely?	Only when the employer has a legitimate reason to suspect this
May an employer ask for "return to work" medical release documentation after a leave due to epilepsy?	Only if there is a legitimate concern regarding their ability to return to work safely
May an employer disclose an employee's condition (epilepsy) to their coworkers in order to explain accommodations made or to explain seizure events?	No. This is at the discretion of the employee themselves

[a]With or without reasonable accommodation.

Section 391.41(b)(8) of the Code of Federal Regulations (Title 49, Part 391) states that the following individuals are prohibited from operating a commercial motor vehicle: "(1) a driver who has a medical history of epilepsy; (2) a driver who has a current clinical diagnosis of epilepsy; or (3) a driver who is taking antiseizure medication" [38]. This sweeping regulation disqualifies a wide range of people with epilepsy, regardless of their seizure type and level of control with medications, and even disqualifies individuals who may be taking an AED for a different indication, such as neuropathic pain. The regulation has been unsuccessfully challenged by many people over the years. The only exceptions considered are for drivers with a history of remitted epilepsy who have been seizure-free *and* off AEDs for 10 years (or 5 years for a single unprovoked seizure) [38].

The Federal Aviation Administration (FAA) is responsible for regulating licensure of pilots. People with a diagnosis of epilepsy or history of seizures are essentially disqualified from obtaining any type of pilot's license. According to Title 14, Part 67 of the Code of Federal Regulations, a person with a disqualifying condition such as epilepsy may obtain a medical certificate from an FAA-approved physician in order to be considered for a pilot's license. As in the case of truckers, individuals are usually only granted exemptions if they have been seizure-free *without* AEDs for at least 10 years [39].

Besides pilot and commercial driver, other jobs with safety concerns for people with epilepsy include air traffic controller, railroad conductor, law enforcement officer, firefighter, border patrol agent, FBI agent, and US mail carrier. These occupations may allow participation by people with epilepsy if the proper documentation of seizure control is provided by a qualified physician, often with recommended limitations on the scope of duties and activities. One employer that is not subject to antidiscrimination laws such as the ADA is the US military. The reasoning behind this exemption is that military personnel should be ready for deployment anywhere at any time, regardless of the availability of medical care at the destination. A person will not be considered for enlistment with a history of seizures or epilepsy unless they have been seizure-free and off AEDs for at least 5 years prior to their application. After enlistment, if a person develops epilepsy, they will likely be given a "disability separation" from the military, although this decision is made on a case-by-case basis [40].

Recreation and socialization

Like employment, recreational and social activities may be limited for people with epilepsy. A primary roadblock is driving restriction, which can impact personal life as much as or more than professional life. In recreational settings, people with epilepsy must also consider the likelihood of a seizure event in any given circumstance and what the outcome would be if a seizure were to occur. Safety issues are of primary concern with activities that involve speed, heights, weapons, water, or heavy machinery, and many other potential hazards. People with epilepsy may also experience real or perceived stigma from peers in their social and recreational pursuits. In the 2002 NHIS, people with self-reported seizures were more likely to be single or divorced, report insufficient leisure-time activity, and have increased levels of psychosocial stress, although this survey did not distinguish between epileptic and nonepileptic "seizures" and therefore was not specific to people with an established diagnosis of epilepsy [24].

The person with epilepsy, their family, other participants, and health care providers should individualize the decision to participate in a particular recreational activity whenever possible. Factors that might be taken into account when making such decisions include: 1) seizure frequency, 2) seizure type, 3) degree of seizure control, 4) the potential dangers posed by the activity, and 5) the actual time spent at risk during the activity. Considering these variables when discussing the possibility of participating in a particular recreational activity often provides a framework for making an appropriate decision.

Conclusion

People with epilepsy are faced with many challenges in their lives beyond the physical impact of their seizures. Driving limitations and other safety concerns may negatively impact their ability to secure and maintain employment and to engage actively in social and recreational activities. Misconceptions about epilepsy's direct and indirect impact continue to challenge QOL for people with epilepsy. There is a danger of people with epilepsy being limited by employers, family, caregivers, and even health care providers to a greater degree than is necessary or lawful. Educating people with epilepsy and others about protective laws and actions that maximize outcomes and ultimate QOL is a crucial mandate for epilepsy care providers, as well as for international epilepsy support and advocacy groups.

References

1 Gilliam F, Kuzniecky R, Faught E et al.: Patient-validated content of epilepsy-specific quality-of-life measurement. *Epilepsia* 1997; **38(2)**:233–236.

2 Longthorne A, Subramanian R, Chen C-L: An analysis of the significant decline in motor vehicle traffic fatalities in 2008. NHTSA Technical Report. US Department of Transportation, National Highway Traffic Safety Administration, Washington, DC, 2010.

3 Drazkowski JF, Sirven JI: Driving and neurologic disorders. *Neurology* 2011; **76(7 Suppl. 2)**: S44–S49.

4 Krumholz A: Driving and epilepsy: a historical perspective and review of current regulations. *Epilepsia* 1994; **35(3)**:668–674.

5 Krauss GL, Ampaw L, Krumholz A: Individual state driving restrictions for people with epilepsy in the US. *Neurology* 2001; **57(10)**:1780–1785.

6 Anon: Consensus statements, sample statutory provisions, and model regulations regarding driver licensing and epilepsy. American Academy of Neurology, American Epilepsy Society, and Epilepsy Foundation of America. *Epilepsia* 1994; **35(3)**:696–705.

7 Bacon D, Fischer RS, Morris JC et al.: American Academy of Neurology position statement on physician reporting of medical conditions that may affect driving competence. *Neurology* 2007; **68(15)**:1174–1177.

8 Epilepsy Foundation: Driving & epilepsy: physician issues. Available from: http://old.epilepsyfoundation.org/about /professionals/medical/drivingphys.cfm?renderforprint=1& (last accessed July 15, 2014).

9 Epilepsy Foundation: Driving laws by state. Available from: https://shop.epilepsyfoundation.org/resources/Driving-Laws-by-State.cfm (last accessed July 15, 2014).

10 Drazkowski JF, Fisher RS, Sirven JI et al.: Seizure-related motor vehicle crashes in Arizona before and after reducing the driving restriction from 12 to 3 months. *Mayo Clin Proc* 2003; **78(7)**:819–825.

11 Sheth SG, Krauss G, Krumholz A, Li G: Mortality in epilepsy: driving fatalities vs other causes of death in patients with epilepsy. *Neurology* 2004; **63(6)**:1002–1007.

12 Krauss GL, Krumholz A, Carter RC et al.: Risk factors for seizure-related motor vehicle crashes in patients with epilepsy. *Neurology* 1999; **52(7)**:1324–1329.

13 Kwon C, Liu M, Quan H et al.: Motor vehicle accidents, suicides, and assaults in epilepsy: A population-based study. *Neurology* 2011; **76(9)**:801–806.

14 Kim LG, Johnson TL, Marson AG et al.: Prediction of risk of seizure recurrence after a single seizure and early epilepsy: further results from the MESS trial. *Lancet Neurol* 2006; **5(4)**:317–322.

15 Bonnett LJ, Tudur-Smith C, Williamson PR, Marson AG: Risk of recurrence after a first seizure and implications for driving: further analysis of the Multicentre study of early Epilepsy and Single Seizures. *BMJ* 2010; **341**:c6477.

16 Hansotia P, Broste SK: The effect of epilepsy or diabetes mellitus on the risk of automobile accidents. *N Engl J Med* 1991; **324(1)**:22–26.

17 Shareef YS, McKinnon JH, Gauthier SM et al.: Counseling for driving restrictions in epilepsy and other causes of

temporary impairment of consciousness: how are we doing? *Epilepsy Behav* 2009; **14(3)**:550–552.

18 Long L, Reeves AL, Moore JL et al.: An assessment of epilepsy patients' knowledge of their disorder. *Epilepsia* 2000; **41(6)**:727–731.

19 Drazkowski JF, Neiman ES, Sirven JI et al.: Frequency of physician counseling and attitudes toward driving motor vehicles in people with epilepsy: comparing a mandatory-reporting with a voluntary-reporting state. *Epilepsy Behav* 2010; **19(1)**:52–54.

20 Coker MF, Bhargava S, Fitzgerald M, Doherty CP: What do people with epilepsy know about their condition? Evaluation of a subspecialty clinic population. *Seizure* 2011; **20(1)**:55–59.

21 Fountain NB, Van Ness PC, Swain-Eng R et al.: Quality improvement in neurology: AAN epilepsy quality measures. *Neurology* 2011; **76(1)**:94–99.

22 Burneo JG, Jette N, Theodore W et al.: Disparities in epilepsy: report of a systematic review by the North American Commission of the International League Against Epilepsy. *Epilepsia* 2009; **50(10)**:2285–2295.

23 Kobau R, Dilorio CA, Price PH et al.: Prevalence of epilepsy and health status of adults with epilepsy in Georgia and Tennessee: Behavioral Risk Factor Surveillance System, 2002. *Epilepsy Behav* 2004; **5(3)**:358–366.

24 Strine TW, Kobau R, Chapman DP et al.: Psychological distress, comorbidities, and health behaviors among US adults with seizures: results from the 2002 National Health Interview Survey. *Epilepsia* 2005; **46(7)**:1133–1139.

25 Wiebe S, Bellhouse DR, Fallahay C, Eliasziw M: Burden of epilepsy: the Ontario Health Survey. *Can J Neurol Sci* 1999; **26**:263–270.

26 Anon: Social aspects of epilepsy in the adult in seven European countries. The RESt-1 Group. *Epilepsia* 2000; **41(8)**:998–1004.

27 Scambler G, Hopkins A: Being epileptic: coming to terms with stigma. *Soc Health Illness* 1986; **8(1)**:26–43.

28 Jacoby A: Felt versus enacted stigma: a concept revisited: evidence from a study of people with epilepsy in remission. *Soc Sci Med* 1994; **38(2)**:269–274.

29 Jacoby A, Gorry J, Baker GA: Employers' attitudes to employment of people with epilepsy: still the same old story? *Epilepsia* 2005;**46(12)**:1978–1987.

30 Fernandes PT, Snape DA, Beran RG, Jacoby A: Epilepsy stigma: what do we know and where next? *Epilepsy Behav* 2011; **22(1)**:55–62.

31 The Americans with Disabilities Act of 1990. Available from: http://www.eeoc.gov/eeoc/history/35th/thelaw/ada.html (last accessed July 15, 2014).

32 Coelho T: The Americans with Disabilities Act. *Neurology* 2007; **68(20)**:1733–1736.

33 Sutton v. United Airlines, Inc. Supreme Court of the United States, 1999. Available from: http://www.law.cornell.edu /supct/html/97-1943.ZS.html (last accessed July 15, 2014).

General health and epilepsy

Toyota Motor Mfg, KY, Inc. v. Williams. Supreme Court of the United States, 2002. Available from: http://www.law.cornell.edu/supct/html/00-1089.ZO.html (last accessed July 15, 2014).

ADA Amendments Act of 2008. Available from: http://www.eeoc.gov/laws/statutes/adaaa.cfm (last accessed July 15, 2014).

Thomas VL, Gostin LO: The Americans with Disabilities Act. *JAMA* 2009; **301(1)**:95–97.

US Equal Employment Opportunity Commission: Questions & answers about epilepsy in the workplace and the Americans with Disabilities Act (ADA). Available from: http://www.eeoc.gov/facts/epilepsy.html (last accessed July 15, 2014).

US Department of Transportation Federal Motor Carrier Safety Administration: Medical. Available from: http://www.fmcsa.dot.gov/regulations/medical (last accessed July 15, 2014).

Epilepsy Foundation: Pilot and other airline positions. Available from: http://www.epilepsy.com/get-help/managing-your-epilepsy/independent-living/employment/safety-sensitive-jobs/pilot-and-other (last accessed July 15, 2014).

Epilepsy Foundation: Military service. Available from: http://www.epilepsy.com/get-help/managing-your-epilepsy/independent-living/employment/safety-sensitive-jobs/military-service (last accessed July 15, 2014).

Index

Note: Page numbers in **bold** refer to illustrations

nonepileptic events and psychological factors, 96
primary cognitive complaints, 97
processing speed, 97–98
cognitive–behavioral therapy (CBT), 200
coma, NCSE in, 41
comorbidities in epilepsy, 7–11, 15–22
and dual diagnoses, 96
health behavior, 9–10
impact, 7–11
and lifestyle factors, 9–10
physician–patient interactions, 9
poverty, 8
psychosocial factors, 7–8
range, 7–11
sleep problems, 9
social support, 8
socioeconomic factors, 8
somatic health issues, 8–9
comorbidity risk factors, AEDs and, 10
complementary and alternative medicine (CAM) in epilepsy,
241–248
biologically-based practices, 243–247
energy medicine, 247–248
herbal remedies, 243–247
mind–body medicine, 242–243
publications reporting use of, **244–245**
in Western countries, 242
whole medical systems, 248
complex etiology of autism, 89
complex partial seizures (CPS), 47, 90
complex partial status epilepticus, 40–41
concentration-related adverse effects of AEDs, **116**
consciousness impairment in epilepsy, 31–35
childhood absence epilepsy (CAE), 32–33
resting-state brain networks, consciousness and, 33–35
Consolidated Standards of Reporting Trials (CONSORT),
247
continuous positive airway pressure (CPAP), 230
continuous spikes and waves during slow-wave sleep syndrome
(CSWS), 70
Cortical mapping, 81
corticotropin-releasing hormone (CRH), 150
courtesy stigma, 16
cryptogenic (nonlesional) epilepsies, 51
C-terminal telopeptide (CTX), 226
cycles of stigma, **17**

D
default networks, 34–35
default-mode network, 49
delaverdine, 114
depression, 19, 197
developmental behavioral disorder (DBD), 90
developmental disorders in epilepsy, 68–71
animal data, 68–69
dietician advice, weight monitoring and, 199–200
differential anticonvulsant effects, **75**
diltiazem, 114
disordered attention and epilepsy, 63–66
donepezil, 55
doxifluridine, 114
Dravet syndrome, 71, 90
driving issues in epilepsy, 258–261
awareness of driving regulation and requirements, 260–261

restrictions, 258–259
risk, 259–260
drug interactions in elderly, 209–210
drug selection principles for minimizing adverse effects, 121–123
drug therapy, initiating and monitoring, 210
drug use in persons with preexisting epilepsy, 256
duration of epilepsy, 46–47
dysexecutive impairments in epilepsy, 45–56

E
education and health promotion, 199
efavirenz, 114
elderly Fall Screening Test (EFST), 219
elderly people, epilepsy in, 203–213
acute seizures, 203–204
AEDs in elderly patients, 207
advantages, **208–209**
disadvantages, **208–209**
aging brain, 203–213
chronic seizures, 204
diagnostic evaluation, 204–205
drug interactions, 209–210
drug therapy, initiating and monitoring, 210
EEG, 205–206
epidemiology, 203–204
etiologies, 203–204
falls and fractures, 210
medication selection, 206–207
neuroimaging, 206
nonmedication therapies, 211
pathophysiology, 203–204
psychosocial implications, 211–212
side effects, 207–209
status epilepticus, 204
therapies selection, 203–213
treatment, 206–211
vascular disease, 203–213
employment issues in epilepsy, 261–264
reasonable accommodations for people with epilepsy, 262
specific job restrictions, 262–264
energy medicine, 247–248
Epilepsy Foundation of America (EFA), 259
epilepticus during slow-wave sleep (ESES), 51
epileptiform EEG abnormalities in autism, 91–92
Epworth Sleepiness Scale (ESS), 163
ertapenem, 114
erythromycin, 114, 209
eslicarbazepine acetate, 75, **116**
ethosuximide, **116**, **128**, 131, 141
European International (EURAP), 137
excessive daytime sleepiness (EDS), 161, 234
executive function in epilepsy, 45–46
exercise, 9–10, 197
extratemporal focal epilepsies, 50–52
Eysenck Personality Questionnaire, 177–178
ezogabine, **128**, 133–134

F
fall risk in patients with epilepsy, 210, 216–221, **220**, *See also*
balance disorders in epilepsy
Falls Efficacy Scale –International (FES-I), 219
Falls Risk Assessment Tool (FRAT), 219
familiarity bias, 17–18
Federal Aviation Administration (FAA), 264